Complications in

SPINAL SURGERY

Richard A. Balderston, M.D.

Clinical Associate Professor, Orthopaedic Surgery and
Director, Spine Fellowship Program,
Jefferson Medical College;
Chief, Scoliosis Services,
Thomas Jefferson University Hospital and
Pennsylvania Hospital, Philadelphia, Pennsylvania

Howard S. An, M.D.

Assistant Professor and Director of Reconstructive Spine Surgery,
Department of Orthopaedic Surgery,
The Medical College of Wisconsin, Milwaukee, Wisconsin

1991
W.B. SAUNDERS COMPANY
Harcourt Brace Jovanovich, Inc.

Philadelphia • London • Toronto • Montreal • Sydney • Tokyo

W. B. SAUNDERS COMPANY
Harcourt Brace Jovanovich, Inc.

The Curtis Center
Independence Square West
Philadelphia, PA 19106

Library of Congress Cataloging-in-Publication Data

Balderston, Richard A.

Complications in spinal surgery / Richard A. Balderston,
Howard S. An.—1st ed.

p. cm.

ISBN 0–7216–3522–9

1. Spine—Surgery—Complications and sequelae.
I. An, Howard S.   II. Title.

[DNLM: 1. Intraoperative Complications.
2. Spine—surgery.   WE 725 B176c]

RD768.B35   1991

617.3'7501—dc20

DNLM/DLC   90-9087

Editor: Ed Wickland
Developmental Editor: Hazel Hacker
Designer: Maureen Sweeney
Production Manager: Bill Preston
Manuscript Editor: Sally Burke
Illustration Coordinator: Peg Shaw
Indexer: Norman Duren

Complications in Spinal Surgery   ISBN 0–7216–3522–9

Printed in the United States of America

Last digit is the print number: 9   8   7   6   5   4   3   2   1

*To our wives, Sue and Claudia,
for their patience and understanding.*

Contributors

Howard S. An, M.D.

Assistant Professor and Director of
Reconstructive Spine Surgery, Department
of Orthopaedic Surgery, The Medical
College of Wisconsin, Milwaukee,
Wisconsin; Attending Staff, The
Milwaukee County Medical Complex, The
Children's Hospital of Wisconsin, and The
Froedert Lutheran Memorial Hospital,
Milwaukee, Wisconsin

*Complications in Scoliosis, Kyphosis, and
Spondylolisthesis Surgery; Complications in
Cervical Disc Disease Surgery;
Complications in Lumbar Disc Disease and
Spinal Stenosis Surgery; Complications of
Spinal Tumor Surgery; Complications of
Treatment of Fractures and Dislocations of
the Thoracolumbar Spine; Complications of
Surgery of the Spine in Rheumatoid
Arthritis and Ankylosing Spondylitis*

Richard A. Balderston, M.D.

Clinical Associate Professor of Orthopaedic
Surgery, Thomas Jefferson University
Medical College, Philadelphia,
Pennsylvania; Chief, Scoliosis Service,
Thomas Jefferson University Hospital, and
Attending Staff, The Pennsylvania
Hospital, Philadelphia, Pennsylvania

*Patient Expectations; Complications in
Scoliosis, Kyphosis, and Spondylolisthesis
Surgery; Complications of Spinal Surgery;
Complications in Cervical Spine Injury;
Complications of Treatment of Fractures*

*and Dislocations of the Thoracolumbar
Spine; Infection in Spine Surgery;
Complications of Surgery of the Spine in
Rheumatoid Arthritis and Ankylosing
Spondylitis*

Kalman Blumberg, M.D.

Assistant Professor, Department of
Orthopaedic Surgery, Thomas Jefferson
University Medical College, Philadelphia,
Pennsylvania

Infection in Spine Surgery

Robert E. Booth, M.D.

Clinical Professor of Orthopaedic Surgery,
Thomas Jefferson University Medical
College, Philadelphia, Pennsylvania; Chief,
Department of Orthopaedic Surgery, The
Pennsylvania Hospital, Philadelphia,
Pennsylvania

*Complications in Lumbar Disc Disease and
Spinal Stenosis Surgery*

Jerome M. Cotler, M.D.

Professor and Vice-Chairman of Orthopaedic
Surgery and Co-Director of Regional
Spinal Cord Injury Center, Thomas
Jefferson University Medical College,
Philadelphia, Pennsylvania

*Complications in Cervical Spine Injury;
Complications of Treatment of Fractures
and Dislocations of the Thoracolumbar
Spine*

v

Michael R. Piazza, M.D.

Attending Staff, Morton Plant Hospital,
    Clearwater, Florida

Complications in Cervical Spine Injury

Richard H. Rothman, M.D.

James Edward Professor and Chairman,
    Department of Orthopaedic Surgery,
    Thomas Jefferson University Medical
    College, Philadelphia, Pennsylvania;
    Attending Staff, Thomas Jefferson
    University Hospital, The Pennsylvania
    Hospital, Philadelphia, Pennsylvania

*Complications in Lumbar Disc Disease and
    Spinal Stenosis Surgery*

Frederick A. Simeone, M.D.

Professor of Neurosurgery, The University of
    Pennsylvania School of Medicine,

Philadelphia, Pennsylvania; Chief of
    Neurosurgery, The Pennsylvania Hospital,
    Philadelphia, Pennsylvania

*Complications in Cervical Disc Disease
    Surgery*

J. Michael Simpson, M.D.

Spine Fellow, Rothman Institute, Thomas
    Jefferson University Medical College,
    Philadelphia, Pennsylvania; Attending
    Staff, The Pennsylvania Hospital, Thomas
    Jefferson University Hospital, Philadelphia,
    Pennsylvania

*Complications of Surgery of the Spine in
    Rheumatoid Arthritis and Ankylosing
    Spondylitis*

Preface

Within the subspecialties of surgery, complications of spinal surgery have some of the greatest potentials for producing catastrophic permanent sequelae for the patient. This book is meant to assist those practitioners who treat spinal disorders in their quest to maximize patient benefit and avoid an unhappy, possibly preventable, poor outcome owing to a complication of treatment. The following chapters represent the philosophy of those surgeons at the Rothman Institute, The Pennsylvania Hospital, and Thomas Jefferson University Hospital in Philadelphia who treat patients with spinal disorders.

The book is organized according to disease entity. The first chapter summarizes some of the unique qualities of the physician-patient relationship as related to spinal surgery. The second chapter covers the subspecialty of surgery for spinal deformities: scoliosis, kyphosis, and spondylolisthesis. Cervical and lumbar disc disease are presented in Chapters Three and Four, whereas the management and complications of spinal tumor surgery are presented in Chapter Five. Complications of trauma to the cervical and thoracolumbar spine are detailed in Chapters Six and Seven. Chapter Eight includes the management of patients with spinal infection, and the last chapter of text summarizes the unique problems of patients with inflammatory disease of the spine.

As much as any other area of surgery, the surgical management of patients with spinal disorders demands that the surgeon consider what harm may be done to the patient before proceeding with an invasive intervention. This book is meant to help the surgeon stay out of trouble and keep the patient as safe as possible.

RICHARD A. BALDERSTON, M.D.
HOWARD S. AN, M.D.

Contents

ONE

Patient Expectations

Richard A. Balderston, M.D.

THE NATURAL HISTORY OF SPINAL DISORDERS

Most orthopedic interventions result in a solution to a particular problem without significant sequelae. Consider the patient who is treated for a distal fibular or nondisplaced ulnar fracture. After a period of immobilization followed by rehabilitation, the patient can expect almost normal function, in most cases, without long-term deterioration in either function or anatomical alignment. Another such circumstance is the uncomplicated medial meniscus tear that is treated arthroscopically. These patients frequently improve almost immediately and have no further disability caused by their knees. Finally, the patient who undergoes total hip replacement for painful degenerative arthritis often considers his operation a miracle and both experiences and expects continued freedom from pain and normal function. In all areas of orthopedics, patients have come to expect a straightforward, uncomplicated solution to a problem—a solution that is not only long lasting, but also preventive for future anatomical deterioration.

Unfortunately, the aging lumbar spine is a structure not yet amenable to this type of treatment. While patients with an extruded herniated lumbar disc may expect dramatic improvement in leg and thigh symptomatology, they frequently complain of low backache at some time during the perioperative and postoperative clinical course.[5] Low back pain occurs with some severity during the lifetime of up to 80 per cent of all persons, and as high as 50 per cent of these patients will have recurrent symptoms.[1, 7, 12] Patients with surgically treated herniated discs who have an excellent early surgical result are certainly at no less risk for low back symptomatology than the general population. The surgeon must acquaint the patient with this fact of life before any surgical procedure is undertaken. Despite continued protestations and education from the operating surgeon, patients will still associate episodic back pain with the suspicion that the surgeon may not have performed the operation correctly. Even though patients may have had a long history of episodic mild back pain before sustaining a herniated lumbar disc, they may perceive that episodic back pain after surgery is a result of operative intervention. Only by acquainting the patient with this possibility preoperatively will the surgeon avoid an unhappy situation in the postoperative period.

Frequently, patients ask if their "arthritis" can be removed at the time of low back surgery. Patients view their lumbar x-ray films and are surprised to see disc degeneration, facet arthritis, and minimal vertebral subluxation and become quite frightened that they will have total, permanent low back disability. Autopsy studies have demonstrated lumbar disc disease in all pathological specimens taken from people over age 50. In addition, numerous authors have demonstrated the lack of clinical correlation with routine degenerative signs on lumbar spine films.[6, 14] Patients are frequently not made aware of this lack of correlation and need to be informed that most abnormalities seen on lumbar spine films do not correlate with low back symptomatology.

One other frequent consideration that patients verbalize early in the course of their treatment for spine disorders is that of prevention of future progression of disease. Specifically, patients will view a contrast study and identify abnormalities of other discs or facet joints that, in the opinion of the surgeon, are not causing their present symptoms. The patient's next question is whether the disc that is almost pathological should be removed as well; and perhaps while the surgeon is performing a multilevel discectomy, a multilevel fusion should be added as well. Patients must understand that the natural history of sequelae of fusion surgery in the lumbar spine is not benign. Given the natural history of the multiple treatment options themselves, often the best plan is one that disrupts the benign anatomy minimally and still effects a significant reduction in present symptomatology.

PSYCHOLOGICAL AND SOCIAL CONSIDERATIONS

As much as 10 per cent of the general population is clinically depressed, and there is no doubt that patients in this group have altered pain perceptions.[10] It must be remembered, however, that depressed patients also will have extruded discs, but their perception of their symptomatology is significantly altered by their depression. The surgeon must recognize this situation, and if discectomy is performed, consideration must also be given to treatment of depression. Ideally, the depression should be treated first, and when this is done, in many cases, leg pain from a chronically herniated disc will be significantly improved to the point that surgery is not needed.

For patients who are at risk for job-related injuries, there are psychological risk factors that have recently been elucidated. Numerous historical, physical, and psychological parameters have been studied in an effort to predict which workers will sustain a low back episode that will cause them to lose time from work. More so than the body habitus, physical conditioning, range of motion of the lumbar spine, and muscle strength, the factor that most often predicts occupational injury is job happiness.

Workers who are happy with the tasks they perform at work have significantly less back injuries than those who are unhappy with their tasks. The surgeon must keep this factor in mind when, after a successful surgery for spinal nerve decompression, the worker returns to his old job in which he was unhappy and has a recurrence of symptoms without objective physical findings.

It has been estimated that as much as 8 per cent of the general population engages in substance abuse. Not only will many of these substances affect doctor-patient communication, but they will also affect the patient's perception of pain. It also must be remembered that alcohol may create a metabolic milieu that does not encourage nerve healing in those patients with chronic compression and inflammation. Substance abuse must be identified before surgery and, ideally, should be treated before surgical intervention is contemplated. Patients with spinal fractures who are under the influence of mind-altering substances will present a difficult pain management problem in the postoperative period.

In most clinical series, treatment of patients who have compensation claims yields a poor result for any given pathological entity when compared with that of noncompensation patients. In many states, patients may receive a significantly higher financial reward for a given entity if they are required to have surgery for that diagnosis as compared with patients who do not require surgery. Thus, if a patient understands that he will get twice as much money if he has an operation and remains disabled, that patient may exaggerate his symptoms and possibly falsify the findings of physical examination in an effort to become a candidate for operation. The surgeon must expect that these patients may continue to have pain, even though the operative pathology reveals that surgery was truly indicated and the problem has been corrected.

A similar situation develops in the field of ongoing litigation. Patients may be rewarded financially for increased symptomatology for a given diagnosis. Even if the surgery is indicated and necessary, the surgeon should expect continuing complaints and dramatic pain behavior until litigation and compensation considerations have been settled.

The same considerations for both natural history and psychological and social factors apply to cervical disc disease as well. Fifty per cent of the population will have an episode of severe neck pain some time during their lives, and in more than 25 per cent, these episodes will recur. Patients who require cervical decompression for radiculopathy may be disappointed with respect to amelioration of their neck pain, even though their arm pain is completely relieved. X-ray changes in the cervical spine are frequently global, and patients should be alerted to the fact that this situation does not mean progressive neck symptomatology. Patients should also be encouraged that the mild, nonpathological roentgenographic changes need not be treated since they occur independently of cervical symptomatology.

SCOLIOSIS AND RELATED DISORDERS

The most common indication for surgical arthrodesis in patients with idiopathic scoliosis is curve progression. Low back symptomatology is usually unrelated to spinal curvature. Cochran and Nachemson and coworkers have shown a relationship between lower extent of fusion and the incidence and severity of low back pain.[3] However, even in those patients who are fused down to the level of the third lumbar vertebra and who are supposed to have no greater chance of low back pain than that of the general population, low back symptoms may occur. Just as in the patient with a herniated lumbar disc, patients with scoliosis may associate the occurrence of low back pain with their scoliosis fusion. Many of these patients had no back pain before surgical arthrodesis and so are disappointed that pain should occur in the general region of their scoliosis operation. These symptoms may occur years after the surgery and be totally unrelated pathoanatomically to the spinal curvature; yet, the patient perceives a connection. Patients must be told before a scoliosis operation about the natural history of low back pain and how they are at risk for a low back event just as any other person in the general population who has a straight spine.

Patients with scoliosis may also have an unrealistic expectation with respect to the cosmetic result. While the details of the cosmetic factors, including shoulder and pelvic symmetry, waistline symmetry, rib hump diminution, and head/trunk/pelvic alignment, may have been discussed with the patient, most patients would like to have a perfectly symmetrical body. The surgeon must take great care to itemize the possible effects of the scoliosis fusion with respect to cosmesis and be very definite, especially with adults, as to the unpredictability of the cosmetic result.

Patients with scoliosis also may not have the correct perception as to the magnitude of their surgery. Most of their acquaintances are familiar with disc surgery and feel that somehow the two entities are related. For this reason, a support group, especially among adult patients, is extremely helpful in dispelling the myths concerning pain after surgery, function in the perioperative and postoperative periods, and cosmetic considerations.

REFERENCES

1. Aiken, A.P., and Bradford, C.H.: End result of ruptured intervertebral discs in industry. Am. J. Surg. 73:365, 1947.
2. Bell, G.R., and Rothman, R.H.: The conservative treatment of sciatica. Spine 9:54, 1984.
3. Cochran, T., Irstam, L., and Nachemson, A.: Long-term anatomic and functional changes in patients with adolescent idiopathic scoliosis treated by Harrington rod fusion. Spine 8:576–584, 1983.
4. Deyo, R.A.: Conservative therapy for low back pain: Distinguishing useful from useless therapy. J.A.M.A. 250(8):1057, 1983.
5. Hakelius, A.: Prognosis in sciatica: A clinical follow-up of surgical and non-surgical treatment. Acta Orthop. Scand. 129(Suppl):1–76.
6. Hitselberger, W., and Witten, R.: Abnormal myelograms in asymptomatic patients. J. Neurosurg. 28:204, 1968.
7. Kelsey, J., and White, A.A.: Epidemiology and impact of low-back pain. Spine 5(2):133, 1980.
8. McGill, C.M.: Industrial back problems: A control program. J. Occup. Med. 10:174, 1968.
9. Nachemson, A., and Morris, J.M.: In vivo measurements of intradiscal pressure: Discometry: A method for determination of pressure in the lower lumbar disc. J. Bone Joint Surg. 46A:1077, 1964.
10. Ransford, A.O., Cairns, D., and Mooney, V.: The pain drawing as an aid to the psychological evaluation of patients with low back pain. Spine 1:127–134, 1976.
11. Southwick, S., and White, A.A.: Current concepts review: The use of psychological tests in evaluation of low-back pain. J. Bone Joint Surg. 65A:560, 1983.
12. Waddell, G., Kummel, E.G., Lotto, W.N., et al.: Failed lumbar disc surgery and repeat surgery following industrial injuries. J. Bone Joint Surg. 61A: 201–207, 1979.
13. Waddell, G., McCulloch, J.A., Kummel, E., et al.: Nonorganic signs of low back pain. Spine 5:117, 1980.
14. Wiesel, S.W., Tsourmas, N., Feffer, H.L., et al.: A study of computer assisted tomography: Part I. The incidence of positive CAT scans in an asymptomatic group of patients. Spine 9:549, 1984.

TWO

Complications in Scoliosis, Kyphosis, and Spondylolisthesis Surgery

Howard S. An, M.D.

Richard Balderston, M.D.

The management of spinal deformities is a challenge to the spinal surgeon, and corrective spinal surgery is a major undertaking. Although there have been significant advances and development of new techniques, pitfalls and complications from treatment of these spinal deformities continue to stay with us today.[81, 103, 120, 121, 150] The risks and complications that occur in the management of scoliosis, kyphosis, and spondylolisthesis are discussed in this chapter.

SCOLIOSIS

PREOPERATIVE PLANNING

Many complications can be prevented by careful preoperative planning before surgical execution. Most structural curvatures seen in the adolescent and adult are idiopathic. However, it is important to consider multiple other possibilities. Table 2–1 shows the classification of structural scoliosis by the Scoliosis Research Society. It is unusual for the adolescent scoliotic patient to complain of back pain, and thus the source of back pain must be sought in this situation. Technetium bone scintigraphy is a useful tool in the diagnosis of a painful tumor such as osteoid osteoma in the spine. On the contrary, pain is the most common presenting symptom in adults with scoliosis, and therefore multiple causes of back pain should be considered in the initial management

of these patients. Nachemson believes that the combination of severe low back pain and lumbar scoliosis is rare.[124] Other investigators cite a higher incidence of significant pain in patients with idiopathic scoliosis.[7, 77, 92, 163] Kostuik has reported that back pain is probably related to scoliosis if the curve is greater than 45 degrees.[92] However, one must be aware of other possible pathology, which may be responsible for back pain, including spondylosis, disc herniation, spinal stenosis, abdominal aneurysm, renal stones, and so forth (Fig. 2–1). Tumors or infections may be sources of back pain in the elderly. The pain in patients with idiopathic scoliosis is usually located over the convexity of the curve initially and then later moves to the concavity of the curve when facet arthrosis and disc degeneration develop.[100, 168] The predominant pain comes from the lumbar region, not the thoracic region. Many studies relate an improvement in pain of 70 to 80 per cent after surgical arthrodesis for adult scoliosis, but residual pain is common and pain relief is not consistent.

Patients with adult lumbar scoliosis may also present with sciatica. As degenerative changes progress with development of disc narrowing, collapsing scoliosis, and vertebral subluxation, the neural elements in the lumbar spine are subject to compression by pedicular kinking, facet hypertrophy, or disc herniation.[14, 22, 51, 66] Trammell and associates have reported that lumbar curves with rotatory olisthesis were

Table 2–1
Classification of Structural Scoliosis (Scoliosis Research Society)

I. IDIOPATHIC
  A. Infantile (0–3 years)
  B. Juvenile (3–10 years)
  C. Adolescent (>10 years)
II. NEUROMUSCULAR
  A. Neuropathic
    1. Upper motor neuron
      a. Cerebral palsy
      b. Spinocerebellar degeneration (Friedreich's disease, Charcot-Marie-Tooth disease, and Roussy-Levy disease)
      c. Syringomyelia
      d. Spinal cord tumor
      e. Spinal cord trauma
      f. Other
    2. Lower motor neuron
      a. Poliomyelitis
      b. Other viral myelitides
      c. Traumatic
      d. Spinal muscular atrophy (Wernig-Hoffmann, Kugelberg-Welander)
      e. Myelomeningocele (paralytic)
    3. Dysautonomia (Riley-Day syndrome)
    4. Other
  B. Myopathic
    1. Arthrogryposis
    2. Muscular dystrophy
      a. Duchenne
      b. Limb-girdle
      c. Fascioscapulohumeral
    3. Fiber type disproportion
    4. Congenital hypotonia
    5. Myotonia dystrophica
    6. Other
III. CONGENITAL
  A. Failure of formation
    1. Wedge vertebra
    2. Hemivertebra
  B. Failure of segmentation
    1. Unilateral (unsegmented bar)
    2. Bilateral
  C. Mixed

IV. NEUROFIBROMATOSIS
V. MESENCHYMAL DISORDERS
  A. Marfan's syndrome
  B. Ehlers-Danlos syndrome
  C. Others
VI. RHEUMATOID DISEASE
VII. TRAUMA
  A. Fracture
  B. Surgical
    1. Postlaminectomy
    2. Post-thoracoplasty
  C. Irradiation
VIII. EXTRASPINAL CONTRACTURES
  A. Postempyema
  B. Postburns
IX. OSTEOCHONDRODYSTROPHIES
  A. Diastrophic dwarfism
  B. Mucopolysaccharidoses (e.g., Morquio's syndrome)
  C. Spondyloepiphyseal dysplasia
  D. Multiple epiphyseal dysplasia
  E. Other
X. INFECTION OF BONE
  A. Acute
  B. Chronic
XI. METABOLIC DISORDERS
  A. Rickets
  B. Osteogenesis imperfecta
  C. Homocystinuria
  D. Others
XII. RELATED TO LUMBOSACRAL JOINT
  A. Spondylolysis and spondylolisthesis
  B. Congenital anomalies of lumbosacral region
XIII. TUMORS
  A. Vertebral column
    1. Osteoid osteoma
    2. Histiocytosis X
    3. Other
  B. Spinal cord

more likely to be associated with radicular pain.[157] Thoracolumbar or lumbar scoliosis may be related to osteoporosis and compression fractures.[70] Every attempt must be made to accurately diagnose the source of pain before proceeding with definitive treatment. Pinpointing the source of pain preoperatively will give better results in terms of pain improvement. Careful history and physical examination along with myelogram, computed tomography, or magnetic resonance imaging are necessary to pinpoint the source of pain. One must be cautious when interpreting computed tomography or magnetic resonance studies since mistaken diagnosis of a herniated nucleus pulposus secondary to three-dimensional deformity is frequently made. Occasionally, injections into the facets, intervertebral discs, or root sleeves may be helpful.[41] If nerve root entrapment is detected by imaging studies, which correlates with symptomatology, neural decompression is indicated.[51, 124] In cases of potentially increased postoperative instability or persistent back complaints, consideration

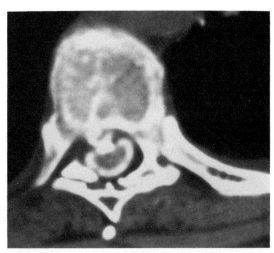

FIGURE 2–1. Computed tomography after myelogram, revealing a calcified herniated thoracic disc in a 45-year-old female patient who presented with a 55-degree nonprogressive thoracic scoliosis with back pain and mild myelopathy.

should be given to augmenting decompressive procedures with instrumentation and fusion.[14, 22, 100] In a relatively younger patient, in whom the lumbar curve is more flexible, anterior instrumentation and fusion may be effective in obtaining curve correction and relief of radiculopathy.[150]

Another important consideration is that of progression. Curves may indeed progress in adulthood.[7, 163] Weinstein and associates reported that the average adult patient with a thoracic or thoracolumbar curve greater than 50 degrees has a 1- or 2-degree progression rate per year over a span of 30 to 40 years.[163] Patients with curves of less than 30 degrees rarely progress more than a degree or two over their lifetime. Progression should be carefully followed and documented in those patients with larger curves.

A rare clinical presentation is respiratory decompensation. Patients with a large curve greater than 60 degrees may develop cardiopulmonary symptoms. Vital capacity reduction, abnormal ventilation perfusion distribution, tachypnea, and tachycardia can be seen later. Patients at risk should have preoperative pulmonary function tests. It should be noted that in patients with respiratory decompensation, anterior surgery from the transthoracic approach may further weaken the patient's precarious pulmonary status postoperatively. Nonetheless, patients with a severe degree of scoliosis and pulmonary compromise are candidates for surgery, as the mortality rate is otherwise significantly higher compared with the general population.[127a]

Cosmesis has not been accepted as a primary indication for adult scoliosis surgery. The clinician must be very careful to determine which of the patient's complaints are based on acceptance of the scoliotic deformity as compared with true disability from back pain, sciatica, progression, or possible respiratory compromise.

Therefore, unrelenting pain, progressive deformity, and cardiopulmonary symptoms are the primary indications for operation in adult scoliosis.[20] The surgical indications for the adolescent scoliotic patient are progressive deformity greater than 40 degrees, failure of brace or electrical treatment, and progressive curvature associated with significant thoracic lordosis. Although it is generally accepted that any patient with scoliosis greater than 60 degrees needs surgical arthrodesis with instrumentation, one must tailor the treatment according to each individual. For example, a greater deformity may be accepted if the curvature is well balanced and nonprogressive in the adult. On the contrary, a lesser but decompensated lumbar curvature with significant psychological and cosmetic concern from the patient should deserve stronger consideration for surgery.

Proper selection of fusion levels is an important determining factor for good surgical outcome. For most idiopathic thoracic curves, King and coworkers recommended that the fusion should only include down to the stable vertebra.[86, 87] The stable vertebra is bisected most symmetrically by the vertical center sacral line, which is drawn perpendicular to the horizontal line connecting the top of the iliac wings. An inadequate fusion length, which does not include the stable vertebra, may result in adding-on of the lower vertebrae into the curve and reoperation may be necessary. On the contrary, if the fusion length is too long, the lumbar segments may be fused unnecessarily, increasing future stress on the remaining unfused segments. Use of Cotrel-Dubousset instrumentation may be complicated by the fact that derotation of the thoracic curve may decompensate the lower lumbar curve, and an unbalanced spine may result.[92, 114, 142] For this reason, two additional levels beyond the stable vertebra may have to be fused if Cotrel-Dubousset instrumentation is used. For example, if T12 is the stable vertebra in a right thoracic curve with left compensatory lumbar curve, fusion should probably extend down to the L2 region to prevent decompensation. Further experience with this instrumentation is necessary to find out its exact role in the surgical treatment of scoliosis.

For combined thoracic and lumbar curves, where the lumbar curve is larger and more rigid, the fusion should include both thoracic and lumbar curves down to the stable vertebra, which is usually L3 or L4. Also, one should include the whole kyphosis in the fusion to prevent junctional instability at the top of the fusion. In general, one should avoid fusion below L4, as late onset of back pain is significantly higher than in the general population.[33, 61] Fusion to the sacrum is not indicated except in the adult patient with severe lumbar oblique take-off and unbalanced lumbosacral curve or with painful lumbosacral segments.[9, 91, 93] For the rare double thoracic scoliosis, the top of fusion should include T2 or T3 in order to level the shoulder as much as possible.

For the isolated short lumbar or thoracolumbar curves, anterior approach should be considered to prevent fusion below L3 or L4. Anterior spine fusion with Zielke instrumentation has been successful, particularly in adolescents.[122, 130, 131] Fusion should extend from the cephalad neutral vertebra to the lowest vertebra that comes within 10 degrees of neutral on the side-bending film. Anterior instrumentation below L3 is not recommended because fusions below L3 are better achieved with posterior instrumentation. Relative contraindications to Zielke instrumentation are the presence of a kyphotic deformity exceeding 10 to 15 degrees, the presence of an unbalanced lumbosacral curve, and a concomitant rigid compensatory thoracic curve above 40 degrees. In adults, the single-stage Zielke instrumentation is associated with a higher incidence of pseudarthrosis and other complications.[74] Combined anterior and posterior fusion has been more successful for adult scoliosis.[78, 90, 130]

The two-stage procedure is also recommended for paralytic scoliotic patients with uncorrectable pelvic obliquity on traction or poor sitting balance.[101, 113, 118, 132] Fusion to the sacrum using the Galveston technique is effective in these cases.[3, 4, 23] Congenital scoliosis should be fused in situ if progression is noted.[169, 170] Preoperative studies should be thorough in these patients to rule out occult intraspinal anomalies such as diastematomyelia, fibrous adhesions, and tumors.[117]

Degenerative lumbar scoliosis presents a special problem. Decompression laminectomy and foraminotomy may be required for radicular pain,[51, 144] but fusion should also be considered to prevent further collapse and progression of the curve.[14, 94, 66, 150] Instrumentation is difficult because of osteoporosis and rotatory deformity in these cases. Pedicle screw fixation is an alternative method of stabilization and fusion in the lumbosacral region.

POSTERIOR APPROACH

OPERATIVE TECHNIQUE

Despite careful preoperative planning and precise selection of fusion levels, pitfalls and complications of scoliosis surgery can be numerous (Tables 2–2 and 2–3). Most feared complications are spinal cord and vascular injuries. In addition, pseudarthrosis, flat back syndrome, instrument failure, and axial pain can develop later. Generally, complications are higher in adults than in adolescents.[20, 103] Surgery in adults is technically more difficult than in children and adolescents, and healing potential is inferior. In order to minimize these potential risks, the surgeon must consider all steps of the operative procedure as possible pitfalls and complications and must approach each with great caution.

The first consideration of a patient's safety begins with the positioning of the patient on the operating table. Our usual spinal deformity frame is the four-poster, or Relton-Hall, frame. By adjusting all posters with regard to the patient's width and height, pressure points are evenly distributed on the chest and anterior thighs while obtaining some reduction of the deformity. One must avoid pressure on the brachial plexus and ulnar nerves for obvious reasons. It is important that the abdomen be free of pressure to allow venous drainage of the lower extremities and to decrease blood loss during surgery. An increased blood loss due to pressure on the vascular system will only decrease the surgeon's vision at surgery and increase the complication rate from excessive blood loss.

Operative blood loss may be increased in patients who take aspirin or nonsteroidal anti-inflammatory medications preoperatively.[5] Therefore, these medications should be stopped several days before surgery. Hypotensive anesthesia should also be employed during major spinal surgery to minimize blood loss.[133] The systolic blood pressure is maintained around 90 mm. Hg to prevent excess blood loss while maintaining perfusion to the vital organs. Normotension should generally be re-

Table 2–2
Complications of Scoliosis Surgery in Adult Patients

AUTHOR	NUMBER OF PATIENTS	OVERALL RATE	NEUROLOGICAL COMPLICATIONS	PSEUDOARTHROSIS	INSTRUMENT PROBLEMS	INFECTION	MORTALITY
Byrd	26	85%	7.7%	0	11.5%	0	0
Court-Brown	32	22%	0	6.2%	12.4%	3.1%	0
Kostuik	107	47%	0.7%	10%	10%	10%	1
Ponder	132	60%	0	17.6%	3.7%	4.6%	2
Sponseller	46	62%	6.5%	8.7%	10.1%	2.2%	1
Swank	222	53%	0.5%	11%	12%	8.0%	3
Van Dam	91	33%	1.1%	15%	5%	1%	0

stored just prior to distraction to minimize vascular compromise to the spinal cord. This point may be arguable. Kling and associates reported on the influence of induced hypotension and spinal distraction on canine spinal cord blood flow.[88] Spinal cord blood flow is reduced by induced hypotension, but it returns to normotensive values in 35 minutes by an autoregulatory mechanism, and spinal distraction does not further decrease spinal cord blood flow once it has returned to normotensive flows. It is then important to remember that spinal distraction should not be applied within 35 minutes of induced hypotension. Patients routinely will donate 3 to 4 units of blood over a period of a few weeks before surgery. Intraoperative blood cell saver system is also used whenever possible. All of the above efforts are to decrease blood loss and minimize transfusion-related complications such as hepatitis, acquired immunodeficiency syndrome, and transfusion reaction.

The lighting of the surgical field is extremely important. The surgeon should wear a headlight when working about the neural elements. In addition, 2.5 to 3.5 power magnification greatly enhances dissection around the spinal nerves or the anterior dura and may help to prevent injuries. For most routine scoliosis cases, however, headlight and magnification are not required. Meticulous operative technique is most important in achieving successful fusion and in preventing both operative and late complications. Initial subperiosteal dissection is done with the Cobb elevator, exposing the spinous processes, lamina, facets, and the tips of the transverse processes. With a right-handed surgeon, the left wrist of the surgeon is always kept on the patient's body and firmly anchored on the instrument. Thus, the left upper extremity forms a block to inadvertent penetration of the instrument anteriorly into the neural elements and provides much greater control of the instrument. Facet excision and decortication can be done with hand instru-

ments such as a Lexcel rongeur or power instruments. Power instruments should again be held in both hands, resting both wrists or forearms on the patient to provide proprioceptive feedback to the surgeon and to minimize the risk of an unexpected wayward deviation of these instruments.

Careful handling of the instruments is the key to avoiding spinal cord injury during scoliosis surgery. Spinal implants such as sublaminar wires and hooks should also be used with great caution. For application of the upper hook, excision of the inferior margin of the inferior facet on the concavity of the curve is done with a ¼-inch osteotome. This osteotome should always be aimed away from the spinal canal if possible, such that the superior cut is made with the osteotome pointing laterally instead of medially, and the sagittal cut is made as parallel to the spine as possible. When the hook is being seated under the lamina, care must be taken that the neural elements underneath are not damaged. Great caution should be taken to avoid dural tear when preparing the inferior hook site. The ligamentum flavum and a section of the superior margin of the lamina are carefully removed with a Lexcel or Kerrison rongeur. Also, seating of the lower hook too laterally on the lamina near the neural foramen runs the risk of root compression. Meticulous decortication and facet excision are performed before inserting a distraction rod (Fig. 2–2A, B).

Harrington or Moe instrumentation corrects the deformity by a distraction force on the concavity of the curve. Distraction should be applied gradually, allowing creep phenomenon to take place. Overdistraction may produce stretching of the spinal cord and neurological deficit. There are numerous situations where distraction force may be dangerous. Certainly in patients with congenital scoliosis, distraction may be detrimental.[117, 169] In cases of diastematomyelia, distraction may produce traction of the neural elements over the bar of cartilage

Table 2-3
Complications of Scoliosis Surgery in Pediatric Patients

AUTHOR	NUMBER OF PATIENTS	SCOLIOSIS TYPE	TREATMENT	OVERALL RATE	NEURO-LOGICAL COMPLI-CATIONS	PSEUD-ARTHROSIS	IMPLANT	INFECTION	MORTALITY
Goldstein	107	Idiopathic	Harrington rod	29%	0.9%	3.7%	4.7%	1.9%	0
Harrington	578	Idiopathic	Harrington rod	32.4%	0	3.3%	21.3%	0.7%	1
Herndon	63	Paralytic	Harrington or Luque with sublaminar wires	50.1%	1.6%	11 with loss of correction and 8 broken rods	23.8%	6.3%	0
Lonstein	107	Paralytic	Harrington with or without anterior fusion	81%	0.9%	17%	23.4%	5%	3
Lovallo	163	Idiopathic	Harrington rod	15.3%	0	1.8%	8.0%	3.4% (superficial)	0
Luque	65	Idiopathic and paralytic	Luque rod with sublaminar wires	18.5%	10.8%	3.1%	9.2%	3.1%	0
Thompson	86	Idiopathic	Harrington or Luque with sublaminar wires	22%	16.3%	0	2.3%	0	0
Winter	66	Congenital	Multiple methods	51.5%	0	20%	3.0%	1.5%	4.5%

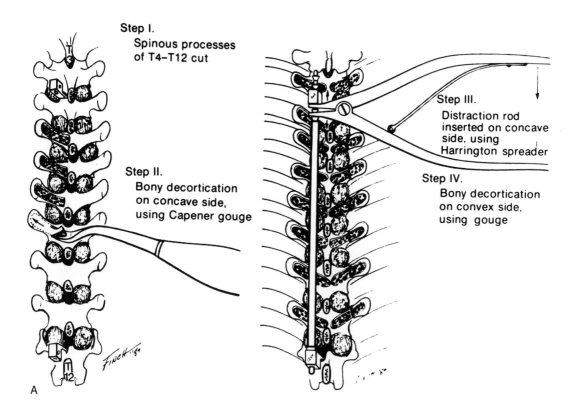

Step I.
  Spinous processes
  of T4–T12 cut

Step II.
  Bony decortication
  on concave side,
  using Capener gouge

Step III.
  Distraction rod
  inserted on concave
  side, using
  Harrington spreader

Step IV.
  Bony decortication
  on convex side,
  using gouge

A

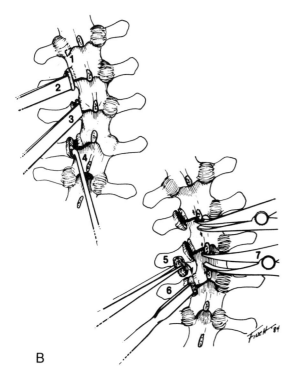

B

FIGURE 2–2. *(A)* Illustration of meticulous bony decortication prior to inserting a distraction rod. (From Bradford, D. S., et al. (eds.): *Moe's Textbook of Scoliosis and Other Spinal Deformities* (2nd ed.). Philadelphia, W. B. Saunders, 1987, p. 145.) *(B)* Illustration of meticulous lumbar facet excision (Moe technique). (From Bradford, D. S., et al. (eds.): *Moe's Textbook of Scoliosis and Other Spinal Deformities* (2nd ed.). Philadelphia, W. B. Saunders, 1987, p. 141.)

or bone, producing neurological deficit. In patients who have relatively stiff spines with osteophyte formation, such as in adults with spinal deformity, distraction as a primary reduction technique may produce an increased risk of neurological deficit. It is important that the distraction rods be contoured for thoracic kyphosis and lumbar lordosis. Distraction forces in the lumbar spine result in loss of lumbar sagittal contours with concomitant changes in posture and gait and late development of back pain.[1, 96, 161] One should avoid instrumentation in the lower lumbar spine if possible. Square-ended Moe rods may be a help to maintain lordosis when distraction rods must be used in the lumbar region. Rod contouring also minimizes the tendency of a straight rod to lever a hook out through the lamina.

Segmental instrumentation with sublaminar wires greatly enhances overall stability of the surgical construct and better maintains sagittal contours. Luque rod with sublaminar wires remains the treatment of choice for patients with paralytic scoliosis.[3, 4, 23, 60] However, the passage of sublaminar wires may be associated with increased neurological risk.[43, 155, 168] Goll and coworkers presented an experiment in which sublaminar wires were observed directly with the use of a television camera pointed axially down the spinal canal.[64] The wire tip must be bent as minimally as possible, and the radius of curvature of the wire should be as maximal as possible to allow easy passage. The sublaminar wire must be held in both hands and upward traction placed on the wire at all times. The wire is then twisted 450 degrees about the lamina to prevent the wire from migrating down the canal (Fig. 2–3). Sublaminar wires should probably be avoided at the same level as a laminar hook as there may not be enough room for both wire and hook in the spinal canal. Under no circumstances should a compression system be used with a sublaminar wire. Tightening of the sublaminar wire produces anterior migration of the compression hook attached to the compression rod and may produce neurological deficit. Interspinous segmental instrumentation is a viable alternative with decreased risk of neurological injury.[44, 71, 135] However, interspinous wiring is not free of danger, as dural penetration by this technique has been documented in the literature.[99] Although segmental instrumentation with either sublaminar or interspinous wires enhances overall stabilization of the surgical construct, the use of postoperative orthosis is important in avoiding problems with fixation or loss of correction.[71, 72]

The Cotrel-Dubousset system has been introduced recently for scoliosis correction and stabilization; its derotating capability allows correction of coronal, sagittal, and axial deformities.[17, 39, 67] The surgical instrumentation and technique are extremely complex, and sufficient training is required for proper use of this system. This system is best used for curves that are relatively more flexible and of less magnitude. In larger and stiffer curves, derotation would be difficult and presents the risk of fracture of the lamina. The Scoliosis Research Society initially reported a higher incidence of neurological injury with use of the Cotrel-Dubousset system compared with other systems.[147] Because of the learning curve, one should obtain hands-on experience and training with other surgeons well versed in the techniques.

For cosmetic purposes and to augment the posterior fusion, rib resection may be performed. The major problem associated with rib resection is prominence of the intact ribs owing to inadequate removal. Inadequate dissection generally occurs medially, inferiorly, or superiorly.[152] A separate vertical incision is usually necessary to remove the rib from the costovertebral junction to beyond the midaxillary line. Depending on the degree of the deformity, one may have to remove ribs from T3 to T12. The transverse processes should be partially removed to avoid prominence on the medial side. Use of the Cotrel-Dubousset system may obviate the need for thoracoplasty if adequate derotation can be achieved.

OPERATIVE COMPLICATIONS OF POSTERIOR APPROACH

Neural Injury

The incidence of spinal cord injury seems to vary depending on the different instrumentation systems. According to the 1987 Morbidity Report from the Scoliosis Research Society, the incidence of cord injury in patients with idiopathic scoliosis was 0.26 per cent.[147] The sublaminar wire was responsible for 39 per cent of the total (0.86 per cent incidence), and Cotrel-Dubousset instrumentation accounted for 33 per cent (0.60 per cent incidence). Use of the Harrington distraction rod showed only a 0.23 per cent incidence. A higher percentage of neurological problems with use of sublaminar wires has been well documented in the literature.[155, 166] Wilber and associates reviewed

Luque wire passage

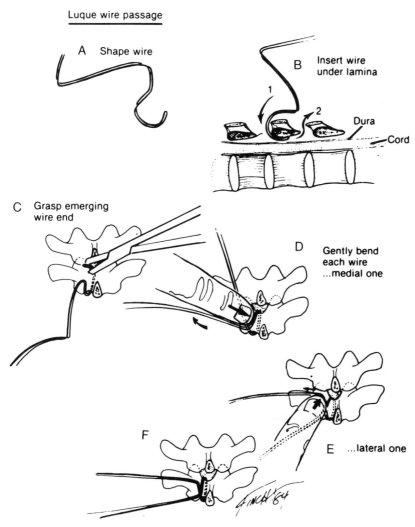

A   Shape wire

B   Insert wire under lamina

Dura

Cord

C   Grasp emerging wire end

D   Gently bend each wire ...medial one

E   ...lateral one

F

FIGURE 2–3. Illustration of Luque wire passage (see text). (From Bradford, D. S., et al. (eds.): *Moe's Textbook of Scoliosis and Other Spinal Deformities* (2nd ed.). Philadelphia, W. B. Saunders, 1987, p. 151.)

69 patients who underwent a posterior spine fusion for scoliosis with segmental wiring and 68 patients who had a Harrington rod inserted without segmental wiring.[166] Neurological complications were significantly higher in the segmentally wired group (17 per cent) compared with the latter group (1.5 per cent). These authors noted that there was definite evidence of a learning process as the incidence of neurological complications was the greatest in the early patients of the series.[166] Recently, the British Scoliosis Society reported an incidence of 1.4 per cent neurological complications in 1,121 patients undergoing segmental wiring for spinal deformity.[43] Because of the complexity of instrumentation, the Cotrel-Dubousset system was initially associated with more neurological problems.[147] Proper and careful han-

dling of these instruments is probably the most important factor in preventing spinal cord injury.

An increased risk of neurological injury is also present in patients with scoliosis of a severe degree, congenital scoliosis, and pre-existing neurological deficit.[11] Certain procedures carry an increased risk of neurological injury. These include distraction instrumentation in congenital scoliosis, skeletal traction, and spinal osteotomy.[111] Another factor related to increased risk for spinal cord injury is intraoperative correction exceeding the preoperative correction.[166] Excessive blood loss should be prevented because accompanying hypotension puts the spinal cord at more risk for circulatory compromise.[137]

The use of the Stagnara wake-up test is a

long and time-honored tradition.[42, 160] However, false-negative wake-up tests have been reported in the literature.[13, 40] Somatosensory-evoked potential (SSEP) monitoring is also helpful in that it gives continuous readouts on cord function during surgery.[16, 50, 127, 143] However, this is not a foolproof method because of false negatives or false positives.[12, 62, 143] At present, we use both SSEP monitoring and wake-up test during scoliosis operation. If a neurological deficit is noted during or after surgery, distraction force must be reduced immediately. Myelogram, computed tomography, or magnetic resonance imaging may also be helpful in looking for epidural hematoma or cord contusion if the neurological deficit is found postoperatively. If hematoma is present, it should be drained expeditiously. The onset of neurological deficit may be delayed for several days owing to edema or cord ischemia.[79, 98] Instrumentation should be removed even in late cases in which the clear etiology of the neurological deficit is not found.[98]

Late neurological complications may be secondary to pseudarthrosis, progression of the curve, bony hypertrophy of the fusion mass,[48] spinal abscess,[111] hook impingement,[19] and syringomyelia.[128] Although rare, one must be aware of these potential complications.

Pseudarthrosis

The development of new instrumentation systems should not detract one from meticulous fusion technique. A long-term good result depends primarily on achieving a solid arthrodesis. The incidence of pseudarthrosis has been decreasing with the use of current surgical procedures, but the incidence is noticeably higher in paralytic and adult scoliotic patients.[101, 153] Swank noted a rate of 17 per cent in the adult population, and solid arthrodesis may be delayed up to 15 months.[153] Paralytic scoliotic patients also have a higher rate of pseudarthrodesis, particularly myelomeningocele patients.[101, 121] Although rigid instrumentations such as Luque or Cotrel-Dubousset systems probably lower the incidence of pseudarthrosis, the meticulous fusion technique cannot be overlooked. There are reports in the literature indicating that combined anterior and posterior procedures are superior to posterior fusion alone in terms of fusion rate.[28] Certainly, large and stiff curves in adults and unbalanced curves in paralytic patients should be approached both anteriorly and posteriorly. Nonetheless, meticulous decortication and facet excision must be stressed. Massive bone

grafts from the iliac crest remain the gold standard. Allografts may be used for augmentation if the autogenous grafts are insufficient. There appears to be no significant difference in the fusion rate between autograft and allograft cases.[8, 89, 115, 126] The more important factor in terms of fusion success may be the amount of bone graft.

Scoliotic pseudarthrosis occurs most commonly at areas of high stress such as the thoracolumbar junction or lumbosacral region.[15, 118, 121] Some argue that facet excision is not necessary in the thoracic spine,[35] but meticulous decortication is necessary in all areas, particularly in the thoracolumbar and lumbar areas to decrease the incidence of pseudarthrosis. Adequate postoperative immobilization is also important to prevent pseudarthrosis and instrumentation failures.[72] In addition, when using the Cotrel-Dubousset system, compression should be applied prior to final distraction in order to provide a better environment for fusion.

Pseudarthrosis is often asymptomatic and difficult to detect with routine radiographs. Loss of correction, instrument failure, and persistent pain are warning signs of pseudarthrosis. Pseudarthrosis may be detected by plain roentgenograms, especially on oblique views. However, tomograms, bone scan, or computed tomography may be necessary in questionable cases.[31, 38, 97] In treating pseudarthrosis, one should first examine the cause. Occult or subclinical infection may be present. Stability may have been compromised by inadequate spinal instrumentation or lack of postoperative immobilization. Cigarette smoking has also been reported to be associated with pseudarthrosis.[24] It is generally accepted that pseudarthrosis in the setting of an attempted scoliotic fusion will eventually lead to failure of internal fixation and subsequent loss of correction and therefore should be treated on detection.[112, 119] Compression instrumentation and copious bone grafts with meticulous exposure of the pseudarthrosis site are usually necessary to repair pseudarthrosis. Direct current stimulation has been used both in primary posterior spinal fusions and in pseudarthrosis repairs with improved results.[45, 83] If the patient is asymptomatic and if there is no significant loss of correction or instrument failure, continued observation is justified.

Instrumentation Problems

Hook dislodgement or instrument failure can be an immediate or late postoperative complication. Hook dislodgement typically involves the proximal distraction hook, which displaces from the thoracic facet joint. Poor placement of the hook, excessive distraction, laminar fracture, and poor contouring are among the main causes of early hook failure. Proper postoperative external immobilization and avoidance of the prone position may prevent some of these complications. Treatment of hook dislodgement is simply replacement of the hook to maintain the initial curve correction. Instrument failure after several months usually indicates the presence of pseudarthrosis. Broken rods, migrating rods, broken wires, and hook dislodgement are well documented in the literature.[30, 52, 72, 136] Instrument failure in the presence of pseudarthrosis requires surgery, especially if loss of correction is noted. Fatigue fractures of the Harrington rod also occur. Erwin found that 2.1 per cent of 888 patients undergoing posterior fusion presented with a fracture of the distraction rod.[52] Most of these failures occurred at the rachet-rod junction, which is biomechanically the weakest part of the rod. Late instrument failure with solid arthrodesis in an asymptomatic patient needs no treatment.

Another complication that may be associated with instrumentation is pain related to the prominence of the implant. Bursitis or skin erosion may develop. This is particularly common in a thin patient. Proper rod contouring is important in this regard. We routinely approximate the skin before closure to examine any prominence caused by the implant. Surgical removal of the offending implant may be necessary in some cases.

Late instrument problems may be associated with neural injuries. Bowen and Ferrer reported a case in which spinal stenosis was caused by a Harrington hook in a neuromuscular disease.[19] A case of meningeal skin fistula secondary to impingement of the lower hook into the cord was reported following Harrington rod instrumentation and segmental wiring.[30] The authors blamed the incorrect placement of the lower sublaminar wire. If the lower wire is placed around the lamina one level above instead of two levels above, the hook would be more stable.

Loss of Lumbar Lordosis

Loss of lumbar lordosis is a significant complication of spinal fusion for scoliosis.[1, 9, 95, 96] Recently, LaGrone and associates reported 55 patients who required corrective osteotomies for symptomatic flat back syndrome.[96] In another paper, the senior author reviewed 43 adult patients with scoliosis who underwent spinal fusion to the sacrum: 16 patients (37 per cent) had loss of lumbar lordosis, and 12 of 16 patients had a pseudarthrosis in the lumbar spine.[9] Of the 25 patients with single-stage posterior surgery, 11 (44 per cent) had loss of lumbar lordosis, but only 2 of 8 patients who underwent two-stage anterior and posterior fusion developed loss of lumbar lordosis.

Patients with a loss of lumbar lordosis present with symptoms that include muscular pain in the upper back and lower cervical area, pain in the knees and inability to stand erect, and gait abnormalities.[96, 161] Without question, the primary etiological factor associated with the development of flat back syndrome is the use of distraction instrumentation in the lower lumbar spine or sacrum without proper rod contouring.[1, 29, 96] Thoracolumbar kyphosis and pseudarthrosis may also contribute to the development of flat back syndrome.[95]

The most effective method of treatment for the flat back syndrome is prevention. As mentioned before, for the King Type II thoracic curves, the lower lumbar spine should not be instrumented or fused as the unfused lumbar curve can compensate and give a balanced spine. If the stable vertebra is below L3 in a double major thoracic-lumbar curve, strong consideration should be given to a two-stage anterior and posterior fusion. If distraction instrumentation is to be used for double thoracic and lumbar curves, proper rod contouring is of utmost importance. The use of squareended Moe rods or segmental fixation will help to maintain lordosis. Compression on the convex side is also a useful technique in preserving lordosis. Another useful technique to preserve lumbar lordosis is to wire the distal two spinous processes together to counteract the localized kyphotic movement at the distal hook insertion site (Fig. 2–4).[167] The Cotrel-Dubousset system allows effective sagittal rod contouring and compression on the convex aspect of the curve plus derotation. This system is encouraging in its ability to correct curvature as well as to preserve lordosis. Fusion to the sacrum is rarely needed except in adult scoliotic patients with significant oblique take-off of the L5 vertebra and markedly degenerated and painful L5-S1 intervertebral disc segment.[91] If fusion to the sacrum is necessary, distraction instrumentation should be avoided. As mentioned before, a high incidence of flat back syndrome and pseudarthrosis is noted when the fusion is carried down to the sacrum.[9] The

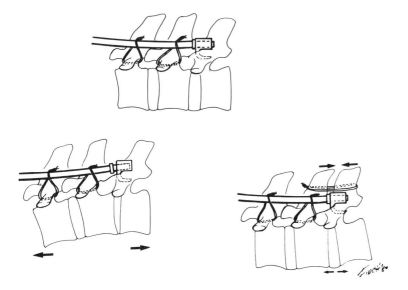

FIGURE 2–4. Illustration of distraction rodding in the lower lumbar spine, which produces a localized kyphotic moment. By tying in the last two spinous processes together, the maintenance of lordosis and better stability of the distal hook are achieved. (From Winter, R. B.: Harrington instrumentation into the lumbar spine (technique for preservation of normal lumbar lordosis). Spine *11*: 633–635, 1986.)

Galveston technique of pelvic fixation with contoured Luque rods and sublaminar wires is preferred. Various pedicular fixation devices are becoming available for sacral fixation. Surgical techniques for corrective osteotomy for symptomatic loss of lumbar lordosis are exacting. Complications are frequent, including neurological injury, pseudarthrosis, and instrument failure. In general, anterior release is done, followed by posterior osteotomy and compression instrumentation to achieve better correction and to improve fusion rate.[96]

Problems in the Juxtafused Segments

Cochran and coworkers reported an increasing incidence of low back pain with fusion below L4, particularly when Harrington rod instrumentation was used without rod contouring.[33] However, Moskowitz and associates reported no correlation between low back pain and the lowest extent of fusion in a long-term study of patients treated before the use of Harrington rod instrumentation.[123] Late onset of back pain may be related to the use of distraction rods in the lower lumbar spine. Accelerated degeneration of unfused segments may also account for back pain. Luk and associates studied the effect on the lumbosacral spine of long spine fusion in adolescent idiopathic scoliosis in 22 patients, with the average follow-up being 12.8 years.[108] The unfused intervertebral spaces were hypermobile distally, which may be a predisposition to early lumbosacral degeneration.

There are reports of acquired spondylolysis and spondylolisthesis following scoliosis surgery.[26, 57, 156] A stress concentration at the im-

mediately adjacent levels is probably responsible for this phenomenon.

Similar to problems arising in the distal unfused segments, proximal unfused segments may give problems. Moskowitz and associates reported a high incidence of neck pain (57 per cent) following fusion to the upper thoracic region. We observed a T1-T2 bilateral facet dislocation in a patient who had had previous instrumentation and fusion up to the T2 region for scoliosis.

Another problem is development of kyphotic deformity or progression of curve above the fusion mass.[37, 56] This is usually related to the improper selection of the fusion areas. All vertebrae responsible for the curve and sagittal deformity should be included in the fusion area to prevent this complication. Progression or lengthening of the curve may occur distally if all rotated vertebrae are not fused. Lengthening of curve or adding-on can occur even with proper selection of the fusion area if continued growth is present. Use of prolonged postoperative immobilization is important in these patients.[103]

SALVAGE AND RECONSTRUCTIVE SURGERY

The complications discussed above are the main reasons why reconstructive surgery may be required in patients who have had previous surgery for scoliosis. These include pseudarthrosis, curve progression, too short a fusion, persistent lateral decompensation, and loss of lumbar lordosis.[104]

Because of extensive scarring and fusion

mass from previous procedures, surgery is more time consuming and difficult. Posterior osteotomy may sometimes be necessary in patients who have had a previous spinal fusion. The purpose of osteotomy is to realign the spine in patients with progression of the curve, imbalance of the trunk, and sagittal deformity. The technique of osteotomy of a posterior fusion involves making a trough cut through the fusion mass between the pedicles, exposing the underlying dura. An osteotomy should be performed at each alternate level rather than at every level, as loosening of the bony elements may compromise the neural structures.[37]

The complication rate in these patients undergoing repeat surgery is high. A total complication rate of 71 per cent has been reported in adults who underwent reconstructive surgery for failed scoliosis fusion.[37] The mortality rate was 3.4 per cent in these series. The most frequent complications were pseudarthrosis (17 per cent), wound infection (17 per cent), wound hematoma (12 per cent), urinary tract infection (8 per cent), loss of lumbar lordosis (8 per cent), and pressure sores (8 per cent). Other complications included neurological deficits, dural lacerations, deep vein thrombosis, instrument problems, and gastrointestinal problems.[37] Floman and associates reported a series of 62 patients who had osteotomy of the fusion mass and refusion, and the rate of complications was 51 per cent.[56] Nine had a postoperative neural deficit, including six patients who developed the complication during halo-femoral traction. Six patients with significant preoperative respiratory decompensation had postoperative respiratory insufficiency. Other complications included pseudarthrosis, urinary tract infection, wound infection, excessive bleeding, gastrointestinal problems, and deep vein thrombosis.[56]

The best way to prevent these complications is to perform the initial surgery well to avoid the necessity for this major reconstructive operation. As stated before, correct levels should be chosen for fusion and instrumentation to achieve overall balance of the spine. The need for meticulous fusion technique cannot be overemphasized.

ANTERIOR APPROACH

OPERATIVE TECHNIQUE

Indications for the anterior surgical approach for idiopathic scoliosis include severe thoracic or thoracolumbar curves or rigid unbalanced lumbar curves greater than 70 to 75 degrees.[20, 146] Adults with a significant kyphotic component to their curve pattern should also have an anterior fusion in addition to posterior fusion with instrumentation. Any patient with paralytic scoliosis whose curve cannot be balanced on traction should also have a combined anterior and posterior procedure.[101, 113, 118, 132] Furthermore, if a posterior procedure necessitates fusion below L4, anterior release and fusion should first be done to save lower lumbar motion segments.[78] The advantages of combined anterior and posterior spinal surgery are improvement of correction and higher fusion rate.[28, 90] Finally, isolated, short, and flexible thoracolumbar or lumbar curves are best managed by primary anterior fusion with instrumentation.[78, 84]

Depending on the level of curve, the anterior procedure may be transthoracic, thoracoabdominal, or retroperitoneal.[21] Great caution should be exercised as potential complications are numerous during anterior exposure of the thoracolumbar spine.[165] Excision of the rib located at the superior end vertebrae is usually done for thoracic or thoracolumbar curves. One should approach from the convex side of the curvature.

For the thoracotomy approach, place the patient in the lateral decubitus position and move the upper arm forward. Insertion of a double-branched endotracheal tube into the right and left main stem bronchi is helpful to allow selective collapse of the lung. An axillary roll under the down arm is important in preventing compression of axillary neurovascular structures. The skin and subcutaneous tissues are opened from the lateral border of the paraspinous musculature to the sternocostal junction over the rib to be resected, usually T5. After the pleura is incised, exposure of the vertebral column is done by deflating the lung with a surgical laparotomy sponge. Remove the lap sponge periodically to prevent atelectasis.

For the thoracolumbar approach, the key to gaining access to the retroperitoneal space is through splitting of the costal cartilage after removal of the appropriate rib, usually T10. The retroperitoneal space is identified by the light areolar tissue of fat, and blunt finger dissection is recommended. Bluntly dissect the peritoneum from the inferior surface of the diaphragm and sweep it medially off the psoas muscle. The diaphragm is detached about 2 cm. from the periphery and suture tags are placed in order to facilitate closure. In order to avoid disruption of the vascular anastomosis located at the intervertebral foramen, the segmental artery must be ligated at the midportion of the vertebral body. For exposure of T12-L1, the crus of the diaphragm is detached. The psoas muscle may also be reflected for exposure.

After the spine is adequately exposed, removal of disc material is completed. All disc tissue must be removed to the posterior annulus and to the annulus on the opposite side. The vertebral end-plates are removed to subchondral bleeding bone, using a fine osteotome or angled curette. Minced rib can be used for the interbody fusion. Anterior instrumentation, such as the Dwyer or Zielke system, may be used, depending on the type and magnitude of the curvature. It is important to realize that Dwyer instrumentation is contraindicated in curves with increased kyphosis. Zielke instrumentation is also difficult in cases with significant kyphosis and curves greater than 80 degrees. Our most common anterior surgical procedure for scoliotic spine is disc removal and interbody fusion, followed by second stage posterior instrumentation and fusion.

OPERATIVE COMPLICATIONS

Neural Injury

Injury to the spinal cord may be due to mechanical damage during removal of the intervertebral disc, insertion of screws into the vertebral bodies or vascular insult. Mechanical damage to the spinal cord is largely preventable. Screw insertion should take place parallel to the posterior longitudinal ligament and in a posteroanterior direction to avoid penetration of the spinal canal. Vascular insult to the spinal cord is minimal if segmental vessels are ligated opposite the midportion of the vertebral body, allowing collateral vessels near the intervertebral foramen to supply blood to the spinal cord. If paraplegia is noted after surgery, x-rays should be taken to rule out penetration of the spinal canal by a screw or bone graft. Spinal cord contusion can be detected by magnetic resonance imaging. Injury to the superior hypogastric plexus or presacral nerve resulting in impotence in the male is largely avoided, as the anterior approach to the L5-S1 region is rarely necessary in scoliosis surgery.

Major Vessel Injury

The aorta or vena cava is at risk of injury during the exposure. Thorough familiarity with their anatomy is obviously important. Great caution should be taken during removal of the

rim of the annulus. It is beneficial to have an assistant hold a Chandler elevator between the vessels and the spinal column during disc removal.[146] It is important to use the appropriate length screw so that it will not extend beyond the opposite cortex. Late hemorrhage due to erosion, leakage, or false aneurysm formation of the vessel is known.[46] If bleeding is encountered during surgery, manual finger pressure or arterial clamp is used to halt bleeding prior to formal vascular repair.

Pseudarthrosis and Instrument Failure

Instrument problems may or may not be related to pseudarthrosis. Early screw pullout, cable failure, tilting of the end screw, and vertebral fracture are related to surgical technique and quality of the bone. Overzealous attempts to correct the deformity should be avoided, especially in the adult scoliotic patient with osteoporotic bone. Late cable or rod breakage is associated with pseudarthrosis (Fig. 2–5). If significant loss of correction is seen and the patient is symptomatic, revision or posterior augmentation instrumentation and

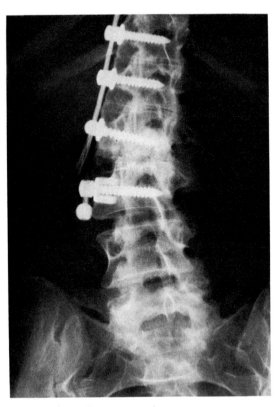

FIGURE 2–5. Anteroposterior roentgenogram revealing a failure of Dwyer cable in an asymptomatic patient who developed a pseudarthrosis after anterior fusion and instrumentation.

fusion are necessary. Problems of pseudarthrosis with or without instrumentation can be avoided if meticulous technique is used for disc removal and interbody fusion. Secondary posterior instrumentation and fusion greatly enhance the overall fusion rate.

Other Complications Related to Anterior Surgery

The most common urological complication during anterior surgery is injury to the ureter. Late hydronephrosis due to retroperitoneal fibrosis has also been reported.[32, 148] Sympathectomy effect is common after an extensive anterior procedure. The patient reports that the opposite leg is colder than the leg on the operated side. The sympathetic trunk should be carefully retracted and preserved as much as possible. Fortunately, this complication is temporary, lasting 3 to 4 months, and is rarely disabling.[149] Injury to the spleen has been reported in a patient who underwent left-sided anterior surgery for scoliosis.[73]

MISCELLANEOUS COMPLICATIONS

INFECTION

The incidence of wound infection in scoliosis surgery varies from 0.1 to 20 per cent.[102] Higher infection rates are noted among adults and paralytic scoliotic patients compared with those of idiopathic scoliotic patients.[102] Use of instrumentation, longer surgery, and previous surgery are associated with an increased infection rate. It should also be noted that the rate of wound infection in posterior procedures is approximately 2½ times greater than the anterior procedures. Lonstein reported a drop in infection rate from 9.3 per cent to less than 2.8 per cent with the use of prophylactic antibiotics.[102] Temperature, white blood cell count, and the sedimentation rate are frequently elevated in patients with wound infection, but these tests are not as reliable as clinical examination of the wound itself. Aspiration of the wound can be done in doubtful cases. If the wound is red, swollen, and tender, suggesting an infectious process, the patient should be taken to the operating room. Thorough debridement and irrigation should be performed. The fascia should be opened unless the infection is clearly localized to the superficial layer only. The bone graft should be removed and washed and may be put back. Instrumentation should not be removed initially. The wound can be closed primarily with a suction-irrigating system or left partially open for delayed primary closure.

CARDIORESPIRATORY COMPLICATIONS

Respiratory complications may include atelectasis, pneumonia, pleural effusion, pneumothorax, chylothorax, hemothorax, acute respiratory distress syndrome, respiratory failure, pulmonary thromboembolism, and fat embolism.[6, 25, 63] A pneumothorax may occur during either an anterior or posterior surgery. The pleura may be violated if the surgeon dissects too deeply between the transverse processes. Thoracoplasty is also associated with development of a pneumothorax. A tension pneumothorax is also possible by respiratory malfunction or rupture of a pulmonary bleb.[103] A tension pneumothorax is a potentially life-threatening problem. Prompt diagnosis and immediate chest tube insertion are required. Chylothorax may follow anterior surgery of the spine.[34, 47, 125, 138] Leakage in the lymphatic system should be recognized during surgery, and the stump should be ligated both proximally and distally. Treatment of chylothorax consists of chest tube drainage and decreasing the patient's fat intake. Postoperative pulmonary problems such as atelectasis and pneumonia are particularly common in adults, patients with nonidiopathic scoliosis or mental retardation, and those who undergo anterior procedures.[6] Preoperative medical consultation should be routine in these patients.

GASTROINTESTINAL COMPLICATIONS

Postoperative ileus may occur following scoliosis surgery, particularly after anterior procedures. Ileus is usually managed with nasogastric suction and delaying oral feeding until bowel sounds return. Use of narcotics should be discouraged as these medications are associated with development of ileus. Ileus may be confused with true mechanical obstruction of the bowels. Particularly in the scoliosis patient, superior mesenteric artery syndrome may occur, which includes symptoms of nausea and vomiting owing to a high intestinal obstruction.[10, 18, 27, 76, 139, 145] This syndrome is due to a mechanical compression of the third part of the duodenum as it passes between the superior mesenteric artery anteriorly and the aorta and vertebral column posteriorly. When the scoliotic patient undergoes casting or instrumentation, resultant correction of the curve narrows the angle between the superior mesenteric artery and the aorta and compresses the duodenum. Upper gastrointestinal studies with barium swallow are diagnostic. The treatment of this syndrome should consist of nasogastric suction, left lateral decubitus positioning, and occasional modification or removal of the cast. Surgical intervention is necessary if conservative treatment fails after several days.

Acute cholecystitis has been seen following spinal fusion.[55, 154] The patient presents with acute abdominal pain in the right upper quadrant in the early postoperative period. Prompt diagnosis with cholecystogram is necessary, and surgery may be required.

GENITOURINARY COMPLICATIONS

Urological complications after spinal fusion for scoliosis may be multiple. In an anterior procedure, dissection of the spine is close to the kidney and ureter. Late hydronephrosis as a result of retroperitoneal fibrosis has been reported.[32, 148] In addition, mechanical correction of severe curves may cause angulation of the ureter with resultant hydronephrosis.[85, 116] Urinary retention and urinary tract infections are common in the postoperative period. The prolonged use of an indwelling catheter is associated with a high rate of urinary tract infection.

OTHER COMPLICATIONS

Proper fluid and electrolyte maintenance is important in patients undergoing major spinal surgery. The syndrome of inappropriate antidiuretic hormone secretion has been reported following fusion.[11, 49] These patients present with hyponatremia, oliguria, and concentrated urine. Fluid intake should be restricted in these patients.

Excessive blood loss during surgery should alert the surgeon to consider disseminated intravascular coagulation (DIC) as a causative factor.[140] The diagnosis of DIC is based on elevated prothrombin and partial thromboplastin times, low platelets, a low fibrinogen level, and high levels of fibrin splint products. Treatment of DIC should include rapid replacement of fresh frozen plasma, cryoprecipitate, and platelets as well as red blood cells.

Complications related to blood transfusions may be blood reaction, hepatitis, and acquired immune deficiency syndrome (AIDS). These problems can be decreased with the use of predeposit autologous transfusions and intra-operative cell saver systems. Careful meticulous surgical technique will minimize blood loss.

The incidence of thromboembolic complications following spinal surgery is relatively lower compared with that of lower extremity surgery.[158] The use of compression stockings or boots both intraoperatively and postoperatively is recommended. Early mobilization is also important in the prevention of thromboembolic complications. Treatment of thrombophlebitis and pulmonary embolism should include prompt heparinization, followed by oral dicumarol anticoagulation. Those patients who require prolonged bedrest should be considered for prophylactic anticoagulation.

COMPLICATIONS RELATED TO DONOR BONE GRAFT SITE

Complications involving the iliac bone graft donor sites are not uncommon. The most serious complication is vascular insult. The superior gluteal artery is a branch of the internal iliac artery, which exits the sciatic notch posteriorly (Fig. 2–6). If dissection is carried down too close to the sciatic notch or if subperiosteal dissection is not maintained, the artery may be injured.[82] In the event of laceration of the superior gluteal artery, the surgeon should first pack the wound. Removal of the upper part of the sciatic notch may be necessary to expose the vessel and ligate it. If the bleeding vessel is not accessible, a retroperitoneal approach

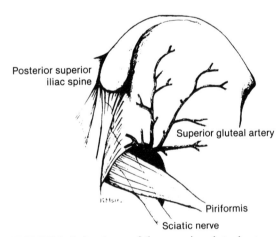

Posterior superior iliac spine

Superior gluteal artery

Piriformis

Sciatic nerve

FIGURE 2–6. Anatomy of the superior gluteal artery in relation to the posterior superior iliac spine. (From Hsu, K., Zucherman, J. F., and White, A. H.: Bone grafts and implants in spine surgery. In: White, A. H., Rothman, R. H., and Ray, C. D. (eds.): *Lumbar Spine Surgery.* St. Louis, C. V. Mosby, 1987, p. 444.)

should be used in order to control bleeding. Arteriogram and embolization may also be considered. The sciatic nerve is also at risk if the dissection is extended to the notch area. A combined traumatic arteriovenous fistula and ureteral injury has also been reported after posterior iliac bone grafting.[53] One should be thoroughly familiar with the anatomy of the sciatic notch and associated neurovascular structures to prevent these complications. The surgeon should stay cephalad to the posterior iliac spine, as an imaginary plumb line dropped from the posterior superior iliac spine passes through the bony rim of the sciatic notch (Fig. 2–7).[75] Also, the gouge should be used in a distal to proximal fashion, instead of in a direct posterior to anterior path, to avoid inadvertent slippage of the instrument deep into the soft tissues. Another complication associated with posterior iliac crest grafting is injury to the sacroiliac joint. Persistent pain or even sacro-iliac instability may result when the sacroiliac joint is significantly violated. Injury to the superior cluneal nerve may result in painful neuritis or anesthesia of the buttocks. Superior cluneal nerves are branches of L1, L2, and L3 dorsal rami and cross over the dorsal aspect of the posterior iliac crest approximately 7 to 12 cm. anterolateral to the posterior superior iliac spine. During the skin incision, care must be taken to stay medial to the superior cluneal nerves. A J-shaped distal incision helps to protect these branches. When the patient is symptomatic from painful buttocks, local anesthetic infiltration or resection of the nerves may be needed to alleviate symptoms.

Anterior iliac crest grafts are used in anterior procedures of the spine. Again, thorough familiarity with the anatomy and meticulous surgical technique will help in the prevention of vessel and nerve injuries. The skin incision should be made parallel to the iliac crest but not over the bony prominence. A skin incision over the bony prominence results in a painful scar, particularly in a thin person. An incision too close to the anterior superior iliac spine may result in meralgia paresthetica.[162] Subperiosteal dissection is important to protect the viscera and vessels medially. The lateral femoral cutaneous, iliohypogastric, and ilioinguinal nerves are at risk during exposure of the anterior iliac crest. Although rare, a hernia through the defect donor site may occur after removal of full-thickness bone.[36, 58, 106] Meticu-

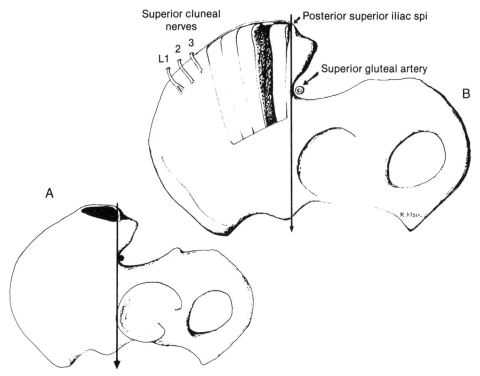

FIGURE 2–7. *(A)* An imaginary vertical line from the posterior superior iliac spine with the patient in the prone position should be the caudal limit of bone removal. *(B)* Bone graft can be removed staying cephalad to the posterior superior iliac spine, sciatic notch, and the imaginary line joining them. (From Hsu, K., Zucherman, J. F., and White, A. H.: Bone grafts and implants in spine surgery. In: White, A. H., Rothman, R. H., and Ray, C. D. (eds.): *Lumbar Spine Surgery*. St. Louis, C. V. Mosby, 1987, p. 444.)

lous closure of the periosteum and fascia prevents this complication. Treatment requires the reduction of the hernia, and the defect may be repaired using soft tissue, methylmethacrylate, or Marlex mesh.

Blood loss, hematoma formation, and infection at the donor sites are largely preventable. Curetting the cancellous bone down to the cortical bone may decrease oozing of the blood. Use of gelfoam or bone wax further minimizes blood loss from the bone. A drain should be placed and removed 1 to 2 days postoperatively. Routine prophylactic antibiotics should decrease the overall incidence of infection. Persistent graft donor site pain is reported to be as high as 37 per cent.[59] We believe that the incidence of pain is less if the posterior cortical portion of the posterior iliac crest is left undisturbed and careful periosteal dissection and closure is performed.

KYPHOSIS

PREOPERATIVE PLANNING

Kyphosis of the spine refers to a sagittal deformity beyond normal limits. The range of normal thoracic kyphosis varies widely, but most are between 21 and 33 degrees, using the Cobb method.[36] Stagnara and associates studied 100 healthy subjects and noted an even wider range of normal kyphosis up to 45 degrees.[41] Any kyphosis at the thoracolumbar junction or in the lumbar spine is abnormal. Kyphosis may be benign such as in postural kyphosis, while at other times it can produce paraplegia if it progresses to a significant degree, particularly in congenital forms.[22] Winter and Hall have classified kyphosis into different groups (Table 2–4).[50] It is important to define the etiology of the kyphotic deformity as treatment will vary accordingly.

Preoperative planning should also include assessment of curve magnitude, curve progression, flexibility, and neurological involvement. The end vertebra of kyphosis should be accurately determined as a short fusion may lead to progression of deformity beyond the fusion site. Myelography is required in congenital cases or in any deformity with neurological involvement. The detection of a tethered cord or cord compression is critical in the successful management of these cases. Preoperative skeletal traction is contraindicated in congenital kyphotic patients as paraplegia may result.

Many patients with postural kyphosis or

Table 2–4
Classification of Kyphosis (Winter and Hall[50])

I. POSTURAL DISORDERS
II. SCHEUERMANN'S KYPHOSIS
III. CONGENITAL DISORDERS
A. Failure of segmentation
B. Failure of formation
IV. PARALYTIC
A. Polio
B. Anterior horn cell disease
C. Upper motor neuron disease (e.g., cerebral palsy)
V. MYELOMENINGOCELE
VI. POST-TRAUMATIC
A. Acute
B. Chronic
C. With or without cord damage
VII. INFLAMMATORY
A. Tuberculosis
B. Other infections
VIII. POSTSURGICAL
A. Postlaminectomy
B. Postexcision (e.g., tumor)
IX. INADEQUATE FUSION
A. Too short
B. Pseudarthrosis
X. POSTIRRADIATION
A. Neuroblastoma
B. Wilm's tumor
XI. METABOLIC
A. Osteoporosis (juvenile or senile)
B. Osteogenesis imperfecta
XII. DEVELOPMENTAL
A. Achondroplasia
B. Mucopolysaccharidosis
C. Other
XIII. COLLAGEN DISEASE (E.G., MARIE-STRÜMPELL)
XIV. TUMOR (E.G., HISTIOCYTOSIS "X")
A. Benign
B. Malignant
XV. NEUROFIBROMATOSIS

Scheuermann's kyphosis respond well to bracing, and surgery is rarely necessary in these patients. The indications of surgery for thoracic Scheuermann's disease may include significant rigid kyphosis above 75 degrees and unrelenting pain despite conservative treatment. The majority of patients who require surgery should have a combined anterior and posterior fusion.[2, 15] Occasionally, surgical correction of kyphosis may be completed through an isolated posterior procedure if the deformity is relatively mild and flexible.[40, 43] Posterior instrumentation and fusion should be adequate if a kyphosis is less than 65 degrees or bending correction is less than 50 degrees.[11] This is a rare circumstance, as most patients with a relatively mild and flexible deformity respond well to bracing.[31] For patients with a large and rigid curve, posterior fusion alone will result in loss of correction and pseudarthrosis in a significant number of cases.[5]

In a congenital kyphosis, a more aggressive approach should be taken as most curves progress to produce grotesque deformities and neurological deficits.[22, 49] Most authors recommend early posterior fusion if the patients are younger than 5 years old and if the deformity is less than 55 degrees.[30, 46] The surgical treatment of congenital kyphosis of a greater magnitude in a patient older than 5 years usually consists of a combined anterior and posterior fusion.[30, 45] Occasionally, anterior cord decompression and strut fusion are necessary in patients with neurological impairment. Decompression of the cord includes removal of bone, disc material, and the posterior longitudinal ligament allowing the spinal cord to move anteriorly.[7] If scoliosis is also present, the spine must be approached from the concavity of the scoliosis to move the cord both forward and toward the concavity. Kyphosis reduction and strut bone grafting should be done in a meticulous manner to avoid graft dislodgement, graft fracture, and loss of correction.[4, 42] Bradford and others reported a series of patients who received a vascularized pedicle rib graft for their kyphotic deformities, and the results are encouraging.[3, 28] Anterior fusions with strut grafts should always include interbody fusions at all levels within the strut, as continued growth at the disc may cause pseudarthrosis. Posterior fusion should not include distraction rods, as distraction of the spine may tether the spinal cord and cause paraplegia. In situ stabilization or in situ fusion is recommended.

Paralytic kyphosis is usually due to neuromuscular diseases such as cerebral palsy, muscular dystrophy, poliomyelitis, and so forth. The deformity tends to be long and frequently associated with scoliosis. The primary problem is related to the lack of the extensor muscles.[6, 37] This lack of muscle control contributes to curve progression beyond skeletal maturity in these patients. Initial management should include spinal bracing to limit progression until early teenage years. Delaying fusion until early teenage years will allow proper trunk height. Most patients with paralytic kyphosis will eventually require a fusion. The entire curve should be included in the fusion, extending from the high thoracic area to the lumbar or sacral area. Luque rods with sublaminar wires and Galveston pelvic fixation techniques are the best methods of stabilization in these long neuromuscular curves. Anterior fusion is also necessary in patients with more severe fixed deformities and in whom traction roentgenograms fail to balance the spine and the pelvis.

Patients with myelomeningocele may have either congenital or paralytic kyphosis. The paralytic type is developmental and increases during growth. Management includes bracing and surgery as in any other paralytic kyphosis. Spinal fusion in patients with myelomeningocele is difficult because of the lack of posterior bony elements, osteopenia, and poor bone stock at the donor site. For these reasons, many patients with myelomeningocele require both anterior and posterior fusions. The congenital type is present at birth and can produce an extreme kyphotic deformity. Excision of two to three vertebral bodies proximal to the apex of the deformity is carried out in patients over 3 years of age.[20] This is a formidable procedure with a significant risk of great blood loss.[8, 13, 17, 19, 23, 27]

Kyphosis may develop secondary to trauma, inflammatory or infectious diseases, laminectomy, irradiation, tumors, metabolic diseases, collagen diseases, skeletal dysplasias, neuropathy, neurofibromatosis, and Klippel-Feil syndrome.[14, 18, 21, 26, 28, 29, 32, 33, 34, 38, 39, 44, 47, 48] Treatment should be individualized according to the curve magnitude, flexibility, and neurological status. A combined anterior and posterior fusion is usually required in severely affected patients in most cases, regardless of the etiology of kyphosis.[12]

OPERATIVE TECHNIQUES

A transthoracic approach is used for anterior exposure, removing the rib corresponding to the upper portion of the kyphosis to be fused.[2] A right- or left-sided approach is feasible, but it should be approached from the convexity of the curvature if scoliosis is also present. If decompression of the spinal cord is planned, the spine should be approached from the concavity of the curvature unless the scoliotic deformity is severe. In general, a scoliotic curve greater than 60 degrees is better exposed from the convex side. The anterior technique for interbody fusion has already been described under scoliosis. A strut graft is placed if anterior decompression is carried out.[2] Rib, iliac crest, fibula, and vascularized rib are all suitable donors.[1, 3, 28, 42] Anterior transthoracic exposure, osteotomy, cord decompression, and strut fusion for congenital or severe kyphosis are techniques that only skillful and experienced spinal surgeons should attempt in well-equipped medical centers with maximum support.

Posterior instrumentation and fusion is most commonly achieved with use of compression Harrington rods; however, Luque rods with sublaminar wires or the Cotrel-Dubousset system may also be used. A posterior fusion with Harrington compression instrumentation is well described in the literature.[5, 43] Harrington compression rods are still commonly used for Scheuermann's kyphosis today. The heavy ¼-inch threaded rods and multiple hooks should be used to increase overall stability. Typically, five upper hooks and five lower hooks are necessary. Upper hooks may be applied to the transverse processes or the laminae. Application of upper hooks over the laminae is slightly more risky but offers better protection against hook dislodgement. The lower hooks are usually applied under the lamina. The threaded contoured rods are then applied, and the hooks are seated with nuts. If associated scoliosis is present, it is recommended that a distraction rod be inserted on the concave side and a compression rod on the convex side. Segmental instrumentation with sublaminar wires has also been used to correct kyphosis. However, the passage of sublaminar wires may be associated with increased neurological risk.[24] In addition, there has been a recent report showing that use of Luque rods and sublaminar wires was associated with greater failures.[9] Under no circumstances should a compression system be used with a sublaminar wire. Tightening of a sublaminar wire may produce anterior migration of the compression hook attached to the compression rod and may produce neurological deficit.

The Cotrel-Dubousset system has been applied to kyphosis surgery. The surgical instrumentation and technique are complex, and sufficient training is required for proper use of this system. This system may be used in a way similar to the Harrington compression rods. Because of heavier rods and interconnecting bars, stability of this construct is better. Using claw hook configuration, the surgeon can compress the apical vertebrae as well as the end vertebrae above and below along the same rod. One should avoid undue force to avoid fracture of the lamina. Because of the learning curve, one should obtain hands-on experience and training with other surgeons well versed in the techniques. Although segmental instrumentation with either sublaminar wires or the Cotrel-Dubousset system enhances the overall stability of the surgical construct, we believe that the use of postoperative orthosis is important in avoiding problems with fixation or loss of correction.

OPERATIVE COMPLICATIONS

The complications discussed under scoliosis are all applicable to kyphosis surgery. Meticulous technique and great care are again important in the prevention of neural injury, pseudarthrosis, instrument failure, and loss of correction. Table 2–5 shows the incidence of various complications of kyphosis surgery from several different series.

NEURAL INJURY

Spinal cord injury is the most feared complication, particularly during cord decompression through an anterior approach. Montgomery and Hall reported neurological deficits in 3 out of 25 patients with Type I congenital kyphosis.[30] Surgical intervention in untreated Type I kyphosis is difficult and complex and is naturally associated with a higher rate of complication. As stated before, early posterior fusion in situ before 5 years of age is therefore recommended in these cases.[46] Neurological impairment may be due to mechanical trauma or vascular insult to the spinal cord. Dural or spinal cord injuries from overly aggressive disc excision or instrument penetration are technical errors that can be avoided. Another important point to remember is to avoid ligating the segmental vessels close to the intervertebral foramen.

Maintaining adequate perfusion to the spinal cord is also important. Malcolm and associates reported four patients with neurological deterioration after combined anterior and posterior fusion for post-traumatic kyphosis.[26] The factors related to postoperative neural deterioration were thoracic location and increased intraoperative blood loss. An anterior procedure between fifth and ninth thoracic vertebrae must not be taken lightly as circulatory compromise to the cord is possible when severe hypotension due to blood loss occurs. Neurological compromise has also been associated with use of skeletal traction. Floman and co-workers reported neurological damage in 4 of 73 patients who underwent combined anterior and posterior fusions for their spinal deformities.[12] All four patients had congenital kypho-

Table 2–5
Complications of Kyphosis Surgery in Different Series

AUTHOR	DIAGNOSIS	NUMBER OF PATIENTS	SURGICAL PROCEDURE	OVERALL COMPLICATION RATE (EXCEPT LOSS OF CORRECTION)	NEURAL PROBLEMS	PSEUDARTHROSIS OR GRAFT PROBLEMS	LOSS OF CORRECTION	INSTRUMENT PROBLEMS
Bradford (1975)	Scheuermann	22	H-rodding & fusion	45%	0	14%	73% (>5°)	23%
Bradford (1980)	Scheuermann	24	A & P fusion with H-rod	58%	0	4.2%	21% (>10°) below fusion	13%
Bradford (1982)	Mixed	48	Anterior, A&P, or H-rod fusion	69%	8%	23%	21% (>10°)	2%
Herndon (1981)	Scheuermann	13	A & P fusion with H-rod	54%	7.6%	0	15%	15%
Lowe (1987)	Scheuermann	24	A & P fusion with Luque	50%	16%	0	17% (>5°) 8% (below fusion)	25%
Malcolm (1981)	Post-trauma	48	Anterior, A&P, or posterior	48%	8.3%	12.5%	42% (>10°)	2%
Montgomery (1982)	Congenital	34	Anterior, A&P, or posterior with or without H-rod	24%	9%	15%	18% (>10°)	0
Speck (1986)	Scheuermann	59	Posterior or A&P	31%	2%	0	15% (>10°)	2%
Taylor (1979)	Scheuermann	27	Posterior H-rod	48%	0%	—	33% (inside fusion) 48% (outside fusion)	7%
Winter (1973)	Congenital	44	Posterior or A&P	80%	4.5%	52% (posterior) 13% (A&P)	—	4.5%
Winter (1985)	Congenital	94	Posterior or A&P	37%	3%	41% (posterior) 8% (A&P)	55% (posterior) 25% (A&P)	3%

sis, and three of them developed neurological deterioration during skeletal traction. The fourth patient suffered paraparesis after Harrington instrumentation that resolved on removal of the rods. Winter and associates reported a similar experience with three cases of neurological injury, of which two were related to halo-femoral traction.[45] Skeletal traction is tempting but should be avoided in congenital scoliosis for this reason.

PSEUDARTHROSIS, LOSS OF CORRECTION, AND INSTRUMENT PROBLEMS

Development of a pseudarthrosis may lead to progression of the kyphosis, loss of correction, or failure of surgical construct. Multiple factors should be considered in the development of pseudarthrosis following kyphosis surgery. Anterior fusion is necessary in many patients with significant kyphosis. In the review by Winter and coworkers it was noted that if the curve was 50 degrees or less, there was a 16.6 per cent rate of pseudarthrosis with posterior fusion alone.[49] However, for curves between 50 and 75 degrees, there was a 75 per cent rate of pseudarthrosis with posterior fusion alone.[49] Combined anterior and posterior fusion for these larger curves resulted in a 12.5 per cent rate of pseudarthrosis in this series.[49] Bradford and associates reported on results in 22 patients with Scheuermann's kyphosis in 1975. They concluded that posterior fusion with Harrington instrumentation relieved pain and improved deformity, but there were 16 patients with loss of correction of more than 5 degrees, 2 pseudarthroses, and 5 instrument problems.[5] Bradford and associates later reported on 24 patients with Scheuermann's kyphosis who underwent a combined anterior and posterior spine fusion.[2] All had a solid arthrodesis with good pain relief. Significant loss of correction was not observed in these patients. They concluded that a kyphosis of more than 70 degrees should have a combined anterior and posterior spine fusion. Herndon and coworkers also recommended a combined anterior and posterior fusion for patients with Scheuermann's kyphosis.[15] Failure to supplement an anterior procedure with a posterior fusion and instrumentation may also lead to a pseudarthrosis and loss of correction.

Fusion techniques must be meticulous. Inadequate length of posterior fusion will lead to failure. Rigid stabilization with Harrington compression rods or the Cotrel-Dubousset sys-

tem is important. The need for meticulous decortication and massive bone grafting cannot be overemphasized. Anterior grafting techniques are even more demanding. Inadequate disc and end-plate removal will lead to pseudarthrosis. Countersinking of the strut graft prevents graft dislodgement. Placing the strut graft too far anteriorly with no bony contact with the apex of the kyphosis will lead to graft fracture. Use of vascularized rib pedicle graft has been described.[1, 3] Postoperative immobilization with a cast or bivalved body jacket is necessary until solid fusion occurs.

Repeat posterior fusion is generally necessary in congenital types as augmentation. A pseudarthrosis should be repaired if it is associated with loss of correction and instrument failure. More rigid constructs, such as Cotrel-Dubousset rods, may enhance fusion rates and lessen instrument failures.

SPONDYLOLISTHESIS

PREOPERATIVE PLANNING

Spondylolisthesis entails the forward displacement of one vertebra on another. The L5-S1 region is most commonly involved, but the upper lumbar spine may also be affected.[23] A pars interarticularis defect without displacement of the vertebra is called spondylolysis. Most authors use Newman's classification of spondylolisthesis (Fig. 2–8). Complications related to spondylolisthesis may stem from incorrect diagnosis, inappropriate treatment, and surgical maloccurrences.

It is important to realize that many patients with spondylolysis or spondylolisthesis are asymptomatic. In other words, symptomatic patients who present with radiographic evidence of spondylolisthesis may actually be suffering from other problems such as neoplasm or a herniated disc. Careful history and examination and thorough work up are mandatory to rule out other pathological processes. In the growing child, back pain with associated hamstring tightness may be due to osteoid osteoma, neurofibroma, or disc space infection. An isthmic spondylolisthesis will rarely progress after the age of 20 and usually produces no symptoms in the adult.[16, 40] Degenerative spondylolisthesis in the older population is commonly associated with symptoms of both back and leg pain. However, spinal infection or metastatic tumor must be considered in the differential diagnosis.

Spondylolisthesis

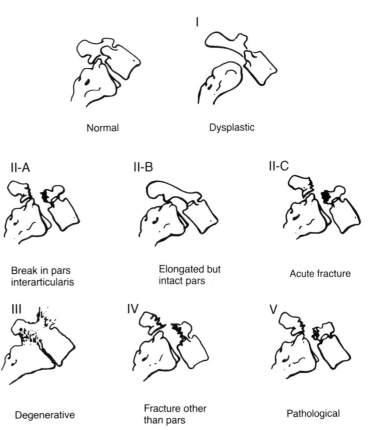

FIGURE 2–8. Newman's classification of spondylolisthesis. (From Bradford, D. S., et al. (eds.): *Moe's Textbook of Scoliosis and Other Spinal Deformities* (2nd ed.). Philadelphia, W. B. Saunders, 1987, p. 404.)

The majority of patients with spondylolisthesis can be managed conservatively. The growing child with mechanical symptoms of back pain, limited motion, and hamstring spasm should restrict his or her activity. If roentgenographic studies or bone scan shows evidence of acute injury to the pars interarticularis, spinal immobilization with a brace should be considered.[47] Brace treatment for symptomatic Grade I and II spondylolisthesis in the child is quite successful in terms of pain relief and prevention of further progression.[3] The adult patient with either isthmic or degenerative spondylolisthesis should receive maximum conservative treatment before surgery is planned. Surgical indications include progressive slippage greater than 50 per cent, particularly in the growing child, and unrelenting pain in any patient. Hanley and Levy reported that unsatisfactory results are higher in males, middle-aged individuals, those with a smoking habit, those with radicular symptoms, compensation cases, and those with a development of

pseudarthrosis.[19] If the child is symptomatic despite conservative treatment, surgery may be offered even with slippage of less than 50 per cent.

The exact method of operative technique depends on the magnitude of slip percentage and slip angle. Although other techniques have been described,[12, 48] the gold standard remains in situ bilateral intertransverse process fusion.[49, 53] This procedure has been successful even in those with a high grade slippage if the slip angle is relatively normal.[24, 37] For mild slips (less than 25 per cent), insertion of screws across the pars defect or passage of wires anterior to the transverse processes that loop over the spinous processes can be done.[8, 34, 36] These procedures may be better for higher lumbar spondylolisthesis distinct from L5-S1 level and if the involved intervertebral disc is relatively normal.

For high-grade slips, a decision must be made whether to fuse in situ or to perform reduction and fusion. Johnson and Kirwan reported on 17 patients with greater than 50 per cent slip: 16 of 17 patients who underwent bilateral-lateral fusion without reduction had an excellent result in terms of pain relief, prevention of progression, and improvement of hamstring tightness.[24] The average follow-up of this study was 14 years. Similarly, Peek and associates reported on eight patients with Grade III or IV isthmic spondylolisthesis who had in situ arthrodesis without decompression.[37] All of these patients had excellent relief of pain with solid arthrodesis at an average follow-up of 5.5 years. Bohlman and associates reported two patients with spondyloptosis who underwent successful posterior decompression and posterolateral and interbody fusion through a posterior approach.[4] An important common denominator of these studies is that significant neural complications were not encountered.

There is great controversy about reduction of the deformity in those with a high slip angle. Bradford recommended reduction in patients with greater than 45-degree slip angle and 75 per cent slippage.[10] There have been a number of reduction techniques reported in the literature.[2, 30, 41, 44] A combined anterior and posterior procedure has also been described to achieve reduction and fusion.[7, 9, 14, 50] A combined procedure is particularly helpful in patients with previous failed posterior fusions.[25] In general, complications are significant when reduction is performed.[7, 14, 30, 32, 43] The advantages of reduction are improvement of posture and gait. Cast reduction by the Scalietti method followed by posterolateral fusion is probably the safest procedure.[18, 41] Gaines and associates reported on the treatment of spondyloptosis by two-stage L5 vertebrectomy and reduction of L4 onto S1.[17] This procedure restores spinal alignment with less likelihood of nerve root stretch.

In the patient with spondylolisthesis and root-related symptoms, the nerve root should be decompressed by laminectomy (Gill procedure) and foraminotomy in addition to fusion.[13] The Gill procedure alone is not adequate for decompression of the involved nerve root and is contraindicated in the growing child.

Bilateral lateral fusions generally can be performed from L5 to the sacrum. For slips greater than 50 per cent, the fusion should include L4 as well. There are many instrumentation techniques that are used in the lumbosacral region to provide additional stability and enhance fusion rates.[7, 9, 14, 15, 27] Use of pedicle screw fixation is probably most advantageous in providing greater stability, achieving some reduction, and perhaps increasing the fusion rate.[28, 30, 33, 44, 45, 46] Disadvantages of pedicle screw instrumentation include added operating time and risk of neurological injury. The technique of bilateral lateral fusion with or without instrumentation is exacting, and each step of the surgical procedure should be done with great care.

OPERATIVE TECHNIQUE

A kneeling position lessens blood loss by reducing the intra-abdominal venous pressure. A midline incision is made, and subperiosteal dissection of the paraspinous muscles is done, exposing the spinous process, lamina, facet joints, pars, and transverse processes. The inferior incision is curved in a J shape for the purpose of obtaining bone grafts from the posterior iliac crest. One must be careful not to destroy the facet capsule above the planned fusion site as degenerative changes or instability may develop later. At this time, laminectomy and foraminotomy are performed if necessary. The facet joints to be fused should be meticulously prepared by excising the cartilage from the joints and removing the cortical bone from the lateral portion of the superior articular process. Decortication of the transverse process, the lateral gutter, and the sacral ala is carefully performed (Fig. 2–9). Morselized bone from the iliac crest or allograft bone is placed in the prepared gutter. A Hemovac drain is used routinely.

The pedicle screw-plate fixation may provide additional stability. Knowledge of pedicular

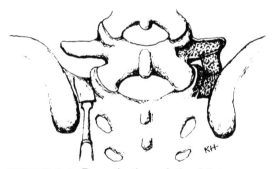

FIGURE 2–9. Decortication of the L5 transverse process and the ala of the sacrum for L5-S1 fusion. (From Hsu, K., Zucherman, J. F., White, A. H., and Wynne, G.: Internal fixation with pedicle screws. In: White, A. H., Rothman, R. H., and Ray, C. D. (eds.): *Lumbar Spine Surgery.* St. Louis, C. V. Mosby, 1987, p. 325.)

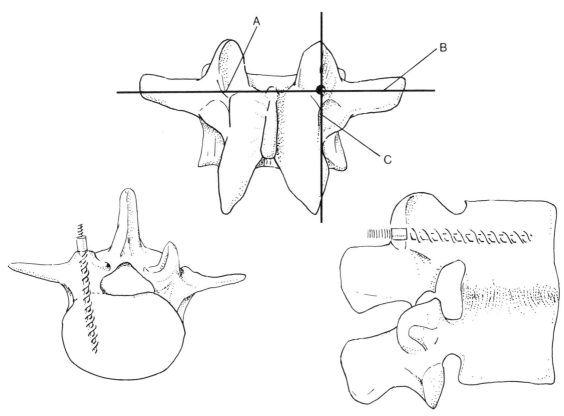

FIGURE 2–10. Pedicle entrance site *(A)* by crossing the horizontal line *(B)* along the midportion of the transverse processes and the vertical line *(C)* along the bony crest or facet. (From Hsu, K., Zucherman, J. F., White, A. H., and Wynne, G.: Internal fixation with pedicle screws. In: White, A. H., Rothman, R. H., and Ray, C. D. (eds.): *Lumbar Spine Surgery.* St. Louis, C. V. Mosby, 1987, p. 326.)

anatomy in relation to neural structures is crucial. The pedicle entrance point is situated at the crossing of two lines (Fig. 2–10). The vertical line is the extension of the facet joint in line with the bony crest coming from the inferior articular facet. The horizontal line passes through the middle of the insertion of the transverse process or 1 mm. below the joint line. The sacral entrance point is at the lower point of the L5-S1 articulation. The nerve root is situated just medial and inferior to the pedicle as it exits into the intervertebral foramen. Therefore, one must avoid the area medial and inferior to the pedicle to prevent damage of the nerve root. A small rongeur or burr is used to decorticate the pedicle entrance (Fig. 2–11). A Steinmann pin and empty drill bits are malleted into each pedicle, penetrating only 1 cm. A lateral x-ray is taken to ensure the correct placement and direction of the pedicular screws. In difficult cases, an antero-posterior view is also recommended for locating the pedicles. A blunt instrument is carefully

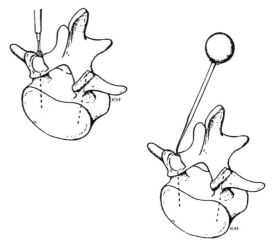

FIGURE 2–11. Preparation for the pedicle screw insertion by power burr and blunt probe. (From Hsu, K., Zucherman, J. F., White, A. H., and Wynne, G.: Internal fixation with pedicle screws. In: White, A. H., Rothman, R. H., and Ray, C. D. (eds.): *Lumbar Spine Surgery.* St. Louis, C. V. Mosby, 1987, p. 327.)

advanced through the pedicle into the vertebral body. The amount of medial angulation varies depending on the level. The pedicle direction is straightforward at L1, and medial angulation is 2.5 degrees at L2, 5 degrees at L3, 10 degrees at L4, and 30 degrees at L5 on the average. One should aim about 25 degrees medially at S1. We do not routinely violate the anterior cortex of the sacrum as the lumbar plexus and vascular structures are at risk of injury. A thin probe is used to feel the walls of the pedicle. Tapping is done, followed by insertion of screws and plates of appropriate diameter and length. The plates must be bent to conform to the lordotic lumbar spine. Decortication of the transverse processes and pars interarticularis is carried out, and bone grafts from the posterior iliac crest are placed. It is important to place some bone graft underneath the plates for improved fusion. Tightening of the plates is completed last.

OPERATIVE COMPLICATIONS

NEURAL INJURY

Nerve root or cauda equina injury is rare during in situ lumbosacral fusion for spondylolisthesis.[31] However, neural injury is a potential concern if laminectomy and foraminotomy are planned or if reduction of slippage is attempted.

The adult patient with severe radiculopathy requires neural decompression in addition to fusion. Dural tears, nerve root injury, and cauda equina syndrome are potential complications. Prevention and treatment of these complications are discussed under lumbar disc disease and spinal stenosis.

Reduction of spondylolisthesis is rarely necessary. Results of in situ fusion for a mild to moderate degree of slippage are satisfactory.[24, 37] Even in patients with a severe degree of slippage, bilateral lateral in situ fusions can be successful if the slip angle is relatively normal. Reduction and stabilization of severe kyphotic lumbosacral junction is one of the most difficult procedures. Complication rates are high, especially L5 nerve root injury (Table 2–6). One should consider cast reduction by Scaglietti[41] and resist the temptation of complete reduction. As long as the slip angle is corrected, the patient will be satisfied with the result.

Table 2–6
Complications of Different Spondylolisthesis Series

AUTHOR	NUMBER OF PATIENTS	SURGERY	NEURAL	NONUNION	OTHERS
Bosworth	73	Gill and PF	0%	15%	none
Boxall	43	PLF, Gill and fusion, or reduction	0.02%	25%	3 infection 2 instrument failure
Bradford (1979)	10	anterior and posterior fusion with reduction	30%	0%	2 deep vein thrombosis
Bradford (1987)	16	anterior and posterior fusion with reduction	31%	38% (delayed unions)	1 DVT 1 bowel obstruction 1 graft slip
Dewald	14	anterior and posterior fusion with reduction	28%	0%	1 instrument failure
Hanley	50	PLF or Gill and PLF	0%	12%	
Harris	21	Posterior fusion	0%	5%	
Hensinger	20	PLF	0%	0%	1 infection
Johnson	17	PLF or posterior fusion	0%	0%	1 wound dehiscence 1 pressure sore
Kaneda	53	Harrington rod and PLF	0%	9%	1 infection
Matthiass	51	Reduction and PLF with pedicle screws	45%	0%	
McPhee	8	anterior and posterior fusion	12%	0%	1 loss of reduction
McQueen	7	PLF with pedicle screws	43%	0%	2 screw breakage 1 screw into the disc
Peek	8	PLF	0%	0%	
Pizzutillo	40	PLF	0%	0%	
Roy-Camille	7	Pedicle screws	14%	0%	
Scaglietti	6	Casting and PLF or Harrington	0%	0%	
Sevastikoglou	10	Traction and anterior fusion	0%	0%	
Van Rens	24	Anterior fusion	0%	4%	
Velikas	36	PLF	0%	17%	

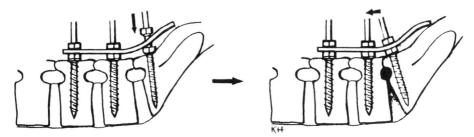

FIGURE 2–12. Hyperlordosis created by the plate and screw may narrow the intervertebral foramen. (From Hsu, K., Zucherman, J. F., White, A. H., and Wynne, G.: Internal fixation with pedicle screws. In: White, A. H., Rothman, R. H., and Ray, C. D. (eds.): *Lumbar Spine Surgery*. St. Louis, C. V. Mosby, 1987, p. 333.)

Pedicle screw fixations are frequently used for stabilization along with fusion. It is important to identify accurately the pedicle entrance point to avoid neural injury. Roentgenographic confirmation of the pedicle is helpful. Avoid drilling into the pedicle. A blunt probe should be used so that the dense cortex of the pedicle will prevent penetrance outside the pedicle. Use of pedicle screws with a correct diameter and length prevents "blow-out fracture" of the pedicle and nerve root injury. When a plate is applied, one should avoid hyperlordosis and compression force between the vertebrae, as resultant narrowing of the intervertebral foramen may compress the nerve roots (Fig. 2–12). Sacral screws may be inserted without penetrating the anterior cortex in most cases. The lumbosacral plexus and vascular structures are at risk when the anterior cortex of the sacrum is perforated, particularly if the screw is too long (Fig. 2–13).

PSEUDARTHROSIS, LOSS OF CORRECTION, AND INSTRUMENT PROBLEMS

Table 2–6 lists different series of patients who underwent surgery for spondylolisthesis. The incidence of pseudarthrosis ranges from 0 to 25 per cent. There are many factors involved in the pathogenesis of pseudarthrosis. Patients who smoke cigarettes are at increased risk for the development of pseudarthrosis.[11, 19] Patients with previous failed fusion, Grade III or IV spondylolisthesis, or multiple level involvement do worse. As mentioned repeatedly, the key to prevention of pseudarthrosis is meticulous surgical technique and massive bone grafting. Adequate postoperative immobilization with a pantaloon cast or brace is also important if rigid internal fixation was not performed. With the advent of rigid internal fixation such as pedicle screw systems, the incidence of pseudarthrosis may decrease. However, this

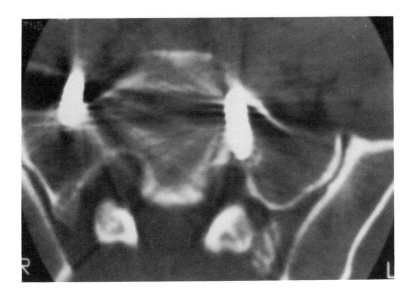

FIGURE 2–13. Computed tomography of the sacrum, showing the left screw penetrating too far anteriorly. (This patient had right L5 radiculopathy, which resolved after changing to a proper length screw.)

device cannot replace the meticulous technique of decortication and bone grafting, as Horowitz reported 32 per cent nonunion rate even with the use of pedicle screwplate system.[22]

Anterior interbody fusion should also be considered in cases where posterolateral bone grafting alone may not be adequate.[42, 45] Those with a high grade slip angle and translation should be considered for anterior interbody fusion. The advantages of anterior or posterior interbody fusion are greater stability of bone graft under compression and probable increased rate of fusion.

Direct current electrical bone growth stimulation has also been used to increase the rate of union. Kane reported 81 per cent radiological union in those who received direct current electrical bone growth stimulation compared with 54 per cent union in control patients.[26] More studies are necessary to further investigate the potential benefits of this device for spinal fusion.

Loss of correction and instrument problems may be related to the development of pseudarthrosis, but they may also occur independently. There seems to be a high incidence of hook dislodgement and instrument failure when a distraction instrumentation is used in the lumbosacral junction. The pedicle screw instrumentation is more rigid and provides a greater stability. However, screw breakage and loss of correction are also reported after pedicle screw instrumentation.[52]

It is important to keep in mind that posterolateral fusion in situ is a safe and reliable procedure with minimal complications for the majority of patients. If reduction with instrumentation is attempted, one must accept a high complication rate. We recommend reduction with instrumentation only if Grade III or more slippage with a high slip angle is present. Reduction should be performed to correct the kyphosis primarily but not translation, and the reduction should be done with the L5 nerves completely exposed and monitored. Partial reduction should be accepted if the nerve root is in danger of stretch. Preoperative traction or casting should be considered to enhance reduction, and pedicle screw instrumentation and interbody fusion can be performed to enhance fusion rate. Postoperatively, the patient can be mobile with a unilateral pantaloon cast in most cases.

REFERENCES

Scoliosis

1. Aaro, S., and Ohlen, G.: The effect of Harrington instrumentation on the sagittal configuration and mobility of the spine in scoliosis. Spine 6:570–575, 1983.
2. Akbarnia, B. A.: Selection of methodology in surgical treatment of adolescent idiopathic scoliosis. Orthop. Clin. North Am. 19:319–328, 1988.
3. Allen, B. L., and Ferguson, R. L.: The Galveston experience with L-rod instrumentation for adolescent scoliosis. Clin. Orthop. 229:59–69, 1988.
4. Allen, B. L., and Fergerson, R. L.: A 1988 perspective on the Galveston technique of pelvic fixation. Orthop. Clin. North Am. 19:409–425, 1988.
5. An, Howard S., Mikhail, W. E., Jackson, W. T., et al.: Effects of hypotensive anesthesia, methylmethacrylate, and nonsteroidal anti-inflammatory medications on bleeding in patients undergoing total hip arthroplasty. Trans. Orthop. 12:724, 1989.
6. Anderson, P. R., Puno, M. R., Lovell, S. L., et al.: Postoperative respiratory complications in non-idiopathic scoliosis. Acta Anaesthesiol. Scand. 29:186–192, 1985.
7. Ascani, E., Bartolozzi, P., Logroscino, C. A., et al.: Natural history of untreated idiopathic scoliosis after skeletal maturity. Spine 11:784–789, 1986.
8. Aurori, B. F., Weierman, R. J., Lowell, H. A., et al.: Pseudoarthrosis after spinal fusion for scoliosis (A comparison of autogeneic and allogeneic bone grafts). Clin. Orthop. 199:153–158, 1985.
9. Balderston, R. A., Winter, R. B., Moe, J. H., et al.: Fusion to the sacrum for nonparalytic scoliosis in the adult. Spine 11:824–829, 1986.
10. Barner, H. B., and Sherman, D. C.: Vascular compression of the duodenum. Surg. Gynecol. Obstet. 117:103, 1963.
11. Bell, G. R., Gurd, A. R., Orlowski, J. P., et al.: The syndrome of inappropriate antidiuretic-hormone secretion following spinal fusion. J. Bone Joint Surg. 68A:720–724, 1986.
12. Ben-David, B., Haller, G., and Taylor, P.: Anterior spinal fusion complicated by paraplegia. A case report of a false-negative somatosensory-evoked potential. Spine 12:536–539, 1987.
13. Ben-David, B., Taylor, P., and Haller, G.: Posterior spinal fusion complicated by posterior column injury: A case report of a false negative wake-up test. Spine 12:540–543, 1987.
14. Benner, B., and Ehni, G.: Degenerative lumbar scoliosis. Spine 4:548–552, 1979.
15. Bialik, K., and Piggott, H.: Pseudoarthrosis following treatment of idiopathic scoliosis by Harrington instrumentation and fusion without added bone. J. Pediatr. Orthop. 7:152–154, 1987.
16. Bieber, E., Tolo, V., and Uematsu, S.: Spinal cord monitoring during posterior spinal instrumentation and fusion. Clin. Orthop. 229:121–124, 1988.
17. Birch, J. G., Herring, J. A., Roach, J. W., et al.: Cotrel-Dubousset instrumentation in idiopathic scoliosis. A preliminary report. Clin. Orthop. 227:24–29, 1988.
18. Bisla, R. S., and Louis, H. J.: Acute vascular compression of the duodenum following cast application. Surg. Gynecol. Obstet. 140:563–566, 1975.

19. Bowen, J. R., and Ferrer, J.: Spinal stenosis caused by a Harrington hook in neuromuscular disease. Clin. Orthop. *180*:179–181, 1983.

20. Bradford, D. S.: Adult scoliosis. Current concepts of treatment. Clin. Orthop. *229*:70–87, 1988.

21. Bradford, D. S.: Techniques of surgery. In: Bradford, D. S., et al. (eds.): *Moe's Textbook of Scoliosis and Other Spinal Deformities*, 2nd ed. Philadelphia, W. B. Saunders Company, 1987, pp. 135–189.

22. Briard, J. L.: Adult lumbar scoliosis. Spine *4*:526–532, 1979.

23. Broom, M. J., Banta, J. V., and Renshaw, T. S.: Spinal fusion augmented by Luque-rod segmental instrumentation for neuromuscular scoliosis. J. Bone Joint Surg. *71A*:32–44, 1989.

24. Brown, C. W., Orme, T. J., and Richardson, H. D.: The rate of pseudoarthrosis (surgical nonunion) in patients who are smokers and patients who are nonsmokers: A comparison study. Spine *11*:942–943, 1986.

25. Brown, L. P., and Stelling, F. H.: Fat embolism as a complication of scoliosis fusion. J Bone Joint Surg. *56A*:1764, 1974.

26. Brunet, J. A., and Wiley, J. J.: Acquired spondylolysis after spinal fusion. J. Bone Joint Surg. *66B*:720–724, 1984.

27. Bunch, W., and Delaney, J.: Scoliosis and acute vascular compression of the duodenum. Surgery *67*:901, 1970.

28. Byrd, J. A., Scoles, P. V., Winter, R. B., et al.: Adult idiopathic scoliosis treated by anterior and posterior spinal fusion. J. Bone Joint Surg. *69A*:843–850, 1987.

29. Casey, M. P., Asher, M. A., Jacobs, R. R., et al.: The effect of Harrington rod contouring on lumbar lordosis. Spine *12*:750–753, 1987.

30. Christodoulou, A. G., Preston, B. J., and Webb, J. K.: Meningeal skin fistula. A complication following Harrington rod instrumentation and segmental wiring. Spine *14*:241–242, 1989.

31. Clader, T. J., Dawson, E. G., and Bassett, L. W.: The role of tomography in the evaluation of the postoperative spinal fusion. Spine *9*:686–689, 1984.

32. Cleveland, R. H., Gilsanz, V., Lebowitz, R. L., et al.: Hydronephrosis from retroper oneal fibrosis and anterior spinal fusion. J. Bone Joint Surg. *60A*:996, 1978.

33. Cochran, T., Irstam, L., and Nachemson, A.: Long-term anatomic and functional changes in patients with adolescent idiopathic scoliosis treated by Harrington rod fusion. Spine *8*:576–583, 1983.

34. Colletta, A. J., and Mayer, P. J.: Chylothorax: An unusual complication of anterior thoracic interbody spinal fusion. Spine *7*:46–49, 1982.

35. Court-Brown, C. M., Stoll, J. E., and Gertzbein, S. D.: Thoracic facetectomy and bone grafting in the surgical treatment of adult idiopathic scoliosis. Spine *12*:992–995, 1987.

36. Cowley, S. P., and Anderson, L. D.: Hernias through donor sites for iliac-bone grafts. J. Bone Joint Surg. *65A*:1023–1025, 1983.

37. Cummine, J. L., Lonstein, J. E., Moe, J. H., et al.: Reconstructive surgery in the adult for failed scoliosis fusion. J. Bone Joint Surg. *61A*:1151–1161, 1979.

38. Dawson, E. G., Clader, T. J., and Bassett, L. W.: A comparison of different methods used to diagnose pseudoarthrosis following posterior spinal fusion for scoliosis. J. Bone Joint Surg. *67*:1153–1159, 1985.

39. Denis, F.: Cotrel-Dubousset instrumentation in the treatment of idiopathic scoliosis. Orthop. Clin. North Am. *19*:291–311, 1988.

40. Diaz, J. H., and Lockhart, C. H.: Postoperative quadriplegia after spinal fusion for scoliosis with intraoperative awakening. Anesth. Analg. *66*:1039–1042, 1987.

41. Dooley, J. F., McBroom, R. J., Taguchi, T., et al.: Nerve root infiltration in the diagnosis of radicular pain. Spine *13*:79–83, 1988.

42. Dorgan, J. C., Abbott, T. R., and Bentley, G.: Intra-operative awakening to monitor spinal cord function during scoliosis surgery. Description of the technique and report of four cases. J. Bone Joint Surg. *66B*:716–719, 1984.

43. Dove, J.: Segmental wiring for spinal deformity. A morbidity report. Spine *14*:229–231, 1989.

44. Drummond, D., Guadagni, J., Keene, J. S., et al.: Interspinous process segmental spinal instrumentation. J. Pediatr. Orthop. *4*:397–404, 1984.

45. Dwyer, A. F.: Direct current stimulation in spinal fusion. Med. J. Aust. *1*:73, 1974.

46. Dwyer, A. P.: A fatal complication of paravertebral infection and traumatic aneurysm following Dwyer instrumentation. In: Proceedings of the Australian Orthopaedic Association. J. Bone Joint Surg. *61B*:239, 1979.

47. Eisenstein, S., and O'Brien, J. P.: Chylothorax—A complication of Dwyer anterior instrumentation. Br. J. Surg. *64*:339–341, 1977.

48. Eismont, F. J., and Simeone, F.: Bone overgrowth (hypertrophy) as a cause of late paraparesis after scoliosis fusion. J. Bone Joint Surg. *63A*:1016–1019, 1981.

49. Elster, A. D.: Hyponatremia after spinal fusion caused by inappropriate secretion of antidiuretic hormone (SIADH). Clin. Orthop. *194*:136–141, 1985.

50. Engler, G. L., Spielholtz, N. I., Bernhard, W. N., et al.: Somatosensory evoked potentials during Harrington instrumentation for scoliosis. J. Bone Joint Surg. *60A*:520–532, 1978.

51. Epstein, J. A., Epstein, B. S., and Jones, M. D.: Symptomatic lumbar scoliosis with degenerative changes in the elderly. Spine *4*:542–547, 1979.

52. Erwin, W. D., Dickson, J. H., and Harrington, P. R.: Clinical review of patients with broken Harrington rods. J. Bone Joint Surg. *62A*:1302–1307, 1980.

53. Escalas, F., and Dewals, R. L.: Combined traumatic arteriovenous fistula and ureteral injury. A complication of iliac bone-grafting. J. Bone Joint Surg. *140*:270, 1977.

54. Evarts, C. M., Winter, R. B., and Hall, J. E.: Vascular compression of the duodenum associated with the treatment of scoliosis. J. Bone Joint Surg. *53A*:431, 1971.

55. Floman, Y., Micheli, L. J., Barker, W. D., et al.: Acute cholecystitis following the surgical treatment of spinal deformities in the adult. Clin. Orthop. *180*:132–134, 1984.

56. Floman, Y., Penny, J. N., Micheli, L. J., et al.: Osteotomy of the fusion mass in scoliosis. J. Bone Joint Surg. 64:1307–1316, 1982.

57. Friedman, R. J., and Micheli, L. J.: Acquired spondylolisthesis following scoliosis surgery. Clin. Orthop. 190:132–134, 1984.

58. Froimson, A. I., and Cumming, A. G.: Iliac hernia following hip arthrodesis. Clin. Orthop. 80:89–91, 1971.

59. Frymoyer, J. W., Howe, J., and Kuhlmann, D.: The long-term effects of spinal fusion on the sacroiliac joints and ilium. Clin. Orthop. 134:196–201, 1978.

60. Gersoff, W. K., and Renshaw, T. S.: The treatment of scoliosis in cerebral palsy by posterior spinal fusion with Luque-rod segmental instrumentation. J. Bone Joint Surg. 70:41–44, 1988.

61. Ginsberg, H. H., Goldstein, L. L., Robinson, S. C., et al.: Back pain in postoperative idiopathic scoliosis. Long-term follow-up study (abstract). Spine 4:518, 1979.

62. Ginsberg, H. H., Shetter, A. G., and Raudzens, P. A.: Postoperative paraplegia with preserved intraoperative somatosensory evoked potentials. Case report. J. Neurosurg. 63:296–300, 1985.

63. Gittman, J. E., Buchanan, T. A., Fisher, B. J., et al.: Fatal fat embolism after spinal fusion for scoliosis. J.A.M.A. 249:779–781, 1983.

64. Goll, S. R., Balderston, R. A., Stambough, J. L., et al.: Depth of intraspinal wire penetration during passage of sublaminar wires. Spine 13:503–509, 1988.

65. Goldstein, L. A.: Treatment of idiopathic scoliosis by Harrington instrumentation and fusion with fresh autogenous iliac bone grafts. J. Bone Joint Surg. 51A:209–222, 1969.

66. Grubb, S. A., Lipscomb, H. J., and Coonrad, R. W.: Degenerative adult onset scoliosis. Spine 13:241–245, 1988.

67. Gurr, K. R., and McAfee, P. C.: Cotrel-Dubousset instrumentation in adults (a preliminary report). Spine 13:510–520, 1988.

68. Harrington, P. R.: Treatment of scoliosis. Correction and internal fixation by spine instrumentation. J. Bone Joint Surg. 44A:591–610, 1962.

69. Harrington, P. R., and Dickson, J. H.: An eleven-year clinical investigation of Harrington instrumentation. A preliminary report on 578 cases. Clin. Orthop. 93:113–130, 1973.

70. Healey, J. H., and Lane, J. M.: Structural scoliosis in osteoporotic women. Clin. Orthop. 195:216–223, 1985.

71. Heilbronner, D. M., and Sussman, M. D.: Early mobilization of adolescent scoliosis patients following Wisconsin interspinous segmental instrumentation as an adjunct to Harrington distraction instrumentation. Clin. Orthop. 229:53–58, 1988.

72. Herndon, W. A., Sullivan, J. A., Yngve, D. A., et al.: Segmental spinal instrumentation with sublaminar wires. A critical appraisal. J. Bone Joint Surg. 69:851–859, 1987.

73. Hodge, W. A., and DeWald, R. L.: Splenic injury complicating the anterior thoracoabdominal surgical approach for scoliosis. J. Bone Joint Surg. 65A:396–397, 1983.

74. Horton, W. C., Leatherman, K. D., Holt, R. T., et al.: Results of Zielke instrumentation of idiopathic thoracolumbar scoliosis. Orthop. Trans. 10:33, 1986.

75. Hsu, K., Zucherman, J. F., and White, A. H.: Bone grafts and implants in spine surgery. In: White, A. H., Rothman, R. H., and Ray, C. D. (eds.): Lumbar Spine Surgery. St. Louis, C. V. Mosby, 1987, pp. 434–458.

76. Hughes, J. P., McEntire, J. D., and Setze, T. K.: Cast syndrome. Arch. Surg. 108:230, 1974.

77. Jackson, R. P., Simmons, E. H., and Stripinis, D.: Incidence and severity of back pain in adult idiopathic scoliosis. Spine 8:749–756, 1983.

78. Johnson, J. R., and Holt, R. T.: Combined use of anterior and posterior surgery for adult scoliosis. Orthop. Clin. North Am. 19:361–370, 1988.

79. Johnston, C. E., Happel, L. T., Jr., Norris, R., et al.: Delayed paraplegia complicating sublaminar segmental spinal instrumentation. J. Bone Joint Surg. 68:556–563, 1986.

80. Jones, E. T., Mathews, L. S., and Hensinger, R. N.: The wake-up technique as a dual protector of spinal cord function during spine fusion. Clin. Orthop. 168:113–118, 1982.

81. Kahanovitz, N., and Levine, D. B.: Iatrogenic complications of spinal surgery. Contemp. Orthop. 9:23–39, 1984.

82. Kahn, B.: Superior gluteal artery laceration, a complication of iliac bone graft surgery. Clin. Orthop. 140:204–207, 1979.

83. Kane, W. J.: Posterior arthrodesis of the thoracolumbosacral spine. In: Chapman, M. W. (ed.): Operative Orthopaedics. Philadelphia, J. B. Lippincott Company, 1988, pp. 1957–1964.

84. Kaneda, K., Fujiya, N., and Satoh, S.: Results with Zielke instrumentation for idiopathic thoracolumbar and lumbar scoliosis. Clin. Orthop. 205:195–203, 1986.

85. Keim, H. A., and Weinstein, J. D.: Acute renal failure—A complication of spine fusion in the tuck position. J. Bone Joint Surg. 52A:1248, 1970.

86. King, H. A.: Posterior scoliosis surgery. In: Chapman, M. W. (ed.): Operative Orthopaedics. Philadelphia, J. B. Lippincott Company, 1988, pp. 1979–1994.

87. King, H. A., Moe, J. H., Bradford, D. S., et al.: The selection of fusion levels in thoracic idiopathic scoliosis. J. Bone Joint Surg. 65A:1302, 1983.

88. Kling, T. F., Jr., Fergusson, N. V., Leach, A. B., et al.: The influence of induced hypotension and spine distraction on canine spinal cord blood flow. Spine 10:878–883, 1985.

89. Knapp, D. R., and Jones, E. T.: Use of cortical cancellous allograft for posterior spinal fusion. Clin. Orthop. 229:99–105, 1988.

90. Korovessis, P.: Combined VDS and Harrington instrumentation for treatment of idiopathic double major curves. Spine 12:244–250, 1987.

91. Kostuik, J. P.: Treatment of scoliosis in the adult thoracolumbar spine with special reference to fusion to the sacrum. Orthop. Clin. North Am. 19:371–380, 1988.

92. Kostuik, J. P., and Bentivoglio, J.: The incidence of low back pain in adult scoliosis. Spine 6:268–273, 1981.

93. Kostuik, J. P., and Hall, B. B.: Spinal fusions to the sacrum in adults with scoliosis. Spine 8:489–500, 1983.

94. Kostuik, J. P., Israel, J., and Hall, J. E.: Scoliosis surgery in adults. Clin. Orthop. 226:225–234, 1973.

95. LaGrone, M. O.: Loss of lumbar lordosis (a complication of spinal fusion for scoliosis). Orthop. Clin. North Am. 19:383–393, 1988.

96. LaGrone, M. O., Bradford, D. S., Moe, J. H., et al.: Treatment of symptomatic flatback after spinal fusion. J. Bone Joint Surg. 70A:569–580, 1988.

97. Lang, P., Genant, H. K., Chafetz, N., et al.: Three dimensional computed tomography and multiplanar reformations in the assessment of pseudoarthrosis in posterior lumbar fusion patients. Spine 13:69–75, 1988.

98. Letts, R. M., and Hollenberg, C.: Delayed paresis following spinal fusion with Harrington instrumentation. Clin. Orthop. 125:45–48, 1977.

99. Liebergall, M., Gomori, M., Porat, S., et al.: Dural penetration by interspinous process segmental spine instrumentation: Case report. J. Spinal Dis. 2:56–58, 1989.

100. Lonstein, J. E.: Adult scoliosis. In: Bradford, D. S., et al. (eds.): Moe's Textbook of Scoliosis and Other Spinal Deformities, 2nd ed. Philadelphia, W. B. Saunders Company, 1987, pp. 369–390.

101. Lonstein, J. E., and Akbarnia, B. A.: Operative treatment of spinal deformities in patients with cerebral palsy or mental retardation. J. Bone Joint Surg. 65A:43–55, 1983.

102. Lonstein, J., Winter, R., Moe, J., et al.: Wound infection with Harrington instrumentation and spine fusion for scoliosis. Clin. Orthop. 96:222–233, 1973.

103. Lonstein, J. E.: Complications of treatment. In: Bradford, D. S. (ed.): Moe's Textbook of Scoliosis and Other Spinal Deformities, 2nd ed. Philadelphia, W. B. Saunders Company, 1987, pp. 465–490.

104. Lonstein, J. E.: Salvage and reconstructive surgery. In: Bradford, D. S. (ed.): Moe's Textbook of Scoliosis and Other Spinal Deformities, 2nd ed. Philadelphia, W. B. Saunders Company, 1987, pp. 391–402.

105. Lonstein, J. E., and Akbarnia, B. A.: Operative treatment of spinal deformities in patients with cerebral palsy or mental retardation. J. Bone Joint Surg. 65A:43–55, 1983.

106. Lotem, M., Maor, P., Haimoff, H., et al.: Lumbar hernia at an iliac bone graft donor site. Clin. Orthop. 80:130–132, 1971.

107. Lovallo, J. L., Banta, J. V., and Renshaw, T. S.: Adolescent idiopathic scoliosis treated by Harrington-rod distraction and fusion. J. Bone Joint Surg. 68:1326–1330, 1986.

108. Luk, K. D., Lee, F. B., Leong, J. C., et al.: The effect on the lumbosacral spine of long spinal fusion for idiopathic scoliosis. A minimum 10-year follow-up. Spine 12:996–1000, 1987.

109. Luque, E. R.: Segmental spinal instrumentation for correction of scoliosis. Clin. Orthop. 163:192–198, 1982.

110. Luque, E. R.: Paralytic scoliosis in growing children. Clin. Orthop. 163:202–209, 1982.

111. MacEwen, G. D., Bunnell, W. P., and Sriram, K.: Acute neurological complications in the treatment of scoliosis. J. Bone Joint Surg. 57A:404–408, 1975.

112. May, V. R., and Mauck, W. R.: Exploration of the spine for pseudoarthrosis following spinal fusion in the treatment of scoliosis. Clin. Orthop. 53:116–122, 1967.

113. Mazur, J., Menelaus, M. B., Dickens, D. R. V., et al.: Efficacy of surgical management for scoliosis in myelomeningocele: Correction of deformity and alteration of functional status. J. Pediatr. Orthop. 6:568–575, 1986.

114. McAllister, J. W., Bridwell, K. H., Betz, R., et al.: Coronal decompensation produced by Cotrel-Dubousset derotation for idiopathic right thoracic scoliosis. Trans. Orthop. 13:79, 1989.

115. McCarthy, R. E., Peek, R. D., Morrissy, R. T., et al.: Allograft bone in spinal fusion for paralytic scoliosis. J. Bone Joint Surg. 68A:370–375, 1986.

116. McMaster, W. C., and Silber, I.: A urologic complication of Dwyer instrumentation. J. Bone Joint Surg. 57A:710, 1975.

117. McMaster, M. J.: Occult intraspinal anomalies and congenital scoliosis. J. Bone Joint Surg. 66A:588–601, 1984.

118. McMaster, M. J.: Anterior and posterior instrumentation and fusion of thoracolumbar scoliosis due to myelomeningocele. J. Bone Joint Surg. 69B:20–25, 1987.

119. McMaster, M. J., and James, J. I. P.: Pseudoarthrosis after spinal fusion for scoliosis. J. Bone Joint Surg. 58B:305–312, 1976.

120. Micheli, L. J., and Hall, J. E.: Complications in the management of adult spinal deformities. In: Epps, C. H. (ed.): Complication in Orthopaedic Surgery. Philadelphia, J. B. Lippincott Company, 1978, pp. 1039–1072.

121. Moe, J. H.: Complications of scoliosis treatment. Clin. Orthop. 53:21–30, 1967.

122. Moe, J. H., Purcell, G. A., and Bradford, D. S.: Zielke instrumentation (VDS) for the correction of spinal curvature. Clin. Orthop. 180:133–153, 1983.

123. Moskowitz, A., Moe, J. H., Winter, R. B., et al.: Long-term follow-up of scoliosis fusion. J. Bone Joint Surg. 62A:364–376, 1980.

124. Nachemson, A.: Adult scoliosis and back pain. Spine 4:513–517, 1979.

125. Nakai, S., and Zielke, K.: Chylothorax—A rare complication after anterior and posterior spinal correction (report of six cases). Spine 11:830–833, 1986.

126. Nasca, R. J., and Whelchel, J. D.: Use of cryopreserved bone in spinal surgery. Spine 12:222–227, 1987.

127. Nash, C. D., Lorig, R. A., Schatzinger, L. A., et al.: Spinal cord monitoring during operative treatment of the spine. Clin. Orthop. 126:100–105, 1977.

127a. Nilsonne, U., and Lundgren, K. D.: Long-term prognosis in idiopathic scoliosis. Acta Orthop. Scand. 39:456, 1968.

128. Norwall, A., and Wikkelso, C.: A late neurological complication of scoliosis surgery in connection with syringomyelia. Acta Orthop. Scand. 50:407–410, 1979.

129. Nuber, G. W., and Schafer, M. F.: Surgical management of adult scoliosis. Clin. Orthop. 208:228–237, 1986.

130. Ogiela, D. M., and Chan, D. P. K.: Ventral derotation spondylodesis (a review of 22 cases). Spine 11:18–22, 1986.

131. Ogilvie, J. W.: Anterior spine fusion with Zielke instrumentation for idiopathic scoliosis in adolescents. Orthop. Clin. North Am. 19:313–317, 1988.

132. Osebold, W. R., Mayfield, J. K., Winter, R. B., et al.: Surgical treatment of paralytic scoliosis associated with myelomeningocele. J. Bone Joint Surg. 64A:841–856, 1982.

133. Patel, N. J., Pater, B. S., Paskin, S., et al.: Induced moderated hypotensive anesthesia for spinal fusion and Harrington-rod instrumentation. J. Bone Joint Surg. 67A:1384–1387, 1985.

134. Phillips, W. A., and Hensinger, R. N.: Control of blood loss during scoliosis surgery. Clin. Orthop. 229:88–93, 1988.

135. Phillips, W. A., and Hensinger, R. N.: Wisconsin and other instrumentation for posterior spinal fusion. Clin. Orthop. 229:44–51, 1988.

136. Ponder, R. C., Dickson, J. H., Harrington, P. R., et al.: Results of Harrington instrumentation and fusion in the adult idiopathic scoliosis patient. J. Bone Joint Surg. 57A:797–801, 1975.

137. Ponte, A.: Postoperative paraplegia due to hypercorrection of scoliosis and drop in blood pressure. J. Bone Joint Surg. 56A:444, 1974.

138. Propst-Proctor, S. L., Riski, L. A., and Bleck, E. E.: The cisterna chyli in orthopaedic surgery. Spine 8:787–792, 1983.

139. Puranik, S. R., Keiser, R. P., and Gilbert, M. G.: Arteriomesenteric duodenal compression in children. Am. J. Surg. 124:334–339, 1972.

140. Raphael, B. G., Lackner, H., and Engler, G. L.: Disseminated intravascular coagulation during surgery for scoliosis. Clin. Orthop. 162:41–46, 1982.

141. Renshaw, T. S.: The role of Harrington instrumentation and posterior spine fusion in the management of adolescent idiopathic scoliosis. Orthop. Clin. North Am. 19:257–267, 1988.

142. Richards, B. S., Birch, J. G., Herring, J. A., et al.: Frontal and sagittal plane balance following Cotrel-Dubousset instrumentation. Trans. Orthop. 13:78, 1989.

143. Roy, E. P., Gutmann, L., Riggs, J. E., et al.: Intraoperative somatosensory evoked potential monitoring in scoliosis. Clin. Orthop. 229:94–98, 1988.

144. San Martino, A., D'Andria, F. M., and San Martino, C.: The surgical treatment of nerve root compression caused by scoliosis of the lumbar spine. Spine 8:261–265, 1983.

145. Scandalakis, J. E., Akin, J. T., Milsap, J. H., et al.: Vascular compression of the duodenum. Contemp. Surg. 10:33, 1977.

146. Schafer, M. F.: The anterior approach to scoliosis. In: Chapman, M. W. (ed.): Operative Orthopaedics. Philadelphia, J. B. Lippincott Company, 1988, pp. 1965–1978.

147. Scoliosis Research Society: Morbidity and Mortality Committee Report, 1987.

148. Silber, I., and McMaster, W.: Retroperitoneal fibrosis with hydronephrosis as a complication of the Dwyer procedure. J. Pediatr. Surg. 12:255, 1977.

149. Simmons, E. H., and Trammell, T. R.: Operative management of adult scoliosis. In: Evarts, M. C. (ed.): Surgery of the Musculoskeletal System. New York, Churchill Livingstone, 1983.

150. Simmons, E. H., and Jackson, R. P.: The management of nerve root entrapment syndromes associated with the collapsing scoliosis of idiopathic lumbar and thoracolumbar curves. Spine 4:533–541, 1979.

151. Sponseller, P. D., Cohen, M. S., Nachemson, A. F., et al.: Results of surgical treatment of adults with idiopathic scoliosis. J. Bone Joint Surg. 69A:667–675, 1987.

152. Steel, H. H.: Rib resection and spine fusion in correction of convex deformity in scoliosis. J. Bone Joint Surg. 65A:920–925, 1983.

153. Swank, S., Lonstein, J. E., Moe, J. H., et al.: Surgical treatment of adult scoliosis. J. Bone Joint Surg. 63A:268–287, 1981.

154. Teele, R. L., Nussbaum, A. R., Wyly, J. B., et al.: Cholelithiasis after spinal fusion for scoliosis in children. J. Pediatr. 111:857–860, 1987.

155. Thompson, G. H., Wilber, R. G., Shaffer, J. W., et al.: Segmental spinal instrumentation in idiopathic scoliosis. Spine 10:623–630, 1985.

156. Tietjen, R., and Morgenstern, J. M.: Spondylolisthesis following surgical fusion for scoliosis. Clin. Orthop. 117:176–178, 1976.

157. Trammell, T. R., Schroeder, R. D., and Reed, D. B.: Rotatory olithesis in idiopathic scoliosis. Spine 13:1378–1382, 1988.

158. Uden, A.: Thromboembolic complications following scoliosis surgery in Scandinavia. Acta Orthop. Scand. 50:175–178, 1979.

159. VanDam, B. E., Bradford, D. S., Lonstein, J. E., et al.: Adult idiopathic scoliosis treated by posterior spinal fusion and Harrington instrumentation. Spine 12:32–36, 1987.

160. Vauzelle, C., Stagnara, P., and Jouvinroix, P.: Functional monitoring of spinal cord during spinal surgery. J. Bone Joint Surg. 55A:441, 1973.

161. Wasylenko, M., Skinner, S. R., Perry, J., et al.: An analysis of posture and gait following spinal fusion with Harrington instrumentation. Spine 8:840–845, 1983.

162. Weikel, A. M., and Habal, M. B.: Meralgia paresthetica: A complication of iliac bone procurement. Plast. Reconstr. Surg. 60:572–574, 1977.

163. Weinstein, S. L., and Ponseti, I. V.: Curve progression in idiopathic scoliosis. J. Bone Joint Surg. 65A:447–455, 1983.

164. West, J. L., Boachie-Adjei, O., Bradford, D. S., et al.: Decompensation following CD instrumentation: A worrisome complication. Trans. Orthop. 13:78–79, 1989.

165. Westfall, S. H., Akbarnia, B. A., Merenda, J. T., et al.: Exposure of the anterior spine. Technique, complications, and results in 85 patients. Am. J. Surg. 154:700–704, 1987.

166. Wilber, R. G., Thompson, G. H., Shaffer, J. W., et al.: Postoperative neurological deficits in segmental spinal instrumentation. J. Bone Joint Surg. 66A:1178–1187, 1984.

167. Winter, R. B.: Harrington instrumentation into the lumbar spine (technique for preservation of normal lumbar lordosis). Spine 11:633–635, 1986.

168. Winter, R. B., Lonstein, J. E., and Denis, F.: Pain patterns in adult scoliosis. Orthop. Clin. North Am. 19:339–345, 1988.
169. Winter, R. B., Moe, J. H., and Lonstein, J. E.: Posterior spinal arthrodesis for congenital scoliosis. J. Bone Joint Surg. 66A:1188–1197, 1984.
170. Winter, R. B., Moe, J. H., and Eiler, V. E.: Congenital scoliosis. A study of 234 patients treated and untreated. J. Bone Joint Surg. 50A:1–47, 1968.

Kyphosis

1. Bradford, D. S.: Anterior vascular pedicle bone grafting for the treatment of kyphosis. Spine 5:318–323, 1980.
2. Bradford, D. S., Ahmed, K. B., Moe, J. H., et al.: The surgical management of patients with Scheuermann's disease. J. Bone Joint Surg. 62A:705–712, 1980.
3. Bradford, D. S., and Daher, Y. H.: Vascularised rib grafts for stabilisation of kyphosis. J. Bone Joint Surg. 68B:357–361, 1986.
4. Bradford, D. S., Ganjavian, S., Antonious, D., et al.: Anterior strut-grafting for the treatment of kyphosis. Review of experience with forty-eight patients. J. Bone Joint Surg. 64A:680–690, 1982.
5. Bradford, D. S., Moe, J. H., Montalvo, F. J., et al.: Scheuermann's kyphosis. Results of surgical treatment by posterior spine arthrodesis in twenty-two patients. J. Bone Joint Surg. 57A:439–448, 1975.
6. Bunch, W. H., Smith, D., and Hakala, M.: Kyphosis in the paralytic spine. Clin. Orthop. 128:107–112, 1977.
7. Chou, S. N.: The treatment of paralysis associated with kyphosis. Clin. Orthop. 128:149–154, 1977.
8. Christofersen, M. R., and Brooks, A. L.: Excision and wire fixation of rigid myelomeningocele kyphosis. J. Pediatr. Orthop. 5:691–696, 1985.
9. Coscia, M. F., Bradford, D. S., and Ogilvie, J. W.: Scheuermann's kyphosis—Results in 19 cases treated by spinal arthrodesis and L-rod instrumentation. Presented at the Scoliosis Research Society, 1987.
10. Daher, Y. H., Lonstein, J. E., Winter, R. B., et al.: Spinal deformities in patients with Friedreich ataxia: A review of 19 patients. J. Pediatr. Orthop. 5:553, 1985.
11. Drummond, D. S.: Kyphosis in the growing child. State of the art review. Spine 1:339–356, 1987.
12. Floman, Y., Micheli, L. J., Penny, N., et al.: Combined anterior and posterior fusion in seventy-three spinally deformed patients. Clin. Orthop. 164:110–122, 1984.
13. Hall, J. E., and Poitras, B.: The management of kyphosis in patients with myelomeningocele. Clin. Orthop. 128:33–40, 1977.
14. Hensinger, R. N.: Kyphosis secondary to skeletal dysplasia and metabolic disease. Clin. Orthop. 128:115–128, 1977.
15. Herndon, W. A., Emans, J. B., Micheli, L. J., et al.: Combined anterior and posterior fusion for Scheuermann's kyphosis. Spine 6:125–130, 1981.
17. Heydemann, J. S., and Gillespie, R.: Management of myelomeningocele kyphosis in the older child by kyphectomy and segmental spinal instrumentation. Spine 12:37–41, 1987.
18. Hsu, L. C., Lee, P. C., and Leong, J. C. Y.: Dystrophic spinal deformities in neurofibromatosis. J. Bone Joint Surg. 66B:495–499, 1984.
19. Leatherman, K. D., and Dickson, R. A.: Congenital kyphosis in myelomeningocele, vertebral resection and posterior spine fusion. Spine 3:22, 1978.
20. Linseth, R. E., and Stelzer, L.: Vertebral excision for kyphosis in children with myelomeningocele. J. Bone Joint Surg. 61A:699–704, 1979.
21. Lonstein, J. E.: Postlaminectomy kyphosis. Clin. Orthop. 128:93–100, 1977.
22. Lonstein, J. E.: Neurologic deficits secondary to spinal deformity. A review of the literature and report of 43 cases. Spine 5:331–355, 1980.
23. Lowe, G. P., and Menelaus, M. B.: The surgical management of kyphosis in older children with myelomeningocele. J. Bone Joint Surg. 60B:40–45, 1978.
24. Lowe, T. G.: Double L-rod instrumentation in the treatment of severe kyphosis secondary to Scheuermann's disease. Spine 12:336–340, 1987.
25. Luque, E. R.: The correction of postural curves of the spine. Spine 7:270–275, 1982.
26. Malcolm, B. W., Bradford, D. S., Winter, R. B., et al.: Post-traumatic kyphosis. J. Bone Joint Surg. 53A:891–899, 1981.
27. Mayfield, J. K.: Severe spine deformity in myelodysplasia and sacral agenesis. Spine 6:498–509, 1981.
28. McBride, G. G., and Bradford, D. S.: Vertebral body replacement with femoral neck allograft and vascularized rib strut graft. A technique for treating post-traumatic kyphosis with neurologic deficit. Spine 8:406–415, 1983.
29. Moe, J. H., and Van Dam, B. E.: Neurofibromatosis. In: Bradford, D. S., et al. (eds.): Moe's Textbook of Scoliosis and Other Spinal Deformities, 2nd ed. Philadelphia, W. B. Saunders Company, 1987, pp. 329–346.
30. Montgomery, S. P., and Hall, J. E.: Congenital kyphosis. Spine 7:360–364, 1982.
31. Montgomery, S. P., and Erwin, W. E.: Scheuermann's kyphosis—Long-term results of Milwaukee brace treatment. Spine 6:5–8, 1981.
32. O'Brien, J. P.: Kyphosis secondary to infectious disease. Clin. Orthop. 128:56–64, 1977.
33. Ogilvie, J. W.: Spine deformity following radiation. In: Bradford, D. S., et al. (eds.): Moe's Textbook of Scoliosis and Other Spinal Deformities, 2nd ed. Philadelphia, W. B. Saunders Company, 1987, pp. 547–554.
34. Piazza, M. R., Bassett, G. S., and Bunnell, W. P.: Neuropathic spinal arthropathy in congenital insensitivity to pain. Clin. Orthop. 236:175–179, 1988.
35. Purnell, M., Drummond, D. S., Keene, J. S., et al.: Hex-nut loosening following compression instrumentation of the spine. Clin. Orthop. 203:172–178, 1986.
36. Propst-Proctor, S. L., and Bleck, E. E.: Radiographic determination of lordosis and kyphosis in normal and scoliotic children. J. Pediatr. Orthop. 3:344–346, 1983.

37. Riddick, M. F., Winter, R. B., and Lutter, L. D.: Spinal deformities in patients with spinal muscle atrophy. A review of 36 patients. Spine 7:476–483, 1982.
38. Riseborough, E. J.: Irradiation induced kyphosis. Clin. Orthop. 128:101–106, 1977.
39. Roberson, J. R., and Whitesides, T. E., Jr.: Surgical reconstruction of late post-traumatic thoracolumbar kyphosis. Spine 10:307–312, 1985.
40. Speck, G. R., and Chopin, D. C.: The surgical treatment of Scheuermann's kyphosis. J. Bone Joint Surg. 68B:189–193, 1986.
41. Stagnara, P., De Mauroy, J. C., Dran, G., et al.: Reciprocal angulation of vertebral bodies in a sagittal plane: Approach to references for the evaluation of kyphosis and lordosis. Spine 7:335–342, 1982.
42. Streitz, W., Brown, J. C., and Bonnett, C.: Anterior fibular strut grafting in the treatment of kyphosis. Clin. Orthop. 128:140–148, 1977.
43. Taylor, T. C., Wenger, D. R., Stephen, J., et al.: Surgical management of thoracic kyphosis in adolescents. J. Bone Joint Surg. 61A:496–503, 1979.
44. Whitesides, T. E., Jr.: Traumatic kyphosis of the thoracolumbar spine. Clin. Orthop. 128:78–92, 1977.
45. Winter, R. B., Moe, J. H., and Lonstein, J. E.: The surgical treatment of congenital kyphosis. A review of 94 patients age 5 years or older, with 2 years or more follow-up in 77 patients. Spine 10:224–231, 1985.
46. Winter, R. B., and Moe, J. H.: The results of spinal arthrodesis for congenital spinal deformity in patients younger than five years old. J. Bone Joint Surg. 64A:419–432, 1982.
47. Winter, R., Moe, J. H., Bradford, D. S., et al.: Spine deformity in neurofibromatosis. J. Bone Joint Surg. 61A:677–694, 1979.
48. Winter, R. B.: Dwarfs. In: Bradford, D. S., et al. (eds.): Moe's Textbook of Scoliosis and Other Spinal Deformities, 2nd ed. Philadelphia, W. B. Saunders Company, 1987, pp. 522–547.
49. Winter, R. B., Moe, J. H., and Wang, J. F.: Congenital kyphosis. Its natural history and treatment as observed in a study of one hundred and thirty patients. J. Bone Joint Surg. 55A:223–256, 1973.
50. Winter, R. B., and Hall, J. E.: Kyphosis in childhood and adolescence. Spine 3:285–308, 1978.

Spondylolisthesis

1. Amundson, G. M., and Wenger, D. R.: Spondylolisthesis—Natural history and treatment. State of the art review. Spine 1:323–338, 1978.
2. Balderston, R. A., and Bradford, D. S.: Technique for achievement and maintenance of reduction for severe spondylolisthesis using spinous process traction wiring and external fixation of the pelvis. Spine 10:376–382, 1985.
3. Bell, D. F., Ehrlich, M. G., and Zaleske, D. J.: Brace treatment for symptomatic spondylolisthesis. Clin. Orthop. 236:192–198, 1988.
4. Bohlman, H. H., and Cook, S. S.: One-stage decompression and posterolateral and interbody fusion for lumbosacral spondyloptosis through a posterior approach. J. Bone Joint Surg. 64A:415–418, 1982.
5. Bosworth, D. M., Field, J. W., Damarst, L., et al.: Spondylolisthesis: A critical review of a consecutive series of cases treated by arthrodesis. J. Bone Joint Surg. 37:767–786, 1955.
6. Boxall, D., Bradford, D. S., Winter, R. B., et al.: Management of severe spondylolisthesis in children and adolescents. J. Bone Joint Surg. 61A:479–495, 1979.
7. Bradford, D. S.: Treatment of severe spondylolisthesis. A combined approach for reduction and stabilization. Spine 4:423–429, 1979.
8. Bradford, D. S., and Iza, J.: Repair of the defect in spondylolysis or minimal degrees of spondylolisthesis by segmental wire fixation and bone grafting. Spine 10:673–679, 1985.
9. Bradford, D. S., and Gotfried, Y.: Staged salvage reconstruction of grade IV and V spondylolisthesis. J. Bone Joint Surg. 69A:191–195, 1987.
10. Bradford, D. S.: Management of spondylolisthesis and spondylolysis. Instructional Course Lectures XXXII. American Academy of Orthopaedic Surgeons, St. Louis, C. V. Mosby, 1983, pp. 151–162.
11. Brown, C. W., Orme, T. J., and Richardson, H. D.: The rate of pseudoarthrosis (surgical nonunion) in patients who are smokers and patients who are nonsmokers: A comparison study. Spine 11:942–943, 1986.
12. Cloward, R. B.: Spondylolisthesis: Treatment by laminectomy and posterior interbody fusion. Review of 100 cases. Clin. Orthop. 154:74–82, 1981.
13. Davis, I. S., and Bailey, R. W.: Spondylolisthesis. Indications for lumbar nerve root decompression and operative technique. Clin. Orthop. 117:129–134, 1976.
14. DeWald, R. L., Faut, M. M., Taddonio, R. F., et al.: Severe lumbosacral spondylolisthesis in adolescents and children. Reduction and staged circumferential fusion. J. Bone Joint Surg. 63A:619–626, 1981.
15. Flatly, T. J., and Derderian, H.: Closed loop instrumentation of the lumbar spine. Clin. Orthop. 196:273–278, 1985.
16. Fredrickson, B. E., Baker, D., McHolick, W. J., et al.: The natural history of spondylolysis and spondylolisthesis. J. Bone Joint Surg. 66A:699–707, 1984.
17. Gaines, R. W., and Nichols, W. K.: Treatment of spondyloptosis by two stage L5 vertebrectomy and reduction of L4 onto S1. Spine 10:680–686, 1985.
18. Garfin, S. R., and Heller, J.: The operative reduction of spondylolisthesis. Indications, results, complications. Semin. Spine Surg. 1:125–132, 1989.
19. Hanley, E. N., Jr., and Levy, J. A.: Surgical treatment of isthmic lumbosacral spondylolisthesis. Analysis of variables influencing results. Spine 14:48–50, 1989.
20. Harris, I. E., and Weinstein, S. L.: Long-term follow-up of patients with grade III and IV spondylolisthesis. J. Bone Joint Surg. 69:960–969, 1987.
21. Hensinger, R. N., Lang, J. R., and MacEwen, G. D.: Surgical management of spondylolisthesis in children and adolescents. Spine 1:207–216, 1976.

22. Horowitch, A., Peek, R. D., Thomas, J. C., et al.: The Wiltse pedicle screw fixation system. Early clinical results. Spine 14:461–467, 1989.
23. Jackson, A. M., Kirwan, E. O'G., and Sullivan, M. F.: Lytic spondylolisthesis above the lumbosacral level. Spine 3:260–266, 1976.
24. Johnson, J. R., and Kirwan, E. O'G.: The long-term results of fusion in situ for severe spondylolisthesis. J. Bone Joint Surg. 65B:43–46, 1983.
25. Jones, A. A. M., McAfee, P. C., Robinson, R. A., et al.: Failed arthrodesis of the spine for severe spondylolisthesis. J. Bone Joint Surg. 70A:25–30, 1988.
26. Kane, W. J.: Direct current electrical bone growth stimulation for spinal fusion. Spine 13:363–365, 1988.
27. Kaneda, K., Satoh, S., Nohara, Y., et al.: Distraction rod instrumentation with posterolateral fusion in isthmic spondylolisthesis. 53 cases followed for 18-89 months. Spine 10:383–389, 1985.
28. Krag, M. H., Beynnon, B. D., Pope, M. H., et al.: An internal fixator for posterior application to short segments of the thoracic, lumbar, or lumbosacral spine. Clin. Orthop. 203:75–98, 1986.
29. Lowe, J., Libson, J. L. E., Nyska, I. Z. M., et al.: Spondylolysis in the upper lumbar spine. A study of 32 patients. J. Bone Joint Surg. 69B:582–586, 1987.
30. Matthiass, H. H., and Heine, J.: The surgical reduction of spondylolisthesis. Clin. Orthop. 203:34–44, 1986.
31. Maurice, H. D., and Morley, T. R.: Cauda equina lesions following fusion in situ and decompressive laminectomy for severe spondylolisthesis. Four case reports. Spine 14:214–216, 1989.
32. McPhee, I. B., and O'Brien, J. P.: Reduction of severe spondylolisthesis. A preliminary report. Spine 4:430–434, 1979.
33. McQueen, M. M., Court-Brown, C., and Scott, J. H.: Stabilisation of spondylolisthesis using Dwyer instrumentation. J. Bone Joint Surg. 68B:185–188, 1986.
34. Nicol, R. O., and Scott, J. H. S.: Lytic spondylolysis. Repair by wiring. Spine 11:1027–1030, 1986.
35. Osterman, K., Lindholm, T. S., and Laurent, L. E.: Late results of removal of the loose posterior element (Gill's operation) in the treatment of lytic lumbar spondylolisthesis. Clin. Orthop. 117:121–128, 1976.
36. Pedersen, A. K., and Hagen, R.: Spondylolysis and spondylolisthesis. Treatment by internal fixation and bone-grafting of the defect. J. Bone Joint Surg. 70A:15–24, 1988.
37. Peek, R. D., Wiltse, L. L., Reynolds, J. B., et al.: In situ arthrodesis without decompression for grade III or IV isthmic spondylolisthesis in adults who have severe sciatica. J. Bone Joint Surg. 71A:62–68, 1989.
38. Pizzutillo, P. D., Mirenda, W., and MacEwen, G. D.: Posterolateral fusion for spondylolisthesis in adolescence. J. Pediatr. Orthop. 6:311–316, 1986.
39. Roy-Camille, R., Saillant, G., and Mazel, C.: Internal fixation of the lumbar spine with pedicle screw plating. Clin. Orthop. 203:7–17, 1986.
40. Saraste, H.: Long-term clinical and radiological follow-up of spondylolysis and spondylolisthesis. J. Pediatr. Orthop. 7:631–638, 1987.
41. Scaglietti, O., Frontino, G., and Bartolozzi, P.: Technique of anatomical reduction of lumbar spondylolisthesis and its surgical stabilization. Clin. Orthop. 117:164–175, 1976.
42. Sevastikoglou, J. A., Spangfort, E., and Aaro, S.: Operative treatment of spondylolisthesis in children and adolescents with tight hamstring syndrome. Clin. Orthop. 147:192–199, 1980.
43. Sijbrandij, S.: Reduction and stabilisation of severe spondylolisthesis. A report of three cases. J. Bone Joint Surg. 65B:40–42, 1983.
44. Steffee, A. D., and Sitkowski, D. J.: Reduction and stabilization of grade IV spondylolisthesis. Clin. Orthop. 227:82–89, 1988.
45. Steffee, A. D., and Sitkowski, D. J.: Posterior lumbar interbody fusion and plates. Clin. Orthop. 227:99–102, 1988.
46. Thalgott, J. S., LaRocca, H., Aebi, M., et al.: Reconstruction of the lumbar spine using AO DCP plate internal fixation. Spine 14:91–95, 1989.
47. Van Dan Oever, M., Merrick, M. V., and Scott, J. H.: Bone scintigraphy in symptomatic spondylolysis. J. Bone Joint Surg. 69B:453–456, 1987.
48. Van Rens, Th. J. G., and Van Horn, J. R.: Long-term results in lumbosacral interbody fusion for spondylolisthesis. Acta Orthop. Scand. 53:383–392, 1982.
49. Velikas, E. P., and Blackburne, J. S.: Surgical treatment of spondylolisthesis in children and adolescents. J. Bone Joint. Surg. 63B:67–70, 1981.
50. Verbiest, H.: The treatment of lumbar spondyloptosis or impending lumbar spondyloptosis accompanied by neurologic deficit and/or neurogenic intermittent claudication. Spine 4:68–77, 1979.
51. Vidal, J., Fassio, J. V. B., Buscayret, C., et al.: Surgical reduction of spondylolisthesis using a posterior approach. Clin. Orthop. 154:156–165, 1981.
52. Whitecloud, T. S., Butler, J. C., Cohen, J. L., et al.: Complications with variable spinal plating system. Spine 14:472–474, 1989.
53. Wiltse, L. L.: Spondylolisthesis in children. Clin. Orthop. 21:156–163, 1961.

THREE

Complications in Cervical Disc Disease Surgery

Howard S. An, M.D.

Frederick A. Simeone, M.D.

One of the most important aspects when dealing with cervical disc disease is making an accurate diagnosis. Many other diagnoses may mimic symptoms of cervical disc disease. Discogenic neck pain should also be differentiated from true radicular pain. Myelopathy should be detected early with careful physical examination. Although there is no consensus on the specific operative treatment of cervical disc disease, a surgical procedure should be completed only with the proper indications and should be approached with great care as potential pitfalls and complications are many.

PREOPERATIVE PLANNING

The patient suffering from cervical disc disease usually presents with one of the five clinical syndromes:

1. Discogenic axial pain with or without referred patterns of pain.
2. Radicular patterns of pain from acute soft lateral herniated disc.
3. Radicular pain from chronic disc degeneration.
4. Acute myelopathic symptoms from central disc herniation.
5. Cervical spondylotic myelopathy from multiple level cervical disc degeneration.[15, 65]

Differential diagnoses included in Table 3–1 should be considered first since an inaccurate diagnosis will lead to inappropriate treatment.

Table 3–1
Differential Diagnosis of Cervical Disc Disease

NEUROLOGICAL

Multiple sclerosis
Amyotrophic lateral sclerosis
Hydrocephalus
Cervical cord tumors
Syringomyelia
Peripheral nerve entrapment neuropathies
Brachial plexus injury or neuritis
Thoracic outlet syndrome

INFLAMMATORY

Rheumatoid arthritis
Fibrositis (trigger-point syndrome)
Polymyalgia rheumatica

NEOPLASTIC

Metastatic disease
Primary bone tumors
Pancoast tumors

INFECTIOUS

Vertebral osteomyelitis/discitis

PRIMARY SHOULDER AND UPPER EXTREMITY PROBLEMS

Subacromial bursitis
Calcific tendinitis
Biceps tendinitis
Impingement syndrome of the shoulder
Rotator cuff tear
Glenohumeral arthritis
Reflex sympathetic dystrophy

CARDIAC ISCHEMIA

For example, primary shoulder and arm problems may be confused with an acute radiculopathy. Multiple sclerosis or amyotrophic lateral sclerosis should also be ruled out in patients in whom cervical spondylosis is not a clear cause for myelopathy. Intraspinal tumors must be excluded in patients with burning pain that is worse at night (Fig. 3–1A, B). For those with neck and referred patterns of pain, conservative measures should be taken as long as possible. In a long-term follow-up study of 205 patients, Gore and associates reported that 79 per cent of patients with neck pain due to cervical spondylosis had a decrease in pain without surgery.[27] Williams and coworkers reported good or excellent results in 73 per cent of patients who had radicular symptoms compared with 27 per cent in those without radicular symptoms.[79] White and associates also reported 75 per cent good results in those with radicular pain but only 57 per cent good results in those with neck pain.[73] Although use of discography is controversial, there are reports that claim better results if pain discography is positive preoperatively.[41, 66] Nonetheless, surgery for degenerated cervical discs without radiculopathy gives unpredictable results, and conservative treatment should be advocated as long as possible.

Radicular symptoms may be caused by a soft lateral disc herniation, chronic disc degeneration with osteophyte formation, or rarely, instability within the spinal motion segment. Most patients will show symptoms and signs of monoradiculopathy, but occasionally, multiple roots may be involved, especially in patients with chronic disc degeneration.

Because radicular pain symptoms are associated with direct mechanical compression of a spinal nerve root, history and neurological examination usually point to the particular nerve root involved. Table 3–2 shows a summary of symptoms and findings seen with individual root irritation or compression.[65] Conservative treatment should be given for at least 6 to 12 weeks before surgical intervention is considered.[15] However, if a profound or progressive motor deficit is found, surgery should be considered early. In particular, impaired shoulder abduction due to C5 root compression or intrinsic weakness of the hand due to C8 root impingement is functionally more disabling. As a general rule, the patient with a significant motor defict should not go untreated beyond three weeks.

When surgery is to be undertaken, the correct symptomatic level should be confirmed by studies such as myelography, computed to-

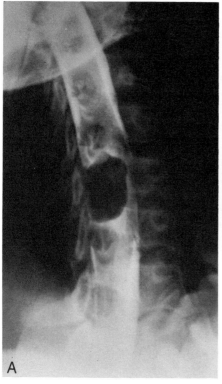

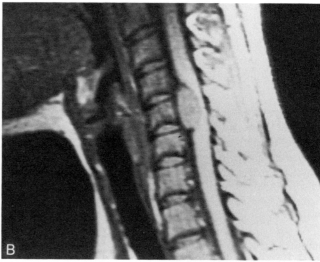

FIGURE 3–1. 35-year-old white female, presenting with cervical radiculopathy, who subsequently underwent surgery for removal of neurofibroma. *(A)* A cervical myelogram revealing an intradural extramedullary spinal neoplasm. *(B)* A magnetic resonance image revealing the tumor size and location.

Table 3–2
Clinical Symptoms and Findings of Cervical Nerve Root Involvement

NERVE ROOT	DISC LEVEL	CLINICAL SYMPTOMS AND FINDINGS
C3	C2–C3	Pain and numbness in back of neck, particularly around mastoid process and pinna of ear; no readily detectable weakness or reflex change
C4	C3–C4	Pain and numbness in back of neck, radiating along levator muscle of scapula and occasionally down anterior chest; no readily detectable weakness or reflex change
C5	C4–C5	Pain radiating from side of neck to shoulder top and numbness over the deltoid muscle; weakness and atrophy of the deltoid muscle; no reflex change
C6	C5–C6	Pain radiating down the lateral side of arm and forearm, often into thumb and index fingers and numbness of tip of thumb or on dorsum of hand over first dorsal interosseous muscle; weakness of biceps muscle and depression of biceps reflex
C7	C6–C7	Pain radiating down middle of forearm, usually to middle finger, although index and ring finger may be involved; weakness of triceps muscle and depression of triceps reflex
C8	C7–T1	Pain radiating down medial aspect of forearm to ring and small finger and numbness of small and medial portion of ring finger; intrinsic muscle atrophy and weakness and no reflex change

mography, or magnetic resonance imaging (Fig. 3–2A–D). Occasionally, multiple tests are necessary to identify the compressive pathology of the nerve root. Clinical correlation is vitally important as a high incidence of false positives is found in these studies.[69]

Chronic disc degeneration with posterior osteophyte formation is the most common cause of spinal cord compression in patients over age 55.[64] Occasionally, a younger patient presents with acute myelopathy caused by a midline soft disc herniation. It is important to recognize the signs and symptoms of myelopathy early, since the results of surgery in patients with prolonged myelopathy are compromised.[39] The patient may report gait disturbance, spasticity of the extremities, and paresthesias or numbness of the extremities.[10] Sphincter abnormalities, motor weakness, and hyperreflexia may also be found. If an imaging study identifies spinal cord compression in the cervical spine, surgery should be done to halt the progression of myelopathy (Fig. 3–3A, B). Early intervention may even reverse many symptoms of myelopathy.

Although rare, vertebral artery compression may occur secondary to chronic cervical disease.[55, 64] The vertebral artery passes through the foramen transversarium in vertebrae C2 through C6 and can be compressed by osteophytes from the lateral portion of the disc margin, zygapophyseal joint, and facet joint, especially if subluxation is present.[64] Symptoms of dizziness and unsteadiness associated with rotary head movement are typical of vertebral artery compression and atherosclerosis.

Selection of the operative approach is controversial in that cervical disc surgery can be performed anteriorly or posteriorly. It is imperative that a conservative approach be taken for a prolonged period of time in the patient for whom pain is the sole presenting complaint. This is especially true for those who believe their injury is compensable, those involved in litigation related to the injury, or those who have a pre-existing history of depression or addiction to narcotics. For patients with radicular arm pain due to either a soft lateral disc or hard spur, our preferred approach has been posterior laminotomy and foraminotomy. The

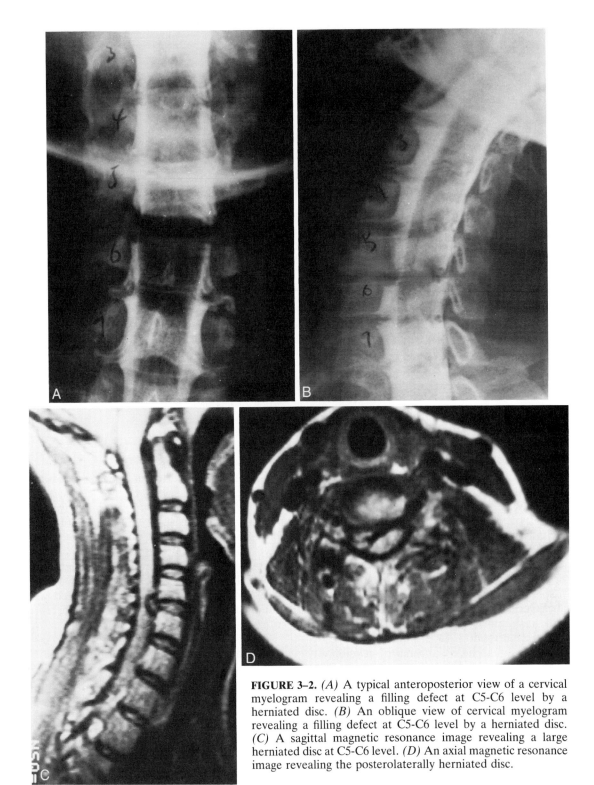

FIGURE 3–2. *(A)* A typical anteroposterior view of a cervical myelogram revealing a filling defect at C5-C6 level by a herniated disc. *(B)* An oblique view of cervical myelogram revealing a filling defect at C5-C6 level by a herniated disc. *(C)* A sagittal magnetic resonance image revealing a large herniated disc at C5-C6 level. *(D)* An axial magnetic resonance image revealing the posterolaterally herniated disc.

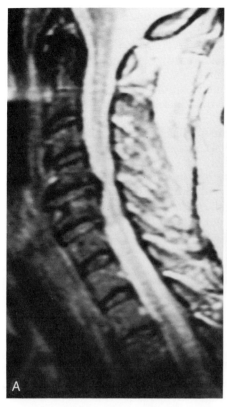
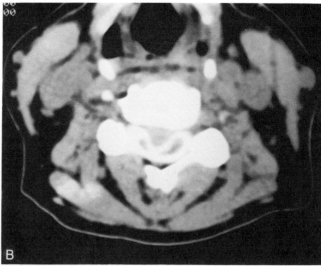

FIGURE 3–3. *(A)* A sagittal magnetic resonance image revealing spinal cord compression in a patient with cervical spondylotic myelopathy. *(B)* An axial magnetic resonance image revealing a large herniated disc with significant spinal cord displacement in a patient with cervical spondylotic myelopathy.

success of posterior approaches for the relief of cervical disc radiculopathy has been well documented in the literature. The anterior approach is a viable alternative for cervical disc radiculopathy with equally good results, but we believe that potential complications may be less with the posterior approach. One definite advantage of the posterior approach is the absence of donor site problems. The incidence of donor site complications is about 20 per cent.[74] The only absolute indication for the anterior approach is central disc herniation. The posterior approach for a central disc herniation makes it difficult to remove the disc sufficiently and may also be associated with an increased risk to the neurological structures in removing the disc material. Although rare, epidural migration of the sequestered disc fragment may occur.[50] Those migrating to the anterior or posterior surface of the spinal canal causing myelopathy should be approached from the appropriate route. If the patient presents with bilateral radiculopathy at the same level, an anterior approach is preferred as bilateral laminotomy and facetectomy at the same level may contribute to late instability or deformity. For patients with multiple level spondylotic radiculopathy, anterior discectomy and interbody fusion or posterior foraminot-

omy at involved levels gives predictable results. For patients with cervical spondylotic myelopathy, we recommend posterior laminectomy if more than three levels are involved. Multiple level discectomy or anterior corpectomy with interbody fusion or strut bone grafting is an alternative, but this formidable operation does not improve results significantly.[39, 76] If the patient has a kyphotic deformity, an anterior procedure should be performed. Posterior facet fusion should be performed after multilevel laminectomy if the patient is young, if instability is present preoperatively, or if a foraminotmy is also completed. An important factor in obtaining better results in cervical myelopathy is early spinal cord decompression before irreversible damage occurs.[19, 39]

ANTERIOR APPROACH

OPERATIVE TECHNIQUE

The anterior surgical approach to the cervical spine allows exposure from C2-C3 through C7-T1. Although the technique is relatively simple and bloodless, potential complications are prodigious (Table 3–3). Currently,

Table 3–3
Potential Complications of Anterior Cervical Fusion

NEURAL INJURY
Spinal cord injury
Nerve root damage
Dural tear
VASCULAR INJURY
Carotid artery
Internal jugular vein
Vertebral artery
VOCAL CORD DAMAGE (RECURRENT LARYNGEAL NERVE INJURY)
ESOPHAGEAL PERFORATION
TRACHEAL INJURY
HORNER'S SYNDROME
PNEUMOTHORAX
BONE-GRAFT COMPLICATIONS
Extrusion
Collapse
Nonunion
Donor site complications
INFECTION
WOUND PROBLEMS (HEMATOMA, DRAINAGE, DEHISCENCE)

anterior cervical spine surgery is one of the most common surgical procedures involved in malpractice litigation. Potential complications such as spinal cord injury, recurrent laryngeal nerve injury, esophageal perforation, vascular injury, and fusion problems may occur.[28]

Meticulous and careful surgical technique is paramount in preventing these complications. The patient is placed in a supine and slight reverse Trendelenburg position to minimize venous pooling in the surgical area. Traction is applied to the head using Gardner-Wells tongs or halter device, and traction to the shoulders is applied caudally using adhesive tape. In order to minimize injury to the recurrent laryngeal nerve, the cervical spine is often approached from the left, but the right-handed surgeon prefers the right-sided approach. On the right side, the recurrent laryngeal nerve may leave the carotid sheath at a higher level, and the surgeon must take caution during dissection, especially below C6. One should remember that the hyoid bone overlies the third vertebra; the thyroid cartilage overlies the C4-C5 intervertebral disc space and the cricoid ring at the C6 vertebra. A useful alternative method involves measuring the distance from the clavicle to the appropriate level on a routine preoperative chest x-ray. Make a transverse incision in line with the skin crease from the midline to the anterior aspect of the sternocleidomastoid muscle. The skin and subcu-

taneous tissue are undermined slightly, and division of the platysma muscle is completed. Retraction of the divided muscle exposes the sternocleidomastoid muscle laterally and strap muscle medially. The deep cervical fascia is divided between the sternocleidomastoid muscle and strap muscles, and blunt finger dissection is done through the pretracheal fascia along the medial border of the carotid sheath (Fig. 3–4). A self-retaining retractor is then positioned to expose the prevertebral fascia and longus colli muscles.

To avoid injury to the carotid artery, internal jugular vein, or vagus nerve, one must be careful not to enter the carotid sheath laterally. Great caution should also be taken medially as the strap muscles surround the thyroid gland, trachea, and esophagus. The surgical dissection should not enter the plane between the trachea and esophagus because the recurrent laryngeal nerve is at risk. A sharp self-retaining retractor should be avoided to prevent perforation of the esophagus medially. It is also important to check for the temporal arterial pulse when the retractor is spread since prolonged occlusion of the carotid artery may cause brain ischemia and stroke.[70] The superior thyroid artery is encountered above C4, and the inferior thyroid artery is seen below C6. These vessels should be identified and ligated as necessary. One should also be aware of the thoracic duct below C7 during the left-sided approach. Further dissection is performed by palpating the prominent disc margins ("hills") and concave anterior vertebral bodies ("valleys"). A bent 18-gauge needle is placed in the disc space and a lateral radiograph is taken to confirm the correct level. The bent needle prevents inadvertent penetration to the spinal cord. In order to minimize bleeding and prevent injury to the sympathetic chain, the pretracheal fascia and the anterior longitudinal ligament must be divided in the midline and subperiosteal mobilization of the longus colli muscles completed. Also, take care not to dissect too far laterally as the vertebral artery and nerve roots are in danger of injury.

Depending on the case, discectomy and interbody fusion at one or more levels or vertebrectomy with strut fusion can be performed. The need for proper technique of discectomy and fusion cannot be overemphasized as neurological consequences may be devastating and bone graft complications are common. Proper lighting and loupe magnification of the surgical field are essential during discectomy. All of the disc material is routinely removed, but the

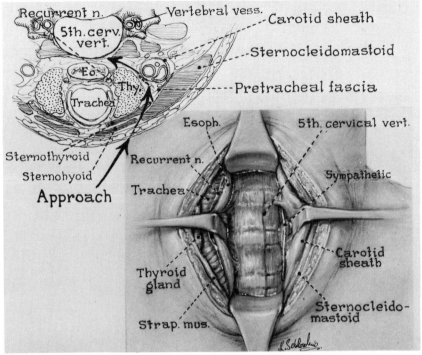

FIGURE 3–4. Anterior approach to the mid and lower cervical vertebrae. (From Southwick, W. O., and Robinson, R. A.: Surgical approaches to the vertebral bodies in the cervical and lumbar regions. J. Bone Joint Surg. *39*A:634, 1957.)

posterior longitudinal ligament is usually left alone. When the posterior longitudinal ligament is perforated by the offending disc material, further decompression should be performed up to the dural margin. Use of an operating microscope and microsurgical instruments is important during dissection around the posterior longitudinal ligament and the dura.

Removal of osteophytic spurs may be associated with an increased risk of neurological injury. Removal of these osteophytes may not be necessary since insertion of the bone graft enlarges the neural foramen and interbody fusion will usually lead to the resorption of the osteophytes.[3, 7, 58] If removal of osteophytes is necessary, meticulous microsurgical technique helps to prevent neural injuries. Somatosensory-evoked potential (SSEP) monitoring should be used during anterior cervical discectomy, particularly in patients with preoperative myelopathy.[71]

A Smith-Robinson interbody fusion is found to be biomechanically superior compared with other counterparts.[73] The graft should be about 8 to 9 mm. in height or 2 mm. greater in height than the degenerated disc space to obtain maximal compressive strength and to enlarge the neural foramina.[7] The graft should not be too thick as overdistraction may result in narrowing of the adjacent neural foramina. Distraction of the intervertebral space can be achieved by skull traction and laminar spreader. Traction with the head halter or Gardner-Wells tongs can also be effective. Graft extrusion can be avoided if the graft is countersunk 2 mm. under the anterior cortical margin of the vertebral body (Fig. 3–5A, B). Obviously, the graft should not be too long since posterior impingement of the spinal cord may be disastrous. Exact measurement of both width and depth of the bone graft slot should be made using a caliper or ruler in each case.

For cervical spondylotic myelopathy, multiple level discectomy and interbody fusion or vertebrectomy with strut grafting is a viable procedure. The iliac crest bone is adequate in most cases, but the fibula may be used in vertebrectomy cases involving more than three levels.[75] A power burr is used to remove bone down to the posterior longitudinal ligament. A strut graft must be countersunk in order to prevent graft dislodgement. We have been satisfied with the slotted technique as shown

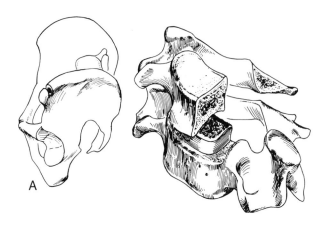

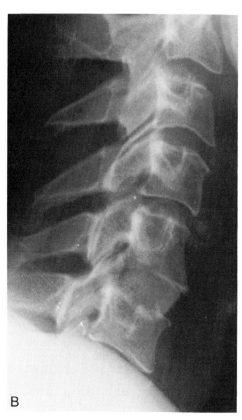

FIGURE 3–5. *(A)* The correct position of the graft introduced into the disc space. (From Simeone, F. A., and Rothman, R. H.: Cervical disc disease. In: Rothman, R. H., and Simeone, F. A. (eds.): *The Spine.* Philadelphia, W. B. Saunders Company, 1982, p. 484.) *(B)* A roentgenogram after anterior interbody fusion with proper position of the graft.

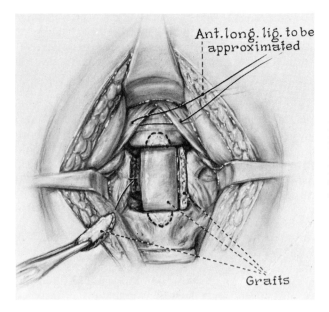

FIGURE 3–6. Anterior view of iliac crest after insertion by slotting method. (From Johnson, R. M., and Southwick, W. O.: Surgical approaches to the spine. In: Rothman, R. H., and Simeone, F. A. (eds.): *The Spine.* Philadelphia, W. B. Saunders Company, 1982.)

in Figure 3–6.[46] Our modification is to place the bone graft against the end-plates to achieve greater stability (Fig. 3–7).

Careful hemostasis is mandatory to prevent wound complications. Hematoma is known to cause cord compression as well.[61] Use of a drain may prevent hematoma complications. The head of the bed should be kept elevated immediately following surgery to minimize venous pooling and bleeding. Postoperative immobilization after anterior fusion depends on the extent of the procedure and stability of the graft at surgery. A Philadelphia collar is most commonly used after routine discectomy and fusion. More rigid braces, such as a halo brace or a Minerva jacket, are recommended after vertebrectomy and strut grafting.

OPERATIVE COMPLICATIONS

NEURAL INJURY

As mentioned before, careful preoperative planning, meticulous surgical technique, and rigid postoperative care are paramount in the prevention of complications. The operative mortality rate associated with anterior procedures is very low. Fatalities are generally related to medical conditions such as cardiac or pulmonary problems. However, mortality may be associated with neural or esophageal injuries. Most spinal cord or nerve root injuries are associated with technical mishaps.[24] The first consideration is anesthesia and positioning. Awake intubation with the aid of a fiberoptic light is helpful to prevent excessive

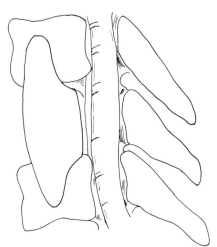

FIGURE 3–7. Lateral view of iliac crest strut graft, which is placed from upper end-plate to the inferior end-plate to provide greater stability.

manipulation during intubation. Awake intubation and SSEP monitoring should be routine in all myelopathic cases. Utmost care should be taken when removing osteophytes and disc material in the lateral corner near the uncovertebral joint to avoid nerve root injury. As stated before, vigorous attempts to remove osteophytes should be avoided.[3, 43] If removal of the posterior longitudinal ligament or osteophytes is necessary because of perforating disc fragments or large osteophytes, great care should be taken and an operative microscope should be used. Tew and Mayfield suggested starting far laterally for spur removal.[70] Unfortunately, plunging of an instrument into the spinal cord has been reported.[11] The depth of the graft should be carefully measured. Gentle tapping is all that is necessary, and stability should be maintained by compressive force on the graft. Krause and Stauffer reported on 10 spinal cord injuries, and 50 per cent of these were directly attributable to the use of instruments and bone-graft insertion.[43] There was one transverse myelitis believed to be secondary to electrocautery on the posterior longitudinal ligament. The etiology was unclear in the remaining patients, but vascular compromise to the anterior arterial system was thought to be pathogenic.[43] The anterior spinal artery is essentially independent with no collateral circulation. An important radicular artery to the cervical cord enters at the C5-C6 or C6-C7 foramen and is second in size only to the artery of Adamkiewicz. Loss of this radicular artery or significant decrease in blood flow may cause ischemic changes in the cervical cord.[43]

The incidence of myelopathic complication is low, ranging from 0 to 1.8 per cent (Table 3–4). Flynn reported that 53 of 70 postoperative myelopathic complications were immediate.[24] If a myelopathic complication is discovered postoperatively, one should administer dexamethasone and take a lateral x-ray to determine the position of the bone graft. Computed tomography or magnetic resonance im-

Table 3–4
Incidence of Myelopathic Complications for Anterior Approach of the Cervical Spine

AUTHOR	PERCENTAGE	REFERENCE
DePalma	1/281 (0.35%)	14
Flynn	0.1%	24
Lesoin	4/800 (0.5%)	45
Simmons	0/154 (0%)	66
Yonenobu	2/95 (1.8%)	81

aging may be valuable in determining hematoma or cord contusion. If hematoma or bone graft is suspected to be the culprit in postoperative myelopathy, expeditious re-exploration is required.[61]

Spinal fluid leaks and dural laceration are rare after anterior cervical surgery since most procedures preserve the posterior longitudinal ligament. Again, the leaks are mainly due to damage caused by the high speed burr or other instruments during disc or bone removal. Intraoperative dural laceration should be repaired if possible, but leaks can be stopped by placing a fascial graft posterior to the bone graft.[70] Postoperative spinal fluid leaks may be managed by catheter drainage to allow the wound to heal. Re-exploration of the wound is necessary in recalcitrant cases.

ESOPHAGEAL PERFORATION

Dysphagia after an anterior cervical surgery is common, but fortunately, it is temporary in most cases. It may be due to postoperative edema, hemorrhage, denervation, or infection.[72] If persistent dysphagia is present, barium swallow or endoscopy should be considered. Consultation with an otolaryngologist is recommended.

Esophageal perforation is a rare but serious complication of anterior cervical spine fusion.[2, 35, 77] It occurs in about 1 of 500 procedures.[70] Sharp retractors must be avoided, and gentle handling of the medial soft structures is necessary. Use of a nasogastric tube may be helpful in identifying the esophagus during surgery. If perforation is suspected during surgery, methylene blue can be injected for better visualization. Often, the perforation is not recognized until the postoperative period when the patient develops an abscess, tracheoesophageal fistula, or mediastinitis. The usual treatment consists of intravenous antibiotics, nasogastric feeding, drainage, debridement, and repair. Early consultation with head and neck surgeons is recommended.

RECURRENT LARYNGEAL NERVE INJURY

Hoarseness or sore throat after anterior cervical fusion may be due to edema or endotracheal intubation and occurs in nearly one-half of patients.[64] However, recurrent laryngeal nerve palsy may be the culprit in persistent hoarseness in a small number of patients. The incidence is about 1 per cent[70] but one report claimed an incidence as high as 11 per cent.[31] The superior laryngeal nerve is a branch of the inferior ganglion of the vagus nerve and travels along with the superior thyroid artery to innervate the cricothyroid muscle. Damage to this nerve may result in hoarseness but often produces only minor symptoms such as easy fatiguing of the voice.[6] The inferior laryngeal nerve is a recurrent branch of the vagus nerve which innervates all laryngeal muscles except the cricothyroid. On the left side, the recurrent laryngeal nerve loops under the arch of the aorta and is protected in the left tracheoesophageal groove. On the right side, the recurrent nerve travels around the subclavian artery, passing dorsomedially to the side of the trachea and esophagus. It is vulnerable as it passes from the subclavian artery to the right tracheoesophageal groove. The recurrent laryngeal nerve should be located when working from C6 downward. The best guideline to its location is the inferior thyroid artery. The nerve usually enters the tracheoesophageal groove where the inferior thyroid artery enters the lower pole of the thyroid. It is also more common for the right inferior laryngeal nerve to be nonrecurrent where it travels directly from the vagus nerve and carotid sheath to the larynx. The incidence of nonrecurrent laryngeal nerve injury on the right side is reported as 1 per cent.[60] If hoarseness persists for more than six weeks following anterior cervical surgery, laryngoscopy should be done to evaluate the vocal cord and laryngeal muscles. Treatment of the inferior laryngeal nerve should include waiting at least six months for spontaneous recovery of function to occur. Further treatment or surgery by the otolaryngologist may be necessary in persistent cases.

HORNER'S SYNDROME

Injury to the sympathetic chain may result in Horner's syndrome. The cervical sympathetic chain lies on the anterior surface of the longus colli muscles posterior to the carotid sheath. Subperiosteal dissection is important to prevent damage to these nerves. Horner's syndrome is usually temporary but may be permanent in some cases.[38] The incidence of permanent Horner's syndrome is less than 1 per cent.[24] Ophthalmologic consultation may be needed for treatment of ptosis.

BLEEDING

Serious bleeding complications following anterior cervical surgery are fortunately rare, but hematoma of the wound is relatively common; one series reported an incidence of 9 per cent.[64] Hematoma may complicate wound healing but is rarely responsible for airway obstruction or spinal cord compression.[61] The patient should have his or her head elevated in the immediate postoperative period as the source of bleeding is frequently venous. Meticulous hemostasis and placement of a drain should be routine to prevent these complications. Arterial bleeding from either superior or inferior thyroid artery can be prevented by careful identification and ligation during surgery. Great caution should be taken not to dissect too far laterally as the vertebral artery is in danger along with the nerve roots. Tears on the vertebral artery should be repaired by direct exposure of the vessel in the foramen, rather than merely packing the bleeding site. Injuries to the carotid artery or internal jugular vein are exceedingly rare.

BONE GRAFT COMPLICATIONS

Complications associated with bone grafting and fusion are more common. Extrusion of graft usually occurs anteriorly away from the spinal cord, and it can be associated with dysphagia, tracheal obstruction, kyphotic deformity, and neurological symptoms. The incidence is reported to be from 1 to 13 per cent (Table 3–5). As mentioned before, meticulous surgical technique is the key to prevention of these problems. Treatment may be observation or reoperation depending on the situation. Graft collapse is another complication, which may or may not require active treatment. The incidence of graft collapse appears to be slightly higher for allograft than autograft.[5] If graft collapse results in a significant kyphosis, especially in patients who have undergone multiple vertebrectomies and strut grafting, revision surgery is required. The incidence of pseudarthrosis after anterior cervical fusion

has been reported to be from 0 to 26 per cent (Table 3–6). Failure of fusion is reported to be greater using the dowel technique, whereas the keystone method described by Simmons had no cases of nonunion in one series.[66, 70] Multiple level fusion has also been associated with a higher rate of nonunion compared with single level fusion.[73] Many patients are asymptomatic despite radiographic evidence of nonunion and require no treatment.[33, 64] Those with symptomatic nonunions may benefit from prolonged immobilization or revision surgery. Posterior foraminotomy is a good procedure following failed anterior cervical fusion for unilateral radiculopathy. Repeat anterior fusion may also be done in these cases with good success.

Degenerative changes above and below fusion masses have been reported in the literature.[14] Altered biomechanics caused by the fused segment puts additional stress on the adjacent segments, and degenerative changes may ensue.[4, 9, 40] Yonenobu reported on patients with neurological deterioration following surgical treatment of cervical myelopathy and partially attributed this to degenerative changes in the juxtafused segments.[81] Williams and associates reported a recurrence rate of 12 per cent at sites adjacent to the fusion.[79]

FAILURE OF ANTERIOR CERVICAL FUSION

Review of the literature reveals up to a 96 per cent success rate after anterior discectomy and fusion (Table 3–7). As mentioned before, single level fusion for radicular symptoms gives a far better result than for neck symptoms only. In general, those patients with compensation or litigation claims and those who are addicted to narcotics do poorly. It is imperative

Table 3–5
Incidence of Graft Extrusion After Anterior Cervical Fusion

AUTHOR	PERCENTAGE	REFERENCE
Depalma	3%	14
Gore	4.1%	26
Lunsford	4.4%	48
Simmons	5.8% (Cloward)	66
	1.5% (Keystone)	
Tew	2%	70

Table 3–6
Pseudarthrosis Rate after Anterior Cervical Fusion

AUTHOR	PERCENTAGE	REFERENCE
Aronson	4%	1
Connolly	21%	12
DePalma	12%	14
Gore	3%	26
Riley	18%	58
Robinson	12%	59
Simmons	18% (Cloward)	66
	0% (Keystone)	
Stuck (Cloward)	5%	68
White	26%	73
Williams	10%	79

Table 3–7
Good to Excellent Results from Anterior Cervical Fusion

AUTHOR	PERCENTAGE	REFERENCE
Connolly	54%	12
DePalma	63%	14
Gore	96%	26
Riley	72%	58
Robinson	73%	59
Simmons	81%	66
Stuck	73%	68
White	67%	73
Williams	63%	79

that the correct diagnosis be made. Other conditions that can simulate a cervical radiculopathy or myelopathy are numerous and must be ruled out. As mentioned before, clinical failures may be associated with graft collapse, pseudarthrosis, and degeneration at the juxtafused segments. If reoperation is necessary, the neck should be approached from the opposite side to avoid scars from the previous surgery. If the patient has persistent or recurrent unilateral radicular symptoms despite solid fusion or stable pseudarthrosis, posterior foraminotomy should be considered.

In summary, anterior discectomy and fusion can be a gratifying procedure if the surgeon makes the correct diagnosis, rules out inappropriate candidates for surgery, and pays attention to surgical details necessary to avoid operative complications.

Results of anterior procedures for cervical spondylotic myelopathy are poorer than those for radiculopathy (Table 3–8). The natural history of this disease is not clearly known, and thus, interpretation of surgical results is difficult.[44] Surgery may be effective in halting the progression of myelopathic symptoms, and therefore, a case in which there is no further change after surgery should not be considered

Table 3–8
Failure Rates after Anterior Procedures for Cervical Spondylotic Myelopathy (No Change or Worse)

AUTHOR	PERCENTAGE	REFERENCE
Galera	60.6%	25
Guidetti	15.6%	30
Lunsford	50%	48
Phillips	26.1%	56
Yonenobu (worse)	18% (Robinson) 5% (vertebrectomy)	81

a therapeutic failure. Yonenobu and associates compared three surgical procedures for multisegmental cervical spondylotic myelopathy and found better results among patients who had undergone subtotal spondylectomy and strut fusion compared with those who had undergone multiple level discectomy and interbody fusion or extensive laminectomy.[80] There was no difference in the results between laminectomy and anterior interbody fusion. However, in terms of direct surgical complications, laminectomy was the safest procedure. These same authors recommend extensive laminectomy if more than three levels are involved.[80] Since no firm statistical evidence exists establishing the superiority of one procedure over another, the surgeon should consider many factors, including the number of levels involved, canal diameter, vertebral alignment and angulation, bone quality, and the surgeon's personal experience. The anterior approach should be done if there is a kyphotic deformity. If less than three levels are involved, the anterior approach is preferred.

POSTERIOR APPROACH

OPERATIVE TECHNIQUE

Compared with an anterior procedure, a posterior foraminotomy for unilateral radicular symptoms caused by a soft herniated or "hard" disc is relatively more benign. Also, multilevel laminectomy for cervical spondylotic myelopathy is less formidable than anterior vertebrectomy and strut grafting. Nonetheless, potential neural injury, recurrence, and cervical instability exist following posterior procedures. Again, meticulous surgical technique is paramount in the prevention of these complications. Mayfield tongs are used to secure the head, and the operating room table is tilted to a 45-degree reverse Trendelenburg position to minimize venous pooling in the surgical area. Some surgeons prefer a sitting position, but air embolism is a potential complication. The neck should be in a flexed position, except in the patient with cervical spondylotic myelopathy as the spondylotic bars may further compress the spinal cord. The neck should be in a neutral position if myelopathy is present.[20] The dissection should stay in the midline and subperiosteally to minimize bleeding. For unilateral foraminotomy, a Taylor retractor is placed just lateral to the edge of the lateral mass. It is important not to place the tip of the retractor too deeply as it may impinge on the exiting nerve root. A Kerrison rongeur is used to remove lateral portions of the inferior lamina above and superior lamina below (Fig. 3–8). Partial facetectomy is carried out by thinning the inferior and superior facets using a power burr. A diamond-tip burr is used to thin the inner cortex. A fine-angled curette is then used to unroof the foramen. Removal of the posterior wall of the neuroforamen accomplishes decompression of the underlying nerve root. Henderson has shown that it is not necessary to remove the soft or hard discs if adequate bony decompression has been performed.[32] Manipulation of the nerve root may cause neurological injuries. If one decides to remove the disc material, the tissue comprising the venous plexus which surrounds the nerve root should be cauterized and peeled off first. The nerve root is then carefully retracted, and discectomy can then be performed (Fig. 3–9). We do not routinely remove the disc material unless the herniated disc is acute, soft, and large.

Laminectomy is our procedure of choice for multilevel cervical spondylotic myelopathy. At the junction of the lamina and facet, a burr is used to thin the cortices, and a small curette or Kerrison rongeur is used to finish the cut. Facet fusion is carried out if indicated. In order to detect trauma to the spinal cord, SSEP monitoring is used routinely in these cases. Meticulous hemostasis is mandatory to prevent hematoma formation. Epidural hematoma may cause spinal cord compression or even death.[45]

OPERATIVE COMPLICATIONS

NEURAL INJURY

Spinal cord injury has almost never been observed in those patients who undergo a foraminotomy for a lateral ruptured disc. However, spinal cord injury is a potential complication during complete laminectomy in myelopathic patients. In fact, according to the Cervical Spine Research Society survey,[28] the overall incidence of neurological complications is higher with posterior than with anterior approaches (an average of 2.18 per cent versus 0.64 per cent). As mentioned before, great caution should be taken during intubation and positioning, and routine SSEP monitoring is recommended. In order to minimize trauma to the cord, an air-driven drill should be used to thin the cortex at the junction of the lamina and lateral mass, and the lamina should be carefully lifted off using an angled curette, rather than inserting an instrument such as a Kerrison rongeur under the lamina. The authors have observed a case of cord contusion in a patient who underwent laminectomy for cervical spondylotic myelopathy. There were no technical difficulties or mishaps during the operation. SSEP monitoring remained unchanged throughout the operation. The patient developed a weakness of the extremities postoperatively, and magnetic resonance imaging revealed cord contusion. Postoperative myelography revealed normal passage of the dye, which was completely blocked preoperatively. The patient gradually improved, regaining independent ambulation over the next several months. Patients with significant myelopathy have poor autoregulation of blood flow, and episodes of hypotension may produce cord anoxia, which is not apparent until the patient awakens from anesthesia.[38]

Root injury resulting in postoperative motor deficit or sensory disturbance may occur during foraminotomy surgery. Root injury in the sensory sphere is rarely of great significance, but motor weakness or paralysis is more serious. This problem may be decreased if decompression of the nerve root is performed by laminotomy and partial facetectomy without excision of disc material or osteophyte. Henderson and coworkers have shown that excision of the disc material is not necessary and foraminotomy alone is compatible with a good result.[32] He reported postoperative sensory deficit in 5.7 per cent and motor deficit in 0.4 per cent of patients.[32] Motor loss of the C5 root and C8 root resulting in deltoid and intrinsic muscle weakness, respectively, is particularly disabling. Most root injuries are traction forces resulting from overzealous manipulation during surgery. Fortunately, most of these deficits are reversible.

Dural tear during a posterior procedure is a definite risk. Cerebrospinal fluid leakage is rare during a unilateral root exposure, but the potential for a dural rent is greater during a complete laminectomy. Using a diamond-tip burr and care during removal of the lamina is essential in preventing this complication. A reverse Trendelenburg position also allows the hydrostatic pressure of the cerebrospinal fluid to be lower.[38] Any dural tear should be repaired in a meticulous manner, and wound closure should be watertight as well. The development of a pseudomeningocele after a cervical laminectomy has been reported in the literature.[38] This patient developed a cyst

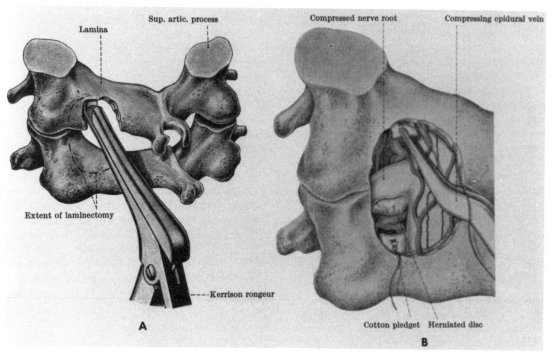

FIGURE 3–8. Posterior cervical laminotomy and partial facetectomy. (From Kempe, L.: *Operative Neurosurgery*. New York, Springer-Verlag, 1972.)

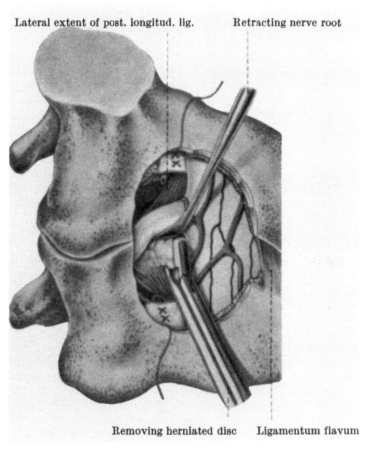

FIGURE 3–9. Removal of herniated disc after posterior cervical laminotomy and partial facetectomy. (From Kempe, L.: *Operative Neurosurgery*. New York, Springer-Verlag, 1972.)

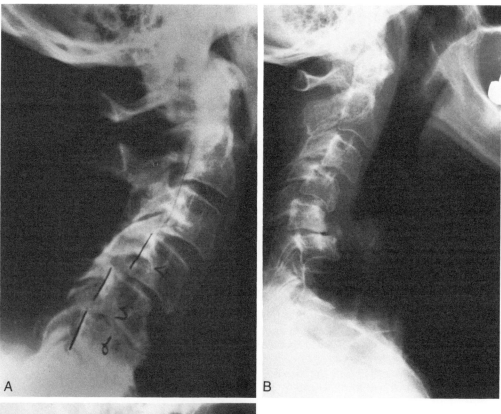

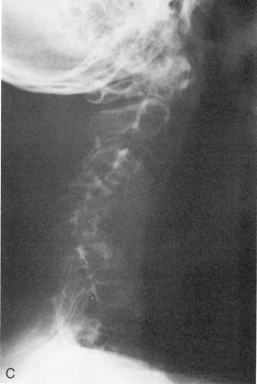

FIGURE 3–10. *(A)* A lateral cervical roentgenogram showing a translational instability after posterior laminectomy. *(B)* A lateral cervical roentgenogram showing a kyphotic deformity after posterior laminectomy. *(C)* A lateral cervical roentgenogram showing solid arthrodesis by anterior fibular strut grafting in a patient who developed postlaminectomy kyphosis.

Table 3–9
Good to Excellent Results after Posterior Cervical Foraminotomy

AUTHOR	PERCENTAGE	REFERENCE
Fager	87.5%	22
Henderson	91.5%	32
Murphy	90%	54
Raaf	94% (soft disc)	57
	67% (hard disc)	
Scoville	97%	62
Williams	96.5%	78

Table 3–10
Failure Rates after Posterior Procedures for Cervical Spondylotic Myelopathy (No Change or Worse)

AUTHOR	PERCENTAGE	REFERENCE
Epstein	15	18
Fager	31	23
Gregorius	67	29
Guidetti	21	30
Magnaes	30	49
Mayfield	19	51
Yonenobu	29 (worse)	81

measuring 1.5 cm., compressing the C7 root dorsally. Recovery was uneventful after amputation of the cyst and closure of the tract.[38]

RECURRENCE

True recurrence at the original operative site is rare. Persistent pain or return of the original pain in the immediate postoperative period suggests inadequate decompression. The highest incidence is 3.3 per cent reported by Henderson and associates, who performed foraminotomy without excision of the disc material or osteophyte.[38] Herniation at other levels is more common, but this cannot be considered a complication from previous surgery. Murphy and coworkers reported a herniation rate at other levels of only 0.5 per cent, but Scoville and associates found 8.0 per cent and Henderson and coworkers found 10.8 per cent who developed a recurrence at other levels.[32, 54, 62] Nonetheless, the recurrence rate at other sites after posterior foraminotomy is generally lower than that following anterior cervical fusion.

INSTABILITY

Cervical instability is a potential complication after extensive laminectomy, particularly in younger patients, patients who had simultaneous partial facetectomy, and those who had previous instability preoperatively (Fig. 3–10 A–C). Laminectomy alone should not be performed in those patients with kyphosis or anterior translational instabilities of the cervical spine. Most patients with cervical spondylotic myelopathy without any risk factor for instability do not develop deformity requiring treatment.[52] Any patient with added risk for developing instability should undergo fusion at the time of laminectomy. Yonenobu and associates reported that 5 of 24 patients who

underwent extensive laminectomy developed instability with clinical deterioration.[81] A similar deteriorating course leading to disability after laminectomy has been reported.[13, 63] Callahan and coworkers treated 42 patients with cervical instability after laminectomy by performing a facet fusion.[8] Another method of facet fusion is Roy-Camille plate and screw fixation, which is biomechanically more rigid.[16] Other procedures, such as laminoplasty, may be considered, particularly if multiple levels are involved.[33, 37, 42, 53]

FAILURE OF POSTERIOR PROCEDURES

The posterolateral foraminotomy with or without use of a microscope has proved successful in high numbers of patients (Table 3–9). Again, a high success rate is possible only with careful patient selection.[21] Those with true radiculopathy who failed conservative treatment are good candidates for surgery. Preoperative imaging studies must confirm the neurocompressive pathology of the particular nerve root. The goals of surgery are to relieve the patient's arm pain and to improve the focal neurological deficits. The patient with pain predominantly in the neck rather than in the arm is a poor candidate for surgery, even in the presence of radiographic abnormalities. Reasons for failures of a posterolateral foraminotomy may include making the wrong diagnosis, exploring an incorrect level, and performing inadequate decompression. Complications such as neural injury, recurrence, and late instability may contribute to poor results. Psychosocial factors have been mentioned repeatedly.

In contrast to results of the posterior approach for decompression of the compromised nerve root, results of posterior laminectomy for myelopathy is generally poorer (Table 3–

10). As mentioned before, the natural history of cervical spondylotic myelopathy is not clearly known, and variability in results is remarkable. Nonetheless, laminectomy serves to improve or halt progression of myelopathy in many patients. However, a significant percentage of patients continues to worsen after posterior decompressive laminectomy. As mentioned before, early detection of progressive cervical myelopathic symptoms and signs is paramount as results are inferior if surgery is performed too late.[17, 39] According to Epstein, the best results are obtained in patients demonstrating early myelopathic symptoms of less than six months' duration.[19] Also, postoperative instability after laminectomy may contribute to clinical deterioration.[81] In order to prevent this complication, a combined laminectomy and fusion should be done in the appropriate patient.

REFERENCES

1. Aronson, N. I.: The management of soft cervical disc protrusion using the Smith-Robinson approach. Clin. Neurosurg. 20:253–258, 1973.
2. Balmaseda, M. T., Jr., and Pellioni, D. J.: Esophagocutaneous fistula in spinal cord injury: A complication of anterior cervical fusion. Arch. Phys. Med. Rehabil. 66:783–784, 1985.
3. Bohlman, H. H.: Cervical spondylosis with moderate to severe myelopathy. Spine 2:151–162, 1977.
4. Braunstein, E. M., Hunter, L. Y., and Bailey, R. W.: Long-term radiographic changes following anterior cervical fusion. Clin. Radiol. 31:201–203, 1980.
5. Brown, M. D., Malinin, T. I., and Davis, P. B.: A roentgenographic evaluation of frozen allografts versus autografts in anterior cervical spine fusions. Clin. Orthop. 119:231–236, 1976.
6. Bulger, R. F., Rejowski, J. E., and Beatty, R. A.: Vocal cord paralysis associated with anterior cervical fusion: Consideration for prevention and treatment. J. Neurosurg. 62:657–661, 1985.
7. Burkus, J. K.: Cervical disc disease. In: Chapman, M. W. (ed.): Operative Orthopaedics. Philadelphia, J. B. Lippincott Company, 1988, pp. 2045–2054.
8. Callahan, R. A., Johnson, R. M., Margolis, R. N., et al.: Cervical facet fusion for control of instability following laminectomy. J. Bone Joint Surg. 59A:991–1002, 1977.
9. Capen, D. A., Garland, D. E., and Waters, R. L.: Surgical stabilization of the cervical spine. A comparative analysis of anterior and posterior spine fusions. Clin. Orthop. 196:229–237, 1985.
10. Clark, C. R.: Cervical spondylotic myelopathy: History and physical findings. Spine 13:847–849, 1988.
11. Cloward, R. B.: New methods of diagnosis and treatment of cervical disc disease. Clin. Neurosurg. 8:93–132, 1962.
12. Connolly, E. S., Seymour, R. J., and Adams, J. E.: Clinical evaluation of anterior cervical fusion for degenerative cervical disc disease. J. Neurosurg. 23:431–437, 1965.
13. Crandall, P. H., and Batzdorf, U.: Cervical spondylotic myelopathy. J. Neurosurg. 25:57–66, 1966.
14. DePalma, A., Rothman, R. H., Lewinnek, G., et al.: Anterior interbody fusion for severe disc degeneration. Surg. Gynecol. Obstet. 134:755–758, 1972.
15. Dillin, W., Booth, R., Cuckler, J., et al.: Cervical radiculopathy (a review). Spine 11:988–991, 1986.
16. Ebraheim, N. A., An, H. S., Jackson, W. T., et al.: Internal fixation of the unstable cervical spine using posterior Roy-Camille plates: Preliminary report. J. Orthop. Trauma 3:23–28, 1989.
17. Epstein, J. A., Carras, R., Epstein, B. S., et al.: Cervical myelopathy caused by developmental stenosis of the spinal canal. J. Neurosurg. 51:362, 1979.
18. Epstein, J. A., Carras, R., Hyman, R. A., et al.: A comparative study of the treatment of cervical spondylotic myeloradiculopathy. Experience with 50 cases treated by means of extensive laminectomy, foraminotomy, and excision of osteophytes during the past 10 years. Acta Neurochir. (Wien) 61:89–104, 1982.
19. Epstein, J. A.: The surgical management of cervical canal stenosis, spondylosis, and myeloradiculopathy by means of posterior approach. Spine 13:864, 1988.
20. Epstein, J. A., and Epstein, N. E.: The surgical management of cervical spinal stenosis, spondylosis, and myeloradiculopathy by means of the posterior approach. In: The Cervical Spine Research Society Editorial Committee (eds.): The Cervical Spine, 2nd ed. Philadelphia, J. B. Lippincott Company, 1989, pp. 625–643.
21. Fager, C. A.: Failed neck syndrome: An ounce of prevention. Clin. Neurol. 27:450–465, 1980.
22. Fager, C. A.: Posterolateral approach to ruptured median and paramedian cervical disk. Surg. Neurol. 20:443–452, 1983.
23. Fager, C. A.: Results of adequate posterior decompression in the relief of spondylotic cervical myelopathy. J. Neurosurg. 38:684, 1973.
24. Flynn, T. B.: Neurologic complications of anterior cervical interbody fusion. Spine 7:536–539, 1982.
25. Galera, R., and Tovi, D.: Anterior disc excision with interbody fusion in cervical spondylotic myelopathy and rhizopathy. J. Neurosurg. 28:305–310, 1968.
26. Gore, D. R., and Sepic, S. B.: Anterior cervical fusion for degenerated or protruded discs: A review of one hundred forty-six patients. Spine 9:667–671, 1984.
27. Gore, D. R., Sepic, S. B., Gardner, G. M., et al.: Neck pain: A long-term follow-up of 205 patients. Spine 12:1, 1987.
28. Graham, J. J.: Complications of cervical spine surgery. In: The Cervical Spine Research Society Editorial Committee (eds.): The Cervical

Spine, 2nd ed. J. B. Lippincott Company, Philadelphia, 1989, pp. 831–837.

29. Gregorius, F. K., Estrin, T., and Crandall, P. H.: Cervical spondylotic radiculopathy and myelopathy: A long-term follow-up study. Arch. Neurol. *33*:618, 1976.

30. Guidetti, B., and Fortuna, A.: Long-term results of surgical treatment of myelopathy due to cervical spondylosis. J. Neurosurg. *30*:714–721, 1969.

31. Heeneman, H.: Vocal cord paralysis following approaches to the anterior cervical spine. Laryngoscope *83*:17–21, 1973.

32. Henderson, C. M., Hennessy, R. G., Shuey, H. M., et al.: Posterior-lateral foraminotomy as an exclusive operative technique for cervical radiculopathy: A review of 846 consecutively operated cases. Neurosurgery *13*:504–512, 1983.

33. Herkowitz, H. N.: A comparison of anterior cervical fusion, cervical laminectomy, and cervical laminoplasty for the surgical management of multiple level spondylotic radiculopathy. Spine *13*:774–780, 1988.

34. Herkowitz, H.: The surgical management of cervical spondylotic radiculopathy and myelopathy. Clin. Orthop. *239*:94–108, 1989.

35. Hilgenberg, A. D., and Grillo, H. C.: Acquired nonmalignant tracheoesophageal fistula. J. Thorac. Cardiovasc. Surg. *85*:492–498, 1983.

36. Hirabayashi, K., Watanabe, K., Wakano, K., et al.: Expansive open-door laminoplasty for cervical spinal stenotic myelopathy. Spine *8*:693, 1983.

37. Hirabayashi, K., and Satomi, K.: Operative procedure and results of expansive open door laminoplasty. Spine *13*:870–876, 1988.

38. Horwitz, N. H., and Rizzoli, H. V.: Herniated intervertebral discs and spinal stenosis. *In*: Horwitz, N. H., and Rizzoli, H. V. (eds.): *Postoperative Complications in Neurosurgical Practice: Recognition, Prevention, Management*. Baltimore, Williams & Wilkins, 1988, pp. 30–98.

39. Hukuda, S., Mochizuki, T., Ogata, M., et al.: Operations for cervical spondylotic myelopathy. J. Bone Joint Surg. *67B*:609–615, 1985.

40. Hunter, L. Y., Braunstein, E. M., and Bailey, R. W.: Radiographic changes following anterior cervical fusion. Spine *5*:399–401, 1980.

41. Kikuchi, S., and Macnab, I.: Localization of the level of symptomatic cervical disc degeneration. J. Bone Joint Surg. *63B*:272–277, 1981.

42. Kimura, I., Oh-Hama, M., Shingu, H., et al.: Cervical myelopathy treated by canal-expansive laminoplasty. J. Bone Joint Surg. *66A*:914–920, 1984.

43. Kraus, D. R., and Stauffer, E. S.: Spinal cord injury as a complication of elective anterior cervical fusion. Clin. Orthop. *112*:130–140, 1975.

44. LaRocca, H.: Cervical spondylotic myelopathy: Natural history. Spine *13*:854, 1988.

45. Lesoin, F., Bouasakao, N., Clarisse, J., et al.: Results of surgical treatment of radiculomyelopathy caused by cervical arthrosis based on 1000 operations. Surg. Neurol. *23*:350–355, 1985.

46. Light, T. R., Wagner, F. C., Johnson, R. M., et al.: Correction of spinal instability and recovery of neurologic loss following cervical vertebral body replacement. A case report. Spine *5*:392–394, 1980.

47. Lindsey, R. W., Newhouse, K. E., Leach, J., et al.: Nonunion following two-level anterior cervical discectomy and fusion. Clin. Orthop. *223*:155–163, 1987.

48. Lunsford, L. D., Bissonette, D. J., Jannetta, P. J., et al.: Anterior surgery for cervical disc disease. Part 1: Treatment of lateral cervical herniation in 253 cases. J. Neurosurg. *53*:1–11, 1980.

49. Magnaes, B., and Hauge, T.: Surgery for myelopathy in cervical spondylosis: Safety measures and reoperative factors related to outcome. Spine *5*:211, 1980.

50. Manabe, S., and Tateishi, A.: Epidural migration of extruded cervical disc and its surgical treatment. Spine *11*:873–878, 1986.

51. Mayfield, F. H.: Cervical spondylosis: A comparison of the anterior and posterior approaches. Clin. Neurosurg. *13*:181–188, 1966.

52. Mikawa, Y., Shikata, J., and Yamamuro, T.: Spinal deformity and instability after multi-level cervical laminectomy. Spine *12*:6–11, 1987.

53. Miyazaki, K., and Kirita, Y.: Extensive simultaneous multisegment laminectomy for myelopathy due to the ossification of the posterior longitudinal ligament in the cervical region. Spine *11*:531–542, 1986.

54. Murphy, F., Simmons, J. C. H., and Brunson, B.: Cervical treatment of laterally ruptured cervical discs: Review of 648 cases, 1939–1972. J. Neurosurg. *38*:679–683, 1973.

55. Nagashima, C.: Surgical treatment of vertebral artery insufficiency caused by cervical spondylosis. J. Neurosurg. *32*:512–521, 1970.

56. Phillips, D. G.: Surgical treatment of myelopathy with cervical spondylosis. J. Neurol. Neurosurg. Psychiatry *36*:879–884, 1973.

57. Raaf, J. E.: Surgical treatment of patients with cervical disc lesions. J. Trauma *9*:327–338, 1969.

58. Riley, L. H., Robinson, R. A., Johnson, K. A., et al.: The results of anterior interbody fusion of the cervical spine. Review of ninety-three consecutive cases. J. Neurosurg. *30*:127–133, 1969.

59. Robinson, R. A., Walker, A. E., Ferlic, D. C., et al.: The results of anterior interbody fusion of the cervical spine. J. Bone Joint Surg. *44A*:1569, 1962.

60. Sanders, G., Uyeda, R. Y., and Karlan, M. S.: Nonrecurrent inferior laryngeal nerves and their association with a recurrent branch. Am. J. Surg. *146*:501–503, 1983.

61. Sang, U. H., and Wilson, C. B.: Postoperative epidural hematoma as a complication of anterior cervical discectomy. J. Neurosurg. *49*:288–291, 1978.

62. Scoville, W. B., and Whitcomb, B. B.: Lateral rupture of cervical intervertebral discs. Postgrad. Med. *39*:174–180, 1966.

63. Sim, F. H., Sivien, H. J., Bickel, W. H., et al.: Swan neck deformity. A review of twenty-one cases. J. Bone Joint Surg. *56A*:564–580, 1974.

64. Simeone, F. A., and Rothman, R. H.: Cervical disc disease. In: Rothman, R. H., and Simeone, F. A. (eds.): *The Spine*. Philadelphia, W. B. Saunders Company, 1982, pp. 440–499.

65. Simeone, F. A., and Dillin, W. A.: Treatment of cervical disc disease: Selection of operative approach. Comtemp. Neurosurg. 8(14):1–6, 1986.

66. Simmons, E. H., and Bhalla, S. K.: Anterior cervical discectomy and fusion. A clinical and biomechanical study with eight-year follow-up. J. Bone Joint Surg. 51B:225–232, 1969.

67. Spencer, D. L.: Anterior cervical fusion. In: Chapman, M. W. (ed.): Operative Orthopaedics. Philadelphia, J. B. Lippincott Company, 1988, pp. 1929–1936.

68. Stuck, R. M.: Anterior cervical disc excision and fusion—Report of 200 consecutive cases. Rocky Mt. Med. J. 60:25, 1963.

69. Teresi, L. M., Lufkin, R. B., Reicher, M. A., et al.: Asymptomatic degenerative disk disease and spondylosis of the cervical spine: MR imaging. Radiology 164:83–88, 1987.

70. Tew, J. M., Jr., and Mayfield, F. H.: Surgery of the anterior cervical spine: Preventions of complications. In: Dunsker, S. B. (ed.): Cervical Spondylosis. New York, Raven Press, 1981, pp. 191–208.

71. Veilleux, M., Daube, J., and Cucchiara, R. F.: Monitoring of cortical evoked potentials during surgical procedures on the cervical spine. Mayo Clin. Proc. 62:256–264, 1987.

72. Welsh, L. W., Welsh, J. J., and Chinnici, J. C.: Dysphagia due to cervical spine surgery. Ann. Otol. Rhinol. Laryngol. 96:112–115, 1987.

73. White, A. A. III, Southwick, W. O., DePonte, R. J., et al.: Relief of pain by anterior cervical fusion for spondylosis—A report of sixty-five patients. J. Bone Joint Surg. 55A:525–534, 1973.

74. Whitecloud, T. S. III: Complications of anterior cervical fusion. In: the American Academy of Orthopaedic Surgeons Instructional Course Lectures. St. Louis, C. V. Mosby, pp. 223–227, 1978.

75. Whitecloud, T. S., and LaRocca, H.: Fibular strut graft in reconstructive surgery of the cervical spine. Spine 1:33–43, 1976.

76. Whitecloud, T. S.: Anterior surgery for cervical spondylotic myelopathy (Smith-Robinson, Cloward, and vertebrectomy). Spine 13:861–863, 1988.

77. Whitehill, R., Sirna, E. C., Young, D. C., et al.: Late esophageal perforation from an autogenous bone graft. Report of a case. J. Bone Joint Surg. 67A:644–645, 1985.

78. Williams, R. W.: Microcervical foraminotomy. Spine 8:708–716, 1983.

79. Williams, J. L., Allen, M. B., Jr., and Harness, J. W.: Late results of cervical discectomy and interbody fusion: Some factors influencing the results. J. Bone Joint Surg. 50A:227, 1968.

80. Yonenobu, K., Fuji, T., Ono, K., et al.: Choice of surgical treatment for multisegmental cervical spondylotic myelopathy. Spine 10:710–716, 1985.

81. Yonenobu, K., Okada, K., Fuji, T., et al.: Causes of neurologic deterioration following surgical treatment of cervical myelopathy. Spine 11:818–823, 1986.

FOUR

Complications in Lumbar Disc Disease and Spinal Stenosis Surgery

Howard S. An, M.D.

Robert E. Booth, M.D.

Richard H. Rothman, M.D., Ph.D.

Approximately 80 per cent of the general population will experience back pain at some time during their lifetimes. However, only 2 to 3 per cent will have sciatica. When approaching these patients, it is important to determine whether the patient's primary complaint is one of low back pain or radicular leg pain. There are numerous causes of back pain, whereas radicular leg pain is usually due to neurocompressive pathology. Accurate diagnosis and proper surgical indications are crucial for the patient's ultimate success. Potential complications of various procedures for lumbar disc disease and spinal stenosis will be discussed in this chapter.

HERNIATED DISC

PREOPERATIVE PLANNING

Patients with lumbar disc disease or spinal stenosis usually present with radicular leg pain with or without neurological deficits. For those with primary back pain, other diagnoses that may cause back or referred pain should be considered first.[7, 75, 122] Table 4–1 lists several etiologies of back pain. Careful history and physical examination along with appropriate laboratory and roentgenographic examination should facilitate making the correct diagnosis. Failure to recognize these entities may lead to inappropriate surgery and the "failed back surgery syndrome"(Fig. 4–1A, B). Also, two

different conditions may coexist in the same individual. For example, cervical spondylosis and lumbar spinal stenosis frequently exist together in the same patient.[34] Spinal stenosis and vascular claudication may also be coexistent.[40]

It is important to emphasize surgical indications and patient selection since these are the most critical factors in terms of the success of a procedure.[110, 122, 137] For those with radiating leg pain, a trial of conservative treatment for two to three months will eliminate most premature surgery.[4, 63, 137] At present, there is no way to predict which individuals will respond to nonoperative therapy. A short period (several days) of bedrest, anti-inflammatory agents, and early mobilization are stressed. On occasion, facet injections or epidural steroid injections may help, but the results are not predictable.[39] Psychological assessment and treatment of depression are also important. One must also be aware of compensation and litigation involvement as these and other social factors have a profound effect on the outcome of surgery.[44] Only after appropriate conservative treatment fails to relieve pain should surgery be considered. Obvious exceptions to this treatment regimen are the cauda equina syndrome and progressive paralysis, which should be dealt with more aggressively.

Above all, patient selection remains the most critical factor in terms of surgical success. The three factors that have the greatest pre-

Table 4–1
Differential Diagnosis of Low Back Pain

CONGENITAL DEFECTS
Facet tropism
Lumbarization or sacralization
Dysplastic spondylolisthesis
NEOPLASMS
Metastatic tumors
Primary bone tumors (benign and malignant)
Intraspinal tumors (spinal cord and nerve root
    tumors)[90]
INFECTIONS
Osteomyelitis
Epidural abscess[3]
Discitis
INFLAMMATIONS
Seronegative spondylitis (ankylosing spondylitis,
    Reiter's syndrome, psoriatic spondylitis, and
    inflammatory bowel diseases)
Sacroiliitis
Isolated disc resorption
METABOLIC DISEASES
Osteoporosis or osteomalacia
Paget's disease
Hyperparathyroidism
Gout
NEUROLOGICAL DISEASES
Neuropathies
Demyelinating diseases
Transverse myelitis
TRAUMA
Muscle strain
Ligamentous sprain
Compression fractures[96]
Spondylolysis and spondylolisthesis
DEGENERATIVE DISEASES
Herniated disc
Spinal stenosis
Mechanical instability
VISCERAL DISEASES
Genitourinary disorders
Uterine and ovarian diseases
Gastrointestinal disorders
Vascular diseases and aortic aneurysm
MISCELLANEOUS DISEASES
Piriformis syndrome
Iliolumbar syndrome
Facet syndrome[92]
Quadratus lumborum syndrome[75]
Meralgia paresthetica[68]
Vertebral sclerosis
POSTSURGICAL PROBLEMS
Osteolysis[14]
Arachnoiditis
Instability
Postfusion stenosis
Recurrent disc herniation
PSYCHONEUROTIC PROBLEMS
Compensation or litigation involvement
Drug addiction
Hysterical conversion state

dictive value in determining disc herniation are the presence of a positive tension sign, a focal and correlative neurological deficit, and a positive radiographic study.[37, 120] A positive radiographic study means an unequivocal x-ray finding which correlates with the patient's symptoms and signs. Myelography, computed tomography, magnetic resonance imaging, or any combination of these may demonstrate the suspected lesion (Fig. 4–2A–D). If all three factors are present, one is almost assured of uncovering mechanical root compression at surgery. Surgical results under these circumstances will be excellent.

Before discussing potential complications associated with various operative procedures, it is important to consider anatomical variations which may directly affect the surgical approach, dissection, and ultimate successful completion of the procedure. Anatomical anomalies include bony or neural variations as well as the anatomical location of disc ruptures. Correct localization of the appropriate level for surgery depends on careful preoperative examination of the radiographs. The intercrestal line crossing the top of the iliac crest usually passes through the L4–L5 disc space, but variations exist among individuals. If the surgeon places his fingertips over the top of the iliac crest when the patient is in a kneeling position, he will be about 1 to 2 cm. higher than the radiographic intercrestal line and must compensate for this accordingly. Also, "lumbarization" or "sacralization" of the last vertebral segments may confuse the surgeon in localizing the appropriate level. By comparing contrast studies with plain radiographs, the surgeon should be able to localize the appropriate level. This is aided intraoperatively by palpation of the sacrum, identification of mobile and immobile segments, and identification of the posterior elements and interlaminar space. However, the only foolproof method is an intraoperative localizing roentgenogram. The best needle placement for localization is the disc space. Intraoperative x-rays should be obtained in those cases where variations in lumbosacral segmentation exist or any case where the surgeon is unsure of the correct level.

Bony variations or anomalies may also relate to posterior element deficiency. Spina bifida occulta is common (Fig. 4–3). Also, the L5–S1 interlaminar space may be unusually wide in some cases. Careful review of the preoperative radiographs will reveal these anomalies. To prevent inadvertent dural tear or neural

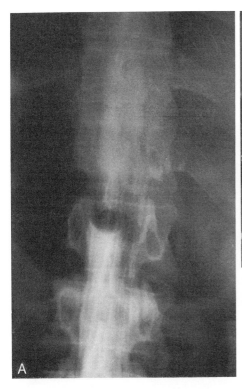

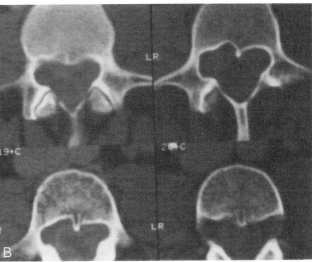

FIGURE 4-1. (*A*) Anteroposterior view of myelogram revealing an intradural extramedullary tumor (neurofibroma) at T12-L1 junction in a patient who underwent two unsuccessful laminotomies and discectomies for apparent herniated discs. (*B*) Computed tomography of a neurofibroma showing the erosion of the pedicle and vertebral body.

injury, one must palpate the bony structures with a finger before using a periosteal elevator. Although herniated lumbar discs typically occur in the posterolateral location, they may rupture laterally, centrally, or axially or migrate as free fragments (Fig. 4–4).[124] Precise preoperative localization of the disc pathology will aid the surgeon in making the proper surgical approach and avoiding neural injury. Preoperative contrast studies must correlate with the patient's symptoms and surgical pathology. Myelography is notoriously inaccurate in demonstrating lateral disc herniation and foraminal stenosis. Computed tomography or magnetic resonance imaging is helpful when myelography has failed to demonstrate a suspected lateral disc herniation. Unlike a posterolateral herniated disc, the lateral herniated disc affects the nerve root numbered one above the ruptured disc. For example, an L4–L5 lateral herniated disc affects the L4 nerve root as it exits into the foramen. A lateral herniated disc in the foramen may be approached either by a medial facetectomy or paraspinal muscle splitting approach. Careful dissection and identification of the involved nerve root are required to avoid neural injury as the herniated disc compresses and pushes the nerve root superiorly against the pedicle. During discectomy the instrument should not reach too deep

as the disc space is very shallow at the lateral margin. A central disc rupture should be approached by a bilateral hemilaminectomy so that the disc can be removed from both sides. A massive central disc rupture presenting as a cauda equina syndrome requires emergency decompression by a midline laminectomy. Axillary disc ruptures are a consequence of disc migration into the axilla of the nerve root. An axillary compression of the L5 nerve root is usually caused by a superiorly migrated disc fragment from the L5–S1 level, but caudal migration from the L4–L5 disc is also possible. A portion of the axillary herniated disc must be removed first in order to retract the nerve root safely for standard discectomy. Free or sequestered fragments are very common. If a free fragment is suspected based on the myelogram or computed tomography, surgical dissection must be modified accordingly. Depending on the location of the free fragment, a complete hemilaminotomy or foraminotomy may be necessary to remove the fragment and decompress the nerve root. Blind probing before complete exposure may dislodge the fragment beyond reach and result in inadequate decompression.

Intradural disc ruptures are very rare.[61, 74, 119] This phenomenon is more common in the failed back surgery syndrome or in patients

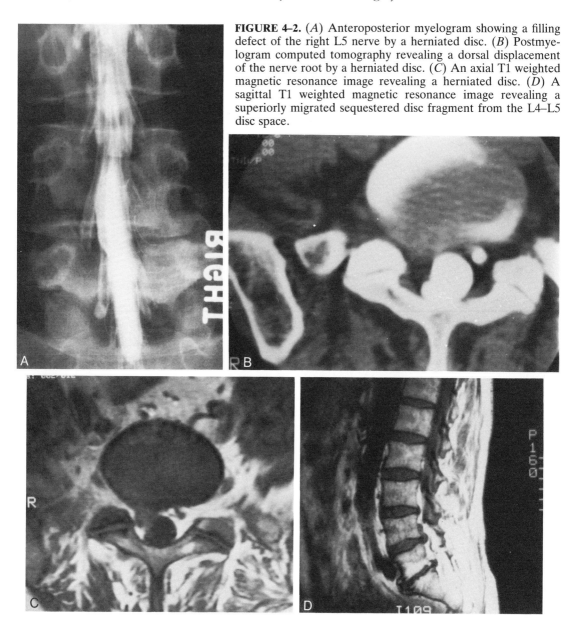

FIGURE 4-2. (*A*) Anteroposterior myelogram showing a filling defect of the right L5 nerve by a herniated disc. (*B*) Postmyelogram computed tomography revealing a dorsal displacement of the nerve root by a herniated disc. (*C*) An axial T1 weighted magnetic resonance image revealing a herniated disc. (*D*) A sagittal T1 weighted magnetic resonance image revealing a superiorly migrated sequestered disc fragment from the L4–L5 disc space.

who have had previous lumbar spine surgery. Anterior rupture of the lumbosacral disc is rare and should not cause radicular leg pain. There is a case report in the literature in which the patient required anterior discectomy and fusion for an anteriorly ruptured disc.[17]

Finally, anatomical anomalies and variation may occur in the nerve roots.[11, 26, 71, 105] Nerve root anomalies can be divided into anatomical variations, enlargement in size, and tumors that mimic symptoms of a herniated disc. Preoperative contrast studies may reveal many of the anatomical variations and anomalies. Cannon classified the anomalous lumbar roots into three types.[26] The most common anomaly

(Type I) is conjoined roots (Fig. 4–5). Type II anomalies are anastomotic, in which the nerve root branches from the dural sleeve of the nerve root that has already left the dural sac. Type III anomalies are the transverse type, which simply have a more horizontal course. Contrast studies may fail to detect these variations, especially Type II, where the anomalies are far lateral. Preoperatively, one should suspect these anomalies if multiple roots are involved and when radiographic and clinical findings do not correlate in a classic manner. Type III anomalies should not be confused with a laterally herniated disc, in which the course of the nerve root runs in a more perpendicular

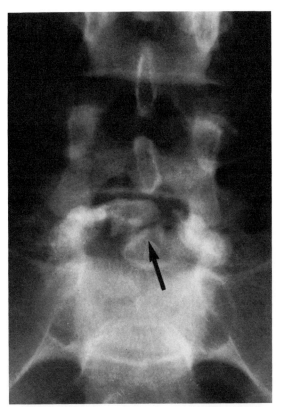

FIGURE 4–3. An anteroposterior roentgenogram showing a spina bifida of L5 lamina (arrow).

direction when the disc elevates the nerve root superiorly in the foramen.[106] Surgical management should respect the principle of exposing the nerve root to its lateral edge before manipulation. Often, more extensive bone removal is necessary to complete exposure and ensure safe decompression in these cases. These patients are not necessarily symptomatic from the anomalous nerve roots, but they are more susceptible to nerve root compression, as a small rupture or fragment can produce significant symptoms. The nerve root may be enlarged for various reasons. Herniated discs may produce inflammation and enlargement of the nerve roots.[126] Most nerve root enlargement from stenosis or compression is reversible upon adequate decompression. Isolated cysts or tumors, such as neurofibroma, may give radicular symptoms. Myelography, computed tomography, and magnetic resonance imaging are helpful in identifying these problems preoperatively. Depending on the pathology, excision or decompression of the nerve root is necessary.

OPERATIVE TECHNIQUE

When surgical indications and patient selection criteria are strictly followed, a standard, limited laminotomy and discectomy for a herniated lumbar disc have been safe and reliable procedures in our hands. The proven success rate is 96 per cent.[63, 137] Meticulous and careful surgical technique is followed to prevent complications.

The patient is placed in a kneeling position to decompress the abdomen (Fig. 4–6). A midline incision rarely exceeds more than 5 to 6 cm. Access to epidural space is achieved by removal of the ligamentum flavum and the inferior margin of the proximal lamina on one side (Fig. 4–7). Packing cottonoid material between the dura and the bony elements of the canal may prevent dural tears. Exposure is carried out laterally so that the lateral edge of the nerve root is visualized before it is retracted (Fig. 4–7). Manipulation of the nerve root before adequate exposure invites neural

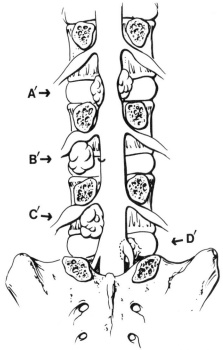

FIGURE 4–4. Pathological variations of lumbar disc herniations: (*A'*) a large central herniation; (*B'*) a left foraminal or far lateral herniation; (*C'*) a left axillary herniation; and (*D'*) a classic posterolateral disc herniation. (From Stambough, J. L.: *Surgical Techniques for Lumbar Discectomy.* Seminars in Spine Surgery *1*:52, Philadelphia, W. B. Saunders Company, 1989.)

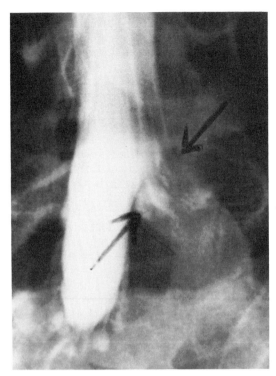

FIGURE 4–5. A myelogram revealing both L5 and S1 nerve roots exiting under the S1 pedicle (conjoined nerve roots). This patient presented with a radiculopathy involving both L5 and S1 nerve roots.

also palpated by a short and long Fraser elevator, recognizing compression in the foramen caused by osteophytic overgrowth, pedicle migration, or bulging or extrusion of the annulus laterally. A systematic approach like this will prevent failure of surgery because of inadequate removal of offending disc material and inadequate evaluation for the presence of concomitant pathology. We have been using spinal anesthesia for routine laminotomy cases. Blood transfusion is rarely indicated, and the patient's recovery is short, requiring three to four days of hospitalization.

CHEMONUCLEOLYSIS, MICRODISCECTOMY, AND PERCUTANEOUS DISCECTOMY

Recently, other procedures have evolved to treat lumbar herniated discs, namely, chemonucleolysis, microdiscectomy, and percutaneous discectomy. Chemonucleolysis is decreasingly popular because of potential disastrous complications, specifically allergic reactions and transverse myelitis.[8, 41, 57] Other complications include dural puncture, infection, bleeding, visceral injuries, an increase in back pain, and so forth.[6, 15, 22, 33, 138] Several

injury. Use of headlight and high-powered loupes (3.5 times magnification and extended field) allows the surgeon to have adequate exposure and to achieve meticulous hemostasis. In addition, this exposure allows the surgeon to remove adequate amounts of the offending disc material, including extruded and sequestered fragments. The surgeon may also undercut the medial aspect of the superior facet in patients with concomitant lateral recess stenosis pathology. By undercutting the superior articular process, the facet joint is largely undisturbed and mechanical stability is maintained in these cases. A large rectangular window of annulus is opened for disc excision to prevent late nerve root compression caused by collapse of the disc space and further buckling of the annulus. The depth of the disc-excising instrument must be kept constant as potential vascular injury can be disastrous. We favor using instruments with a mark 2.5 cm. from the tip to remind us of the depth of the instrument during disc evacuation. It is not necessary to remove the entire nucleus pulposus vigorously, as good results are obtainable with limited disc excision.[121] The excursion and course of the nerve root into the foramen is

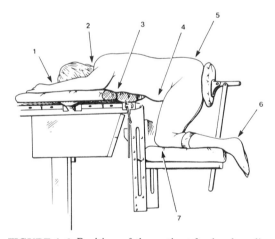

FIGURE 4–6. Position of the patient for lumbar disc and spinal stenosis surgery. The patient is prone in a kneeling posture. The arm is positioned at 90 degrees or less of abduction (1), and the neck is not hyperextended (2). The ulnar nerves and axillae are padded (3). The abdomen is hanging free (4). The lumbar spine is slightly hyperextended (5). Antithrombotic stockings are worn (6). The patient rests on the chest and both knees, providing three-point stability (7). (From Stambough, J. L.: *Surgical Techniques for Lumbar Discectomy.* Seminars in Spine Surgery *1*:48, Philadelphia, W. B. Saunders Company, 1989.)

FIGURE 4-7. (A) The inter-laminar exposure starts with removal of the ligamentum flavum. (B) Further removal of laminar bone is done until the lateral portion of the nerve root is visualized with a punch, working parallel to the lumbar nerve roots. (C) The nerve root is protected by placing cotton surgical patties cephalad and caudad to the nerve root, and the nerve root is retracted medially to expose the herniated disc. (From Stambough, J. L.: *Surgical Techniques for Lumbar Discectomy*. Seminars in Spine Surgery *1*:50, Philadelphia, W. B. Saunders Company, 1989.)

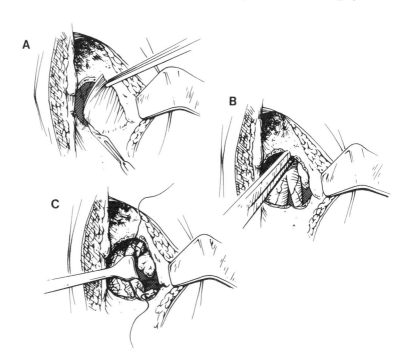

studies reported higher failure rates compared with those of standard discectomy.[20, 31, 99, 115] A microsurgical discectomy involves the use of the operating microscope during all or a portion of the procedure. The proponents cite small incisions, decreased blood loss, and short hospital stay as the main advantages.[27, 54, 66, 73, 116, 134] Percutaneous discectomy has recently captured the public interest as chemonucleolysis did several years ago.[35, 72, 65, 47] Despite the advantages of smaller incision and reduced hospital stay by microdiscectomy or percutaneous discectomy, one must look at more important factors which ultimately determine the outcome of surgery:

1. Adequate removal of disc material including extruded and sequestered fragments.

2. Evaluation for concomitant pathology.

3. Minimal retraction or trauma of the nerve root.

4. Meticulous hemostasis and prevention of perineural fibrosis.

The poor results of lumbar disc surgery are not from incisional morbidity but from a failure to consider the above factors.[136] Also, as a result of advances in anesthesia, particularly spinal and epidural, the patient's recovery is short, even after a standard laminotomy and discectomy.

As mentioned before, a patient undergoing surgery for a herniated lumbar disc should be one whose leg pain was not relieved by conservative treatment. The majority in this category will have extruded disc material at surgery. The clinical result after an excision of extruded disc is superior to results following excision of a bulging disc alone.[120] It is not unusual for extruded disc material to migrate and also become sequestered. The extruded disc material may be adherent to the nerve root or annulus fibrosus. Often, manipulation of this disc material is necessary for adequate removal and decompression. Adequate exposure with standard laminotomy makes this part of the procedure less complicated than attempts through a "keyhole" incision with microdiscectomy and is simply not possible with percutaneous discectomy.

Inadequate lateral decompression and persistent foraminal compression account for some of the failures seen after microdiscectomy. Microdiscectomy without adequate bone removal will fail to recognize bony pathology such as facet encroachment and foraminal compression, and it will lead to failures in a significant percentage of patients. Adequate decompression and maintenance of stability is possible if one undercuts the superior articular process to preserve the facet joint as much as possible.

As mentioned before, the single most important measure of safety during discectomy is clear identification of the lateral border of the root. The root may be stretched and tightly compressed or adherent to an extruded disc fragment, making identification difficult. The use of the microscope without bone removal does not allow room for manipulation of the nerve root, and traction injuries to the nerve and inadequate decompression may result. Exposing a greater area of dura and nerve root permits more gentle retraction and more adequate decompression.

Meticulous hemostasis, atraumatic technique, and the placement of fat grafts are important in the prevention of perineural fibrosis. With 3.5 times magnification loupe, the small arteries and veins coursing along the nerve root and epidural space can be identified and protected or coagulated with a bipolar cautery if bleeding is encountered. Also, coaxial illumination provided by a fiberoptic headlight is a must for adequate visualization during intraspinal surgery. The epidural fat can be saved and placed over the dura at the end of the procedure, or a thin fat graft can be obtained if the epidural fat is inadequate in amount.

Above all, we emphasize proper surgical indications and patient selection, since they are of prime inportance in terms of ultimate success. Microdiscectomy or percutaneous discectomy may offer certain advantages, such as smaller incision and shorter recovery, but potential disadvantages outweigh advantages so greatly that we cannot recommend its routine use in a patient with a herniated disc. Limited exposure microsurgery may prove adequate if a herniated disc is the sole problem. Likewise, percutaneous discectomy may be adequate in a patient with a contained, nonextruded herniated disc. As mentioned before, variations in the location and extent of disc pathology are very common. A precisely accurate preoperative diagnosis is absolutely necessary for these procedures to be successful. Even with today's technology and radiographic studies, one is never certain of all the pathology that may contribute to the patient's radiculopathy. Potential failure to remove extruded or sequestered disc material, failure to evaluate for concomitant pathology such as lateral recess stenosis, or potential injury to the nerve root by blind percutaneous technique are among the main reasons why microdiscectomy or percutaneous discectomy should be approached with caution by the lumbar spine surgeon. Furthermore, the percutaneous technique is not without risk, as potential injuries to vital structures and infection are possible.[12]

SPINAL STENOSIS

PREOPERATIVE PLANNING

The great majority of spinal stenosis cases result from degenerative changes in the intervertebral disc and facet joints with resultant constriction of the spinal canal and neural foramina. The onset of symptoms is usually insidious. Complaints such as fatigue, weakness, low back pain, and numbness in the lower extremities are frequent. The classic symptom of spinal stenosis is claudicating leg pain, aggravated by standing and walking and relieved by forward flexion or sitting. The differential diagnoses of low back pathology and sciatica should always be considered in older patients. Particularly, vascular claudication should be ruled out, and these conditions may coexist in some individuals.[40] Also, many patients with spinal stenosis have concurrent herniated discs, and preoperative studies should identify these lesions.

In the patient with severe spinal stenosis, myelography typically will show hourglass constrictions or complete obstruction of the dye. Computerized tomography shows anatomical narrowing of the lateral recesses and facet hypertrophy. In most cases of significant spinal stenosis with neurogenic claudication, conservative treatment is usually unsuccessful. Nonetheless, rest, exercise, orthosis, physical therapeutic modalities, or epidural injections should be tried to abate the symptoms. When properly performed, excellent results can be obtained in these individuals. It is important to realize that the nerve root or roots to be decompressed should be clinically determined. Imaging studies are used as confirmatory tests.

OPERATIVE TECHNIQUE[13]

As stated before, the kneeling position reduces intra-abdominal pressure and minimizes operative bleeding (see Fig. 4–6). This position also hyperextends the lumbar spine, which most nearly reproduces the axial and appendicular symptoms of nerve root compression. Thus, if the spine is decompressed in this hyperextended posture, complete relief of pain when the patient is erect should be expected. The midline skin incision is followed by a careful subperiosteal dissection of the paraspinous muscle. A self-retaining retractor serves to compress the paraspinous muscles, thereby reducing hemorrhage. Before opening the canal itself, the operating physician should identify the location of the pedicles, which are the key to the subsequent dissection. The nerve root courses under the pedicle to exit into the foramen. The location of the pedicle and corresponding nerve root to be decompressed should be firmly established by the surgeon before proceeding with further dissection.

After the ligamentum flavum has been cleanly exposed, a small curette is used to dissect gently the insertion of the ligament from the undersurface of the superior vertebra. When the inferior edge of the lamina has been exposed, a Kerrison punch or Lexcel rongeur is used to remove the bone of lamina itself. This step is started in the midline, where the canal is most capacious, and then carried to the lateral sides of the spinal canal. When using the Kerrison punch, pressure should be directed dorsally, and the punch should not be rocked from side to side to keep from damaging the dura underneath. The cottonoid material can also be used to displace the dural sac from the posterior elements. It is important to free adhesions between the anterior surface of the lamina and the dura as the dissection is carried out proximally. Any epidural bleeding should be controlled with bipolar cautery. This dissection is carried out to make a central trough extending in a distal-proximal direction over the symptomatic levels to be decompressed and extending laterally to the medial edge of the facet joint. In patients with a central spinal stenosis secondary to congenitally short pedicles, midline dissection alone is adequate.

In the majority of patients, the area of stenosis extends to the lateral recess or foramen, and further dissection is necessary. A 45-degree Kerrison punch is used to undercut portions of the superior facet, thus freeing the lateral recess. Dissecting instruments should always be parallel to the nerve root, thereby minimizing grasping or transecting the nerve roots. Undercutting the facet allows decompression of the lateral recess without jeopardizing spinal instability.

At this juncture, this dissection eliminates symptoms of spinal stenosis in the vast majority of patients. The nerve root should move at least 1 cm. from a medial to lateral direction. The intervertebral discs should be examined to rule out concurrent herniated discs. Further foraminal or extraforaminal decompression should be performed if the nerve is not loose at this time. The facet joint should be removed more laterally to look for the entrapment of the spinal nerve between the superior facet of the vertebra below and the posterolateral aspect of the vertebral body or pedicle of the vertebra above. The nerve can be decompressed by excising the tip of the superior facet or the entire facet joint. Another common place for nerve root entrapment is between the laterally bulging annulus or herniated disc and the pedicle of the supra-adjacent vertebra. In this case, decompression of the nerve root is performed by excising the lateral annulus. The inferomedial aspect of the vertebral pedicle should be relieved if necessary. As mentioned before, the nerve root affected in these lateral syndromes is the one numbered above the disc. In other words, foraminal stenosis or a laterally herniated disc at the L4–L5 level affects the L4 nerve root. Also, the nerve root is frequently seen exiting in a perpendicular direction instead of on a normal oblique course because the laterally bulging disc pushes the nerve root in a cephalad direction against the pedicle.[106]

Another pattern of neural compression at the foraminal level occurs in degenerative spondylolisthesis. The L5 nerve root is commonly caught between the vertebral body of L5 and the advancing inferior facet of L4, which has eroded through the superior facet of the subjacent vertebra. Wiltse described a "far-out syndrome," in which the L5 nerve root is impinged between the transverse process of L5 and the ala of the sacrum.[135] This syndrome occurs mainly in the elderly person with degenerative scoliosis and in the adult patient with isthmic spondylolisthesis. The involved nerve root should be decompressed as far as necessary. Stabilization and fusion are frequently necessary in these cases.

Nerve root constriction within the dural sac is rare. Tsuji and associates recommend durotomy in certain cases where redundant nerve roots are compressed within the dural sac.[129] We have not encountered this situation so far.

A systematic approach like this will prevent failed back surgery syndrome because of inadequate decompression of the involved root. Spinal fusion should be considered after decompressive laminectomy if more than equivalent to one facet joint is excised. Those patients with a "dynamic spinal stenosis" as seen on flexion-extension x-rays or degenerative spondylolisthesis should probably undergo fusion after decompressive laminectomy, although this point is controversial.[45, 60] The technique of lumbar spinal fusion is discussed under spondylolisthesis. The exact role of pedicle screws and plate fixation is not clear at this time.[118]

OPERATIVE COMPLICATIONS RELATED TO DISC AND STENOSIS SURGERY

NEURAL INJURY

Perforations of the dura may occur with or without nerve root damage and may lead to pseudomeningocele formation, cerebrospinal fluid fistula, meningitis, or wound healing problems. The incidence of dural tears is about 4 per cent,[70] but in reoperations it may be as high as 17.6 per cent.[125] Dural tears may occur during excision of the ligamentum flavum, but more commonly, they occur during manipulation of the dural sac to free adhesions, particularly in a stenotic canal. Gentle handling of the dural sac largely avoids this complication. Dural tears should be primarily closed using a 6:0 silk or nonabsorbable suture in such a way that it does not produce constriction of the cauda equina. A fascial or free fat graft may be used to augment the repair.[42] The paraspinous muscle, overlying fascia, subcutaneous tissue, and skin should be closed in multiple layers in a watertight manner. Drains should be avoided.

Postoperative leakage of cerebrospinal fluid may be troublesome. Strict bedrest and antibiotic treatment are recommended for a few days. Insertion of a subcutaneous drain or epidural catheter may be of help. If persistent leakage is present, surgery is required to repair the dural defect.

Injuries to the nerve roots may result in sensory alteration, a motor deficit, or even sphincter dysfunction. As mentioned before, exposing the lateral aspect of the nerve root prior to manipulation is the key to prevention of nerve root damage. Excessive retraction with metallic instruments can be avoided by packing the nerve roots with cotton pledgets. Repeated manipulation and stretching of the nerve may result in the "battered root syndrome."[9] Lacerations of the nerve root may occur if adequate visualization or identification of the nerve root is not achieved. A flattened nerve root over an extruded disc, excessive bleeding, and inadequate bony exposure may be the reasons for difficulty in identification of the nerve root. Also, failure to recognize nerve root anomalies may lead the unwary surgeon to injure the nerve root. Kadish and Simmons showed a 14 per cent incidence of various forms of nerve root anomalies that affect the patient's symptoms and the surgeon's decompressive technique.[71] When using bipolar electrocautery for hemostasis, the current level should be set low and the nerve root should be retracted and protected in order to prevent thermal burns. Nerve root injuries are more common during reoperation.

The incidence of cauda equina syndrome after lumbar surgery is considerably lower. McLaren and associates reported 6 cases of acute postdiscectomy cauda equina syndrome in a series of 2,842 lumbar discectomies.[91] Five of six patients were thought to have inadequate decompression of coexisting spinal stenosis. Free epidural fat graft was blamed for postoperative cauda equina syndrome in another report.[101] If the cauda equina syndrome is identified after surgery, urgent decompression is mandatory. Recovery of bowel and bladder function and motor and sensory deficits is variable. Spangfort reported on five patients with complications of cauda equina syndrome, only two of whom recovered completely.[120]

Scar formation about the dura and nerve roots may or may not cause recurrent symptoms of sciatica. Since there is no effective surgical treatment for epidural fibrosis, prevention is of utmost importance.[133] Careful hemostasis and gentle handling of the neural tissue will decrease the amount of scar tissue formed. A free fat graft or pedicle fat graft is superior to other materials such as gelfoam.[53, 67, 104, 134] The thickness of the free fat graft should be less than 5 mm. to prevent possible compression of the cauda equina and also to enhance vascularization of the graft.[101]

Adhesive arachnoiditis is a nonspecific inflammatory process, resulting in fibrosis and adherence of the nerve roots to the dura.[5, 23, 102] The myelographic agent Pantopaque has been implicated in the majority of cases of arachnoiditis in the past. Again, surgery is futile for these patients. Physical therapy, chronic pain rehabilitation, or neurostimulators may be effective in some patients.[24, 36]

The superior hypogastric plexus of the sympathetic nervous system is the major innervation of the urogenital system. In anterior exposures of the lower lumbar spine, injury to this structure may result in retrograde ejaculation or sterility in males.[48] Fortunately, anterior discectomy and fusion for lumbar disc surgery is rarely indicated.

VASCULAR AND VISCERAL INJURIES

The abdominal structures anterior to the intervertebral disc are at risk of damage if the anterior annulus is violated during disc removal.[58, 64, 93] The aorta bifurcates into the common iliac arteries at the L4–L5 disc level. The right common iliac artery crosses the anterior surface of the L4–L5 disc and fixes the left common iliac branch of the vena cava against the vertebral column (Fig. 4–8). The structures lateral to the vessels are the ureters, and the terminal ileum lies anterior to the vessels. The injuries to the intra-abdominal structures may be catastrophic. In addition to reducing venous bleeding and giving better exposure of the disc space, the kneeling position allows the intra-abdominal contents to fall anteriorly, away from the vertebral column. One should avoid overzealous attempts to remove the entire nucleus. Many patients with degenerative disc disease have fissuring of the annulus, and penetration of the annulus is possible if the surgeon pushes the instrument forward until resistance is met. The surgeon should always be aware of the depth of the instrument in the disc space. By maintaining contact with the vertebral end-plates, the surgeon has better depth perception. The pituitary rongeur with a depth marking is helpful in avoiding excessively deep penetration. Preoperative lateral lumbar spine roentgenograms should also be reviewed carefully to measure the depth of the intervertebral disc space.[55]

Injuries to the great vessels, including the aorta, inferior vena cava, and iliac vessels, lead to shock and death unless prompt diagnosis is made and repair performed. The mortality rate reported in the recent literature varies from 23 per cent to 55 per cent.[30, 49, 62, 63] With partial injury to the vessel wall, delayed hemorrhage, false aneurysm, or arteriovenous fistula may result.[10] The patients with arterio-venous fistula may present with an increase in pulse pressure, tachycardia, dyspnea, and cardiac enlargement months or years after back surgery.[10, 88, 112] Symptoms include high-output circulatory failure, and vascular repair is necessary in these patients.

Bowel injuries during lumbar disc surgery are uncommon.[113] Injuries to the ileum and appendix are described in the literature.[93, 117] Patients may develop abdominal distention, rigidity, and peritonitis. Prompt diagnosis and treatment are important. Ureteral injuries are again mostly caused by the pituitary rongeur.

INFECTION

Spangfort reviewed more than 10,000 laminectomies and reported an operative laminectomy infection rate of approximately 2.9 per cent.[120] More recent series indicate that the infection rate may be somewhat lower with preoperative prophylaxis.[87] Wound infection should be suspected when persistent temperature elevation occurs several days after surgery. The wound should be examined for erythema, swelling, tenderness, and drainage. Management should include needle aspiration, immediate Gram's stain and culture, and antibiotic treatment if the clinical suspicion is strong. In the presence of probable infection or persistent infection despite antibiotic treatment, the patient should be returned to the operating room and the wound reopened, thoroughly debrided, and irrigated. The wound is usally managed open, with frequent dressing changes.

Postoperative intervertebral disc space infec-

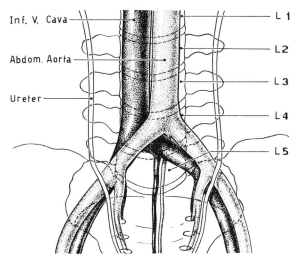

FIGURE 4–8. Relationship between the great vessels and the lumbar disc spaces. (From Montorsi, W., and Ghiringhelli, C.: Genesis, diagnosis, and treatment of vascular complications after intervertebral disc surgery. Int. Surg. 58:233, 1973.)

tion is uncommon.[43, 85, 103] The incidence was 0.75 per cent in one series.[85] Persistent back pain several weeks after removal of the intervertebral disc is a sign of postoperative discitis. Elevated erythrocyte sedimentation rates are observed in most patients with discitis. Bone scan, tomogram, or magnetic resonance imaging is helpful in identifying changes associated with discitis earlier than plain roentgenographic films.[56, 103] The bacteria responsible for postoperative discitis are identified in less than 50 per cent.[127] The most common organisms cultured are Staphylococcus species. Early diagnosis and prompt treatment are important in the prevention of chronic infection. Occasionally, lumbar epidural abscesses may develop and frank paresis or paralysis may occur.[3] Under these circumstances, immediate decompressive laminectomy is indicated.

INSTABILITY

The incidence of postdecompression spondylolisthesis is reported to be from 2 to 10 per cent[79, 114, 131] (Fig. 4–9A, B). The incidence of progressive slippage after decompression laminectomy in patients with preoperative degenerative spondylolisthesis is even higher.[69, 131] The contributing factors for postdecompression slippage have been reported to be age under 40 years, normal disc heights, and extent of surgery.[59, 114] The extent of surgery is probably the most important factor in the development of postoperative instability. Concomitant operation on the disc at the time of laminectomy may contribute to additional instability. Total laminectomy and bilateral facetectomy will make the spine unstable. Although there is no evidence in the literature, in general, if one retains the total of one facet joint at each spinal level, fusion may not be necessary. For routine spinal stenosis surgery, by undercutting the superior facet, one can perform a bilateral hemifacetectomy to leave enough facet joint to prevent postoperative spondylolisthesis.

COMPLICATIONS RELATED TO FUSION

Before discussing specific complications related to lumbar fusion, we emphasize strict patient selection criteria. Lumbar fusion is almost never indicated in patients undergoing routine lumbar disc surgery. There is no randomized prospective study in the literature supporting fusion for lumbar disc disease.

White and coworkers compared 38 patients who received Knodt rod and fusion with 31 patients who had laminectomy with no fusion for a herniated disc.[132] The general success rate of both groups was 87 per cent, but excellent results were higher in the nonfusion group. Lumbar fusion is also not indicated in patients who have nonspecific low back pain without clear radiographic instability. Performing indiscriminate lumbar fusion will result in many failures in that postoperative pain relief is not predictable and complications of fusion are numerous. The indication for lumbar fusion is therefore unrelenting mechanical low back pain due to instability, which is clearly demonstrable by flexion-extension roentgenograms. Another indication for fusion is spinal instability created by surgical dissection, as discussed above.[95]

Performing fusion in addition to neural decompression obviously entails more operative time, increased blood loss, and greater risk of complications.[78, 100] Posterior interlaminar fusion is an abandoned procedure, since it may cause iatrogenic stenosis of the spinal canal by bony hypertrophy.[16] Lateral intertransverse process fusion is the gold standard today. Various other techniques of fusion have surfaced in the literature.[47, 81, 84, 118] Further research is needed to sort out the advantages of these techniques over fusion in situ. Potential operative risks of this procedure were mentioned in the section on spondylolisthesis. These include bleeding, nerve root injury, and retroperitoneal visceral injury. Potential injuries associated with pedicular screw and plate implants were also discussed. Donor site complications may range from trivial incisional discomfort to potentially fatal gluteal artery laceration.[77]

Pseudarthrosis is a complication that may stem from technical faults by the surgeon or from biological deficiency of the patient[19, 29, 128] (Fig. 4–10). The incidence of pseudarthrosis varies depending on the number of levels fused, the techniques employed, and whether the patient smokes.[19, 38] The overall rate of pseudarthrosis is higher in two-level fusion compared with that in one-level fusion.[38] In particular, the lumbosacral junction presents a challenge. Cigarette smoking has been implicated as a risk factor in the development of pseudoarthrosis.[19] Adequate postoperative immobilization by cast or brace is also important. The effects of various implants on the rate of fusion in the lumbar spine are not clearly known at this time. Meticulous decortication

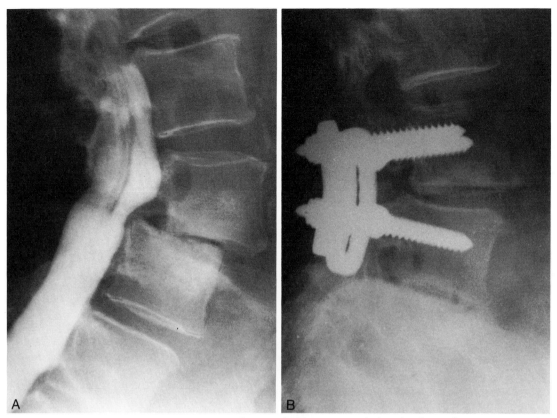

FIGURE 4–9. (*A*) Lateral myelogram revealing an impingement of the dural sac from postoperative spondylolisthesis. This patient developed unrelenting back pain three years after laminectomy. (*B*) Lateral roentgenogram of this patient after stabilization and fusion. This patient had an excellent result afterward.

and massive bone grafts favor solid fusion. The ala of the sacrum must be well exposed and decorticated, as the lumbosacral junction is the most common region of pseudarthrosis. There seems to be no statistical difference between use of autograft versus allograft in the overall fusion rate.[2, 76, 89, 94]

Although the goal of spinal fusion is to achieve eventually a solid bony bridge between the motion segments, the presence of pseudarthrosis does not translate to clinical failure.[38, 50, 108] DePalma and Rothman compared patients who developed pseudarthrosis with the group who had a solid fusion.[38] Little difference was found between the pseudarthrosis and solid fusion groups in terms of pain relief, subjective rating of surgery, and residual back pain. Pseudarthrosis may represent a fibrous stabilization as effective as bony fusion. One should avoid reoperating to achieve union when the cause of the patient's symptoms is not clearly pseudarthrosis or instability.

Motion segments adjacent to the fused spine may undergo accelerated degeneration.[80] Increased stress is expected at the segment next to fusion. Lee reported 18 patients who developed new symptoms from the segment adjacent to a fusion after an average symptom-free interval of 8.5 years.[80] The most common pathological conditions at the adjacent segments were hypertrophic facet joints and disc degeneration. Spondylolysis and spondylolisthesis are also reported after lumbar fusion.[21] It is difficult to assess the overall incidence of this late complication. Frymoyer and associates reviewed 96 patients who had undergone disc excision and midline fusion with a follow-up of more than 10 years; 2.5 per cent developed symptomatic spondylolysis, but symptomatic degenerative disc disease at levels above the spinal fusions was uncommon.[50, 51] Lehmann and coworkers reported patients who had undergone lumbar fusion with a 33-year median follow-up.[82] They concluded that, although these patients were generally satisfied with the results of their surgery, they had a

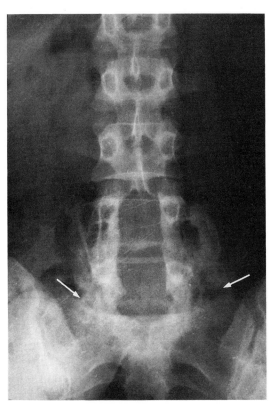

FIGURE 4–10. Anteroposterior roentgenogram revealing a probable pseudarthrosis at the L5–S1 junction, particularly on the left side. This patient had a recurrence of unrelenting back pain and had a pseudarthrosis on surgical exploration.

higher incidence of pain and more radiographic evidence of instability and stenosis than the general population.[82]

MISCELLANEOUS COMPLICATIONS

Pulmonary atelectasis is seen frequently in patients who have had endotracheal anesthesia. It is detected in the first three days after surgery and is a common cause of temperature elevations. Spinal anesthesia should obviate the problem of pulmonary atelectasis to a great degree. Ventilation exercise, discontinuation of smoking, breathing treatment, and early mobilization are all important in the prevention of this complication.

Intestinal ileus may cause the patient to become nauseated and to vomit in the early postoperative period. Bowel sounds are hypoactive on auscultation. Electrolyte imbalance must be ruled out early. Treatment includes nasogastric suctioning and intravenous fluids and electrolytes. Urinary retention may present with lower abdominal pain. Early mo-

bilization or intermittent catheterization should resolve the symptoms. Use of narcotics will aggravate urinary retention. If persistent symptoms are present, nerve root injury should be suspected. Postoperative thrombophlebitis or pulmonary embolism occurs in about 1 per cent of patients after laminectomy.[120] There was a 3.2 per cent incidence of thrombophlebitis in patients undergoing posterior lumbar fusion.[100] Postoperative calf pain may be confused with persistent radiculopathy secondary to inadequate decompression. Pulmonary embolism must be diagnosed and treated promptly. Careful physical examination and clinical suspicion lead to correct diagnosis and proper treatment.

FAILURE OF LUMBAR SURGERY

As mentioned before, patient selection is the key to surgical success. When the three diagnostic factors (the presence of a positive tension sign, a focal and correlative neurological deficit, and a positive radiographic study) are present, one is almost assured of uncovering mechanical root compression at surgery. Surgical results under these circumstances will be excellent, provided that complications are avoided.

There are many other reasons for the failed back surgery syndrome.[28, 32, 46, 52, 83, 86, 98, 107, 108, 109, 123, 130] One of the most common pitfalls during nerve root decompression is the failure to recognize lateral foraminal or extraforaminal compression. Analyzing more than 800 failed back surgery patients, Burton reported that concomitant conditions of lateral recess or central stenosis accounted for 65 to 71 per cent of failures.[25] Spengler has reported that in his series of discectomy patients there is a 30 per cent incidence of lateral recess stenosis, requiring a limited medial foraminotomy at the time of surgery.[123] At the end of any nerve root decompression, with the possible exception of a case of severe spondylolisthesis, the nerve root should have excursion of at least 1 cm. If this is not the case, further bony decompression should be performed to uncover a laterally herniated disc or hypertrophic superior facet in the foramen. In some cases, the entire facet joint or even the pedicle may have to be sacrificed in order to free the nerve. Sequestered and retained disc fragments may also contribute to persistent nerve root compression. Since the primary purpose of the operation is to relieve nerve root compression, surgery is not finished until adequate de-

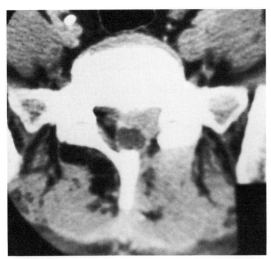

FIGURE 4–11. Computed tomography revealing a recurrent herniated disc in a patient who underwent laminotomy and discectomy one month before. A large extruded fragment was recovered on re-exploration, and the patient has been symptom free since.

compression is accomplished. If the spine is rendered unstable, concomitant fusion is indicated.

Recurrent disc herniation and reoperation rate following lumbar discectomy was as high as 11.8 per cent in one study[130] (Fig. 4–11). In this study, 60 per cent of recurrences were at the same side and level, and the rest were same level, opposite side, or different level. It is difficult to predict who is at risk for recurrence. It is not known whether the amount of disc tissue removed will influence the recurrence rate. It is sometimes difficult to distinguish recurrent disc herniation from scar. Return of symptoms after prolonged symptom-free interval favors the diagnosis of recurrence. Intravenous-enhanced computed tomography or gadolinium-enhanced magnetic resonance imaging may help to distinguish between scar tissue and recurrent herniated disc. The results of reoperation are good if the same strict clinical and radiographic criteria are followed. More complications are expected from reoperation, particularly dural tear.[125]

REFERENCES

1. Altman, R. D., Brown, M., and Gargano, F.: Low back pain in Paget's disease of bone. Clin. Orthop. 27:152–161, 1987.
2. Aurori, B. F., Weierman, R. J., Lowell, H. A., et al.: Pseudoarthrosis after spinal fusion for scoliosis (a comparison of autogeneic and allogeneic bone grafts). Clin. Orthop. 199:153–158, 1985.
3. Baker, A. S., Ojemann, R. G., Schwarts, M. N., et al.: Spinal epidural abscess. N. Engl. J. Med. 293:463, 1975.
4. Bell, G. R., and Rothman, R. H.: The conservative tre ment of sciatica. Spine 9:54, 1984.
5. Benoist, M., Ficat, C., Baraf, P., et al.: Postoperative lumbar epiduro-arachnoiditis: Diagnostic and therapeutic aspects. Spine 5:432, 1980.
6. Berkson, B., Zakhary, M. G., Primack, M. L., et al.: Urological complications following chemonucle ysis. J. Urol. 133:1065–1066, 1985.
7. Bernard, T. N., Jr., and Kirkaldy-Willis, W. H.: Recognizing specific characteristics of nonspecific low back pain. Clin. Orthop. 217:266–280, 1987.
8. Berstein, I. L.: Adverse effects of chemonucleolysis. JAMA 250:1167, 1983.
9. Bertrand, G.: The "battered" root problem. Orthop. Clin. North Am. 6:305, 1975.
10. Birkeland, I. W., and Taylor, T. K. F.: Major vascular injuries in lumbar disc surgery. J. Bone Joint Surg. 51B:4–19, 1969.
11. Bernini, P. M., Wiesel, W. W., and Rothman, R. H.: Metrizamide myelography and the identification of anomalous lumbosacral nerve roots. J. Bone Joint Surg. 62A:1203–1208, 1980.
12. Blankstein, A., Rubinstein, E., Ezra, E., et al.: Disc space infection and vertebral osteomyelitis as a complication of percutaneous lateral discectomy. Clin. Orthop. 225:234–237, 1987.
13. Booth, R. E.: Spinal stenosis. In: Anerson, L. D. (ed.): The American Academy of Orthopaedic Surgeons Instructional Course Lectures, St. Louis, C. V. Mosby Company, 1986, pp. 420–435.
14. Bradford, D. S., and Gotfried, Y.: Lumbar spine osteolysis: An entity caused by spinal instability. Spine 11:1013–1019, 1986.
15. Brian, J. E., Jr., Weterman, G. R., and Chadduck, W. M.: Septic complications of chemonucleolysis. Neurosurgery 15:730–734, 1984.
16. Brodsky, A. E.: Post-laminectomy and post-fusion stenosis of the lumbar spine. Clin. Orthop. 115:130–139, 1976.
17. Brooks, S., Dent, A. R., and Thompson, A. G.: Anterior rupture of the lumbosacral disc: Report of a case. J. Bone Joint Surg. 65A:1186–1187, 1983.
18. Brooks, M. E., Moreno, M., Sidi, A., et al.: Urologic complications after surgery on lumbosacral spine. Urology 26:202–204, 1985.
19. Brown, C. W., Orme, T. J., and Richardson, H. D.: The rate of pseudoarthrosis (surgical nonunion) in patients who are smokers and patients who are nonsmokers: A comparison study. Spine 11:942–943, 1986.
20. Brown, M. D., and Tompkins, J. S.: Chemonucleolysis (discolysis) with collagenase. Spine 11:123–129, 1986.
21. Brunet, J. A., and Wiley, J. J.: Acquired spondylolysis after spinal fusion. J. Bone Joint Surg. 66B:720–724, 1984.
22. Buchman, A., Wright, R. B., Wichter, M. D., et al.: Hemorrhagic complications after the lum-

bar injection of chymopapain. Neurosurgery 16:222–224, 1985.

23. Burton, C. V.: Lumbosacral arachnoiditis. Spine 3:24, 1978.

24. Burton, C. V.: Safety and efficacy: Session on spinal cord stimulation. Neurosurgery 1:214–215, 1977.

25. Burton, C.V., Kirkaldy-Willis, W. H., Yong-Hing, K., et al.: Causes of failure of surgery on the lumbar spine. Clin. Orthop. 157:191, 1981.

26. Cannon, B. W., Hunter S. E., and Picaza, J. A.: Nerve root anomalies in lumbar disc surgery. J. Neurosurg. 19:208–214, 1961.

27. Cares, H. L., Steinberg, R. S., Robertson, E. T., et al.: Ambulatory microsurgery for ruptured lumbar discs: Report of ten cases. Neurosurgery 22:523, 1988.

28. Cauchoix, J., Ficat, C., and Girard, B.: Repeat surgery after disc excision. Spine 3:265, 1978.

29. Cleveland, M., Bosworth, D. M., and Thompson, F. R.: Pseudoarthrosis in the lumbosacral spine. J. Bone Joint Surg. 30A:302–312, 1948.

30. Connaly, J. F., and Brooks, A. L.: Vascular problems in orthopaedics. In: The American Academy of Orthopaedic Surgeons Instructional Course Lectures, St. Louis, C. V. Mosby Company, 22:12, 1973.

31. Crawshaw, C., Frazer, A., and Merriam, W. F.: A comparison of surgery and chemonucleolysis in the treatment of sciatica: A prospective randomized trial. Spine 9:195, 1984.

32. Crock, H. V.: Observations on the management of failed spinal operations. J. Bone Joint Surg. 58B:193, 1976.

33. Dabezies, E. J., and Murphy, C. P.: Dural puncture using the lateral approach for chemonucleolysis. Spine 10:93–96, 1985.

34. Dagi, T. F., Tarkington, M. A., and Leech, J. J.: Tandem lumbar and cervical spinal stenosis. Natural history, prognostic indices and results after surgical decompression. J. Neurosurg. 66:842–849, 1987.

35. Davis, G. W., and Onik, G.: Clinical experience with automated percutaneous lumbar discectomy. Clin. Orthop. 238:98, 1989.

36. De LaPorte, C., and Siegfried, J.: Lumbosacral spinal fibrosis (spinal arachnoiditis): Its diagnosis and treatment by spinal cord stimulation. Spine 8:593, 1983.

37. DePalma, A., and Rothman, R.: Surgery of the lumbar spine. Clin. Orthop. 63:162, 1969.

38. DePalma, A., and Rothman, R. H.: The nature of pseudoarthrosis. Clin. Orthop. 59:113–118, 1968.

39. Destouet, J. M., Bilula, L. A., Murphy, W. A., et al.: Lumbar facet injection: Indication, technique, clinical correlation and preliminary results. Radiology 145:321, 1982.

40. Dodge, L. D., Bohlman, H. H., and Rhodes, R. S.: Concurrent lumbar spinal stenosis and peripheral vascular disease. A report of nine patients. Clin. Orthop. 230:141–148, 1988.

41. Dyck, P.: Paraplegia following chemonucleolysis. A case report and discussion of neurotoxicity. Spine 10:359–362, 1985.

42. Eismont, F. J., Wiesel, S. W., and Rothman, R. H.: The treatment of dural tears associated with spinal surgery. J. Bone Joint Surg. 63A:1132, 1981.

43. El-Gindi, S., Aref, S., Salama, M., et al.: Infec-tion of the intervertebral discs after surgery. J. Bone Joint Surg. 58B:114, 1976.

44. Fager, C. A., and Freiberg, S. R.: Analysis of failures and poor results of lumbar spine surgery. Spine 5:87–94, 1980.

45. Feffer, H. L., Wiesel, S. W., Cuckler, J. M., et al.: Degenerative spondylolisthesis. To fuse or not to fuse. Spine 10:287–289, 1985.

46. Finnegan, W. J., Fenlin, J. M., Marvel, J. P., et al.: Results of surgical intervention in the symptomatic multiple-operated back patient: Analysis of sixty-seven cases followed for three to seven years. J. Bone Joint Surg. 61A:1077, 1979.

47. Flately, T. J., and Derderian, H.: Closed loop instrumentation of the lumbar spine. Clin. Orthop. 196:273–278, 1985.

48. Flynn, J. C., and Price, C. T.: Sexual complications of anterior fusion of the lumbar spine. Spine 9:489, 1984.

49. Freeman, D. G.: Major vascular complications of lumbar disc surgery. West. J. Surg. Obstet. Gynecol. 69:175, 1961.

50. Frymoyer, J. W., Hanley, E., Howe, J., et al.: A comparison of radiographic findings in fusion and nonfusion patients. Ten or more years following lumbar disc surgery. Spine 4:435–440, 1979.

51. Frymoyer, J. W., Hanley, E., Howe, J., et al.: Disc excision and spine fusion in the management of lumbar disc disease. A minimum ten-year follow-up. Spine 3:1–6, 1978.

52. Frymoyer, J. W., Matteri, R. E., Hanley, E. N., et al.: Failed lumbar disc surgery requiring second operation: A long-term follow-up study. Spine 3:7, 1978.

53. Gill, G. G., Sakovich, L., and Thompson, E.: Pedicle fat grafts for the prevention of scar formation after laminectomy. Spine 5:59–64, 1980.

54. Goald, H. J.: Microlumbar discectomy. Spine 3:183, 1978.

55. Gower, D. J., Culp, P., and Ball, M.: Lateral lumbar spine roentgenograms: Potential role in complications of lumbar disc surgery. Surg. Neurol. 27:316–318, 1987.

56. Guyer, R. D., and Flemming, J. E.: Laminectomy—indications, techniques and complications. Spine 3:91–101, 1989.

57. Hall, B. B., and McCulloch, J. A.: Anaphylactic reactions following the intradiscal injection of chymopapain under local anesthesia. J. Bone Joint Surg. 65A:1215, 1983.

58. Harbison, S. P.: Major vascular complications of intervertebral disc surgery. Ann. Surg. 140:342, 1954.

59. Hazlett, J. W., and Kinnard, P.: Lumbar apophyseal process excision and spinal instability. Spine 7:171, 1982.

60. Herron, L. D., and Trippi, A. C.: L4–5 degenerative spondylolisthesis. The results of treatment by decompressive laminectomy without fusion. Spine 14:534, 1989.

61. Hodge, C. J., Binet, E. F., and Kieffer, S. A.: Intradural herniation of lumbar intervertebral discs. Spine 3:346, 1978.

62. Hofh, R. P.: Arterial injuries occurring during orthopaedic operations. Clin. Orthop. 28:21–37, 1963.

63. Holmes, H. E., and Rothman, R. H.: The Penn-

sylvania plan: An algorithm for the management of lumbar degenerative disc disease. Spine 4:15, 1979.

64. Holscher, E. C.: Vascular and visceral injuries during lumbar disc surgery. J. Bone Joint Surg. 50A:383–393, 1968.

65. Hoppenfeld, S.: Percutaneous removal of herniated lumbar discs. Clin. Orthop. 238:92, 1989.

66. Hudgins, W. R.: The role of microdiscectomy. Orthop. Clin. North Am. 14:589, 1983.

67. Jacobs, R. R., McClain, O., and Neff, J.: Control of post laminectomy scar formation: An experimental and clinical study. Spine 5:223–229, 1980.

68. Jiang, G. X., Xu, W. D., and Wang, A. H.: Spinal stenosis with meralgia paresthetica. J. Bone Joint Surg. 70B:272–273, 1988.

69. Johnsson, K. E., Willner, S., and Johnsson, K.: Postoperative instability after decompression for lumbar spinal stenosis. Spine 11:107–110, 1986.

70. Jones, A. M., Stambough, J. L., Balderston, R. A., et al.: Long-term results of lumbar spine surgery complicated by unintended incidental durotomy. Spine 14:443, 1989.

71. Kadish, L., and Simmons, E. H.: Anomalies of the lumbosacral nerve roots and anatomical investigation and myelographic study. J. Bone Joint Surg. 66B:411, 1984.

72. Kambin, P., and Schaffer, J. L.: Percutaneous lumbar discectomy. Clin. Orthop. 238:24, 1989.

73. Kahanovitz, N., Viola, K., and McCulloch, J.: Limited surgical discectomy and microdiscectomy. A clinical comparison. Spine 14:79–81, 1989.

74. Kataoka, O., Nishibayashi, Y., and Sho, T.: Intradural lumbar disc herniation. Report of three cases with a review of the literature. Spine 14:529, 1989.

75. Kirkaldy-Willis, W. H., and Hill, R. J.: A more precise diagnosis for low-back pain. Spine 4:102–109, 1979.

76. Knapp, D. R., and Jones, E. T.: Use of cortical cancellous allograft for posterior spinal fusion. Clin. Orthop. 229:99–105, 1988.

77. Kurz, L. T.: Harvesting autogenous iliac bone grafts: Complications and techniques. Presented at the annual meeting of the Western Orthopaedic Association, San Francisco, California, September 28–October 2, 1986.

78. Laasonen, E., and Soini, J.: Low-back pain after lumbar fusion. Surgical and computed tomographic analysis. Spine 14:210–213, 1989.

79. Lee, C. K.: Lumbar spinal instability (olisthesis) after extensive posterior spinal decompression. Spine 8:429–433, 1983.

80. Lee, C. K.: Accelerated degeneration of the segment adjacent to a lumbar fusion. Spine 13:375–377, 1988.

81. Lee, C. K., and deBari, A.: Lumbosacral spinal fusion with Knodt distraction rods. Spine 11:373–375, 1986.

82. Lehmann, T. R., Spratt, K. F., Tozzi, J. E., et al.: Long-term follow-up of lower lumbar fusion patients. Spine 12:97–104, 1987.

83. Lehmann, T. R., and LaRocca, H. S.: Repeat lumbar surgery: A review of patients with failure from previous lumbar surgery treated by spinal canal exploration and lumbar spinal fusion. Spine 6:615, 1981.

84. Lin, P. M.: Posterior lumbar interbody fusion technique: Complications and pitfalls. Clin. Orthop. 193:90–102, 1985.

85. Lindholm, T. S., and Pylkanen, P.: Discitis following removal of intervertebral disc. Spine 7:618–622, 1982.

86. Long, D. M., Filtzer, D. L., BenDebba, M., et al.: Clinical features of the failed-back syndrome. J. Neurosurg. 69:61–71, 1988.

87. Malis, L. I.: Prevention of neurosurgical infection by intraoperative antibiotics. Neurosurgery 5:339–343, 1979.

88. May, A. R. L., Brewster, D. C., and Darling, R. C., et al.: Arteriovenous fistula following lumbar disc surgery. Br. J. Surg. 68:41, 1981.

89. McCarthy, R. E., Peek, R. D., Morrissy, R. T., et al.: Allograft bone in spinal fusion for paralytic scoliosis. J. Bone Joint Surg. 68A:370–375, 1986.

90. McGuire, R. A., Brown, M. D., and Green, B. A.: Intradural spinal tumors and spinal stenosis. Report of two cases. Spine 12:1062–1066, 1987.

91. McLaren, A. C., and Bailey, S. I.: Cauda equina syndrome: A complication of lumbar discectomy. Clin. Orthop. 204:143–149, 1986.

92. Mooney, V., and Robertson, J.: The facet syndrome. Clin. Orthop. 115:149–156, 1976.

93. Moore, C. A., and Cohen, A.: Combined arterial venous and urethral injuries complicating disc surgery. Am. J. Surg. 115:574, 1968.

94. Nasca, R. J., and Whelchel, J. D.: Use of cryopreserved bone in spinal surgery. Spine 12:222–227, 1987.

95. Nasca, R.: Rationale for spinal fusion in lumbar spinal stenosis. Spine 14:451–454, 1989.

96. Natelson, S. E.: The injudicious laminectomy. Spine 11:966–969, 1986.

97. Onik, G., Marron, J., Helms, C., et al.: Automated percutaneous diskectomy: Initial patient experience. Work in progress. Radiology 162:129–132, 1987.

98. Pheasant, H. C., and Dyck, P.: Failed lumbar disc surgery: Cause, assessment, treatment. Clin. Orthop. 154:14, 1982.

99. Postacchini, F., Lami, R., and Massobrio, M.: Chemonucleolysis versus surgery in lumbar disc herniations: Correlation of the results to preoperative clinical pattern and size of the herniation. Spine 12:87–96, 1987.

100. Prothero, S. R., Parke, J. C., and Stinchfield, F. E.: Complications after low-back fusion in 1000 patients. J. Bone Joint Surg. 48A:57–65, 1966.

101. Prusick, V. R., Lint, D. S., and Bruder, W. J.: Cauda equina syndrome as a complication of free epidural fat-grafting. A report of two cases and a review of literature. J. Bone Joint Surg. 70:1256–1258, 1988.

102. Ransford, A. O., and Harries, B. J.: Localized arachnoiditis complicating lumbar disc lesions. J. Bone Joint Surg. 54B:656–665, 1972.

103. Rawlings, C. E., Wilkins, R. H., Gallis, H. A., et al.: Postoperative intervertebral disc space infection. Neurosurgery 13:371–376, 1983.

104. Ray, C. D.: Epidural fat grafts for the prevention of postoperative adhesions in the lumbar

spine. In: White, A. H. (ed.): *Lumbar Spine Surgery: Techniques and Complications*. St. Louis, C. V. Mosby Company, 1986.

105. Reynolds, F. C.: Complications in disk surgery. Clin. Orthop. 53:13–19, 1967.

106. Rosenblum, B. R.: The perpendicular nerve root sign. Spine 14:118–119, 1989.

107. Rothman, R. H., and Tarlov, E.: Failed back surgery syndrome. JAMA 251:657, 1984.

108. Rothman, R. H., and Booth, R.: Failures of spinal fusion. Orthop. Clin. North Am. 6:299–304, 1975.

109. Rothman, R. H., and Bernini, R. H.: Algorithm for salvage surgery of the lumbar spine. Clin. Orthop. 154:14, 1981.

110. Rothman, R. H., and Simeone, F. A.: *The Spine*, 2nd ed. Philadelphia, W. B. Saunders Company, 1982.

111. Schwartz, A. M., and Brodkey, J. S.: Bowel perforation following microsurgical lumbar discectomy. Spine 14:104, 1989.

112. Serrano Hernando, F. J., Paredero, V. M., Solis, J. V., et al.: Iliac arteriovenous fistula as a complication of lumbar disc surgery. Report of two cases and review of literature. Cardiovasc. Surg. 27:180–184, 1986.

113. Shaw, E. D., Scarborough, J. T., and Beals, R. K.: Bowel injury as a complication of lumbar discectomy: A case report and review of the literature. J. Bone Joint Surg. 63A:478, 1981.

114. Shenkins, H. A., and Hash, C. J.: Spondylolisthesis after multiple bilateral laminectomies and facetectomies for lumbar spondylosis. Follow-up review. J. Neurosurg. 50:45–47, 1979.

115. Shields, C. B., Reiss, S. J., and Garretson, H. D.: Chemonucleolysis with chymopapain: Results in 150 patients. J. Neurosurg. 67:187–191, 1987.

116. Silvers, H. R.: Microsurgical versus standard lumbar discectomy. Neurosurgery 22:837, 1988.

117. Simmons, E. H., and Wilber, R. G.: Complications of spinal surgery for discogenic disease and spondylolisthesis. In: Epps, C. (ed.): *Complications of Orthopaedic Surgery*. Philadelphia, J. B. Lippincott Company, 1978, pp. 1181–1214.

118. Simmons, E. H., and Capicotto, W. N.: Posterior transpedicular Zielke instrumentation of the lumbar spine. Clin. Orthop. 236:180–191, 1988.

119. Smith, R. V.: Intradural disc rupture: Report of two cases. J. Neurosurg. 55:117, 1981.

120. Spangfort, E. V.: The lumbar disc herniation—A computer-aided analysis of 2504 operations. Acta Orthop. Scand. (Suppl.) 142:52, 1971.

121. Spengler, D.M.: Lumbar discectomy: Results with limited disc excision and selective foraminotomy. Spine 7:604–607, 1982.

122. Spengler, D. M., and Freeman, C. W.: Patient selection for lumbar discectomy. Spine 4:129, 1979.

123. Spengler, D. M., Freeman, D., and Westbrook, R.: Low back pain following multiple lumbar spine procedures. Spine 5:356, 1980.

124. Stambough, J. L.: Surgical techniques for lumbar discectomy. Sem. Spine Surg. 1:47–53, 1989.

125. Stolke, D., Sollmann, W., and Seifert, V.: Intra and postoperative complications in lumbar disc surgery. Spine 14:56–59, 1989.

126. Takata, K., Inoue, S., Takahashi, K., et al.: Swelling of the cauda equina in patients who have herniation of a lumber disc. A possible pathogenesis of sciatica. J. Bone Joint Surg. 70A:361–368, 1988.

127. Thibodeau, A. A.: Closed space infection following removal of lumbar intervertebral disc. J. Bone Joint Surg. 50A:400–410, 1968.

128. Thompson, W. A., and Ralston, E. L.: Pseudoarthrosis following spine fusion. J. Bone Joint Surg. 31A:400–405, 1949.

129. Tsuji, H., Tamaki, T., Itoh, T., et al.: Redundant nerve roots in patients with degenerative lumbar spinal stenosis. Spine 10:72–82, 1985.

130. Weir, B. K. A., and Jacobs, G. A.: Reoperation rate following lumbar discectomy. An analysis of 662 lumbar discectomies. Spine 5:366–370, 1980.

131. White, A. A. III, and Wiltse, L. L.: Spondylolisthesis after extensive lumbar laminectomy. Presented at the 43rd Annual Meeting of the American Academy of Orthopaedic Surgeons, New Orleans, February 1976.

132. White, A. H., Rogov, P. V., Zucherman, J., et al.: Lumbar laminectomy for herniated disc: A prospective controlled comparison with internal fixation fusion. Spine 12:305–307, 1987.

133. Wiesel, S. W., and Rothman, R. H.: Lumbar disc disease and spinal stenosis. In: Evarts, C. M. (ed.): *Surgery of the Musculoskeletal System*. New York, Churchill Livingstone, 1983, pp. 57–84.

134. Williams, R. W.: Microlumbar discectomy. Spine 3:175, 1978.

135. Wiltse, L. L., Guyer, R. D., Spencer, C. W., et al.: Alar transverse process impingement of the L5 spinal nerve: The far-out syndrome. Spine 9:31–41, 1984.

136. Wisneski, R. J., and Rothman, R. H.: Microdiscectomy and percutaneous discectomy: Indications, history and results. In: White, A. H., Rothman, R. H., and Ray, C. D. (eds.): *Spine Surgery*. St. Louis, C. V. Mosby Company, 1987, pp. 115–122.

137. Wisneski, R. J., and Rothman, R. H.: The Pennsylvania plan II: An algorithm for the management of lumbar degenerative disc disease. The American Academy of Orthopaedic Surgeons Instructional Course Lectures, St. Louis, C. V. Mosby Company, 34:17–36, 1985.

138. Zeiger, H. E., Jr., and Zampella, E. J.: Intervertebral disc infection after lumbar chemonucleolysis: Report of a case. Neurosurgery 18:616–621, 1986.

FIVE

Complications of Spinal Tumor Surgery

Howard S. An, M.D.

Richard A. Balderston, M.D.

Frederick A. Simeone, M.D.

Complications of treatment for spinal neoplasms may arise from failure to correctly diagnose the lesion and from surgical procedures themselves. Careful history and physical examination along with appropriate laboratory investigations lead to the correct diagnosis. In general, once a suspected lesion is found, a biopsy should be undertaken to make a definitive diagnosis. Exact techniques of biopsy or surgery should be tailored to the nature and location of the lesion and the patient's general condition. In this chapter, complications and pitfalls of treatment of spinal tumors are presented.

PREOPERATIVE PLANNING

History is often quite helpful in separating neoplastic processes from other causes of back pain. Pain associated with tumors is characteristically persistent and worse at night and usually not relieved by rest. The patient's age is of importance in that metastatic tumors and multiple myeloma usually occur after the fifth decade. Eosinophilic granuloma, osteoid osteoma, and osteoblastoma are found in children and young adults. Leukemia and neuroblastoma are malignancies found in the younger child.

Physical examination should include a general survey, because primary tumors from breast, prostate, lung, rectum, or thyroid may be detected. Rectal examination may detect chordoma in the sacrum. Careful neurological examination is mandatory to detect early signs of cord compression. Any elderly patient with a new onset of persistent back pain should have a work-up to rule out tumors or infections. A complete blood count with a differential white blood cell count and an erythrocyte sedimentation rate will suggest or rule out an infectious process. Calcium, phosphorus, and alkaline phosphatase levels are altered in metabolic diseases such as osteomalacia, Paget's disease, and hyperparathyroidism. Roentgenographically, severe osteoporosis is often difficult to distinguish from multiple myeloma. Paget's disease also mimics osteoblastic tumors such as prostate carcinoma or lymphoma. If multiple myeloma is suspected, serum immunoglobulin electrophoresis should be ordered. Acid phosphatase testing should be ordered for patients suspected of prostate carcinoma. Further studies such as mammography, thyroid studies, intravenous pyelography, and chest or abdominal computed tomography should be obtained according to the suspected primary carcinoma. Although metastatic lesions are the most common tumors of the spine, primary tumors including benign and malignant bone tumors, intraspinal tumors, and cysts should be considered in the differential diagnosis (Tables 5–1 through 5–4). Metabolic disorders such as osteoporosis and Paget's disease should also be considered in the differential diagnosis.[44] Spinal infections should be ruled out, particularly in older patients with diabetes mel-

Table 5–1
Benign Bone Tumors

TUMOR	AGE	SEX	LOCATION	X-RAY	TREATMENT	COMMENTS
Osteoid osteoma	<30	M>	posterior elements	nidus & sclerosis	excision	painful scoliosis
Osteoblastoma	<30	M>	posterior elements	radiolucent	excision	painful scoliosis
Hemangioma	>30	M=F	body	vertical trabeculae	none, radiation or surgery	most are asymptomatic
Giant cell tumor	>20	F>	body & sacrum	radiolucent	excision (radiation?)	recurrence is common
Aneurysmal bone cyst	<25	M=F	posterior elements	lytic & expansile	excision (radiation?)	may involve next vertebra
Eosinophilic granuloma	<20	M>	body	radiolucent or collapse	orthosis	self-limiting process
Osteochondroma	10–20	M>	posterior elements	exophytic	excision if symptomatic	most are asymptomatic

Table 5–2
Malignant Bone Tumors

TUMOR	AGE	SEX	LOCATION	X-RAY	TREATMENT	COMMENTS
Multiple myeloma	>50	M>	body	osteopenia & collapse	chemotherapy & radiation	surgery if instability
Chordoma	30–70	M>	sacrum, C1–2	radiolucent destructive	aggressive excision	recurrence is common
Lymphoma	>20	M>	body	lytic or sclerotic	radiation and chemotherapy	non-Hodgkin's type
Neuroblastoma	<3	M>	body	osteopenia, destructive	excision & chemotherapy/radiation	rosette on histology
Chondrosarcoma	50–70	M=F	body	calcified & destructive	excision	chemotherapy/radiation not helpful
Osteosarcoma	10–20	M>	body	destructive	debulk, chemotherapy, and radiation	rare de novo in spine
Metastatic tumors	>40	M,F	body	lytic or blastic	radiation, surgery	breast, lung, prostate, etc.

Table 5–3
Intraspinal Neoplasms or Cysts

CYST	AGE	SEX	X-RAY	TREATMENT	COMMENTS
INTRADURAL EXTRAMEDULLARY					
Neurilemmoma (schwannoma)	30–40>	M=F	circular filling defect on myelogram	excision	commonest intraspinal tumor
Neurofibroma			circular defect, dumbbell shape	excision	associated with neurofibromatosis
Meningioma	50–60>	F>	circular defect with dural attachment	excision	80% in thoracic spine
INTRADURAL INTRAMEDULLARY					
Ependymoma	20–60>	M>	cord widening and dye defect	excision	50% in the filium terminale
Astrocytoma	20–50>	M>	cord widening	excision (radiation ?)	higher grades worse prognosis

Table 5–4
Cystic Lesions

CYST	AGE	SEX	X-RAY	TREATMENT	COMMENTS
Arachnoid cyst			multiple dye defects	excision if symptoms	most common in thoracic
Syringomyelia	>20	M = F	cord widening and MRI is +	laminectomy or syringostomy	multiple causes
Perineural cyst			cystic dilatation of sacral roots	observation, decompress	many are asymptomatic

litus and urinary tract infections. Occasionally, an infection and tumor may exist in the same individual.[29]

Metastatic malignancies significantly outnumber primary axial tumors of the spine. Metastatic tumors are principally extradural, since the dura mater forms a natural barrier. Pain is the first symptom in the majority of cases. The pain is characteristically axial, but radiating pain may develop and mislead the physician. As the neoplasm increases in size, specific neurological deficit can result. The rapidity of development of subsequent neurological findings after onset of axial pain differentiates this tumor from intradural neoplasms. The manifestations of cord compression include difficulty in maintaining balance, wide-based gait, fatigue after a short walk, urinary symptoms, paresthesia, and weakness of the extremities. It is important to detect these signs and symptoms early to prevent irreversible neurological deficits.

Symptoms from primary bone tumors vary considerably depending on the nature of the tumor. For example, pain secondary to osteoid osteoma is characteristically throbbing, worse at night, and relieved by aspirin, while most patients with hemangioma are asymptomatic. Primary malignant bone tumors are rare except for multiple myeloma and chordoma. Rapid progression of the patient's symptoms and destructive process as seen on a roentgenogram are typically present in these cases. Early diagnosis is important to prevent late sequelae such as neurological compromise and deformity.

Intradural extramedullary tumors are mostly benign, and they frequently grow in relation to a nerve root, resulting in radicular symptoms (Fig. 5–1). The pain is typically worse at night. It may take months or years for these tumors to compress the spinal cord. Often, a slowly evolving neurological syndrome is attributed to other causes such as diabetic neu-

ropathy, primary lateral sclerosis, or cervical spondylosis. Intramedullary tumors are rare, may progress insidiously, and are often painless. Because the fibers controlling pain and temperature are located centrally in the spinal cord, centrally placed tumors can affect pain and temperature sensation only in segmental fashion without affecting light touch or position sense. This "segmental differential sensory deficit," or "dissociated sensory loss," is characteristic of an intramedullary tumor.[83] The most common location of intramedullary tumors is the cervical cord, and therefore, the hands are frequently affected early. Subsequently, long tract signs, weakness, and incontinence may develop. The evolution of these symptoms is almost invariably slow, and this fact, associated with the absence of pain, is responsible for misdiagnoses such as multiple sclerosis and cervical spondylosis.

At present, there are many imaging modalities. The surgeon should decide which of these

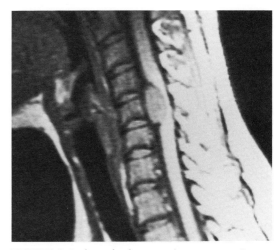

FIGURE 5–1. A sagittal magnetic resonance image revealing an intradural extramedullary tumor (neurofibroma) in a 35-year-old white female.

imaging modalities is necessary to the evaluation. Conventional high-quality roentgenographs should be obtained in all cases. These roentgenographs should suggest whether the lesion is benign or malignant and provide a most likely diagnosis. Computed tomography can usually demonstrate bony involvement, while magnetic resonance imaging provides additional information on soft tissue and neural involvement[7] (Fig. 5–2). Technetium bone scan provides information on both local and systemic involvement. It is important to realize that multiple myeloma and metastatic thyroid carcinoma do not show up on bone scan in approximately 50 per cent of cases.[4] Myelography can be helpful in making the diagnosis of epidural metastasis,[75] but magnetic resonance imaging may replace myelography in the future (Fig. 5–3).

Preoperative angiography is invaluable for tumors with significant vascularity. Metastatic renal cell carcinoma is particularly vascular. Preoperative Gelfoam injection during angiography may be effective in reducing blood loss.[42, 49, 76] Angiography also identifies the feeding artery to the spinal cord, which may be involved by tumor. In addition, if the tumor is close to a major artery, angiography will be helpful in defining the relationship between the tumor and the artery.

BIOPSY

Biopsy of a spinal lesion may be necessary before definitive treatment, because histological diagnosis of the lesion may be required.

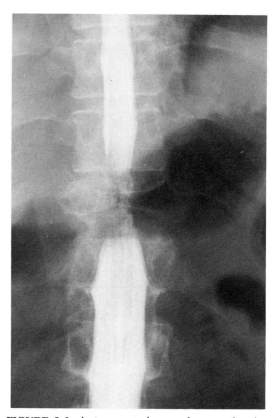

FIGURE 5–3. Anteroposterior myelogram showing a significant block of the dye owing to epidural infiltration of a plasmacytoma in a 60-year-old female.

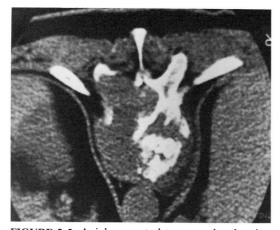

FIGURE 5–2. Axial computed tomography showing tumor destroying the vertebral body, pedicle, and lamina on the left side in a 60-year-old female with T11-T12 plasmacytoma.

Biopsy may be done through a percutaneous needle approach or open surgery[70] (Fig. 5–4). Disadvantages of percutaneous needle biopsy include the risks of damaging vital structures and totally missing the lesion.[37] According to Boland and associates, percutaneous biopsies yielded positive results in 65 per cent of lytic lesions but in only 20 to 25 per cent of blastic metastases.[10] On the other hand, open biopsies had a positive yield of greater than 85 per cent in both types of lesions.[10] Open biopsy is preferred in many cases, particularly in thoracic and cervical lesions. The technique of closed or open biopsy is not simple, and associated complications are not uncommon.

Technique of closed needle biopsy for the lower thoracic and lumbar spine employs the lateral or prone position. Local anesthesia minimizes injury to neural structures, as the patient can communicate if the needle is in close proximity to the neural structures. The point of needle insertion varies depending on the level of the spinal lesions and the size of the patient. One can estimate it by pointing a

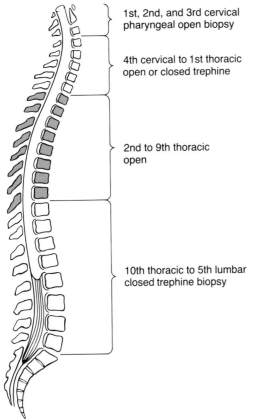

1st, 2nd, and 3rd cervical pharyngeal open biopsy

4th cervical to 1st thoracic open or closed trephine

2nd to 9th thoracic open

10th thoracic to 5th lumbar closed trephine biopsy

FIGURE 5–4. Regional consideration of vertebral biopsy. (From Evarts, C. M.: Diagnostic techniques: Closed biopsy of bone. Clin. Orthop. *107*:100, 1974.)

Steinmann pin vertically at the center of the lesion. The distance from the tip of the Steinmann pin to the surface of the body should equal the distance of the needle insertion from the midline if a 45-degree angle is used for the needle path[2] (Fig. 5–5A,B). This distance is usually 8 to 10 cm. in the lumbar spine, 6 to 7 cm. in the thoracolumbar junction, and only 4 to 5 cm. in the thoracic spine.[8, 38, 57] A local anesthetic is infiltrated using a long 22-gauge needle. The needle should point at an angle of 45 degrees, and a C-arm fluoroscope monitors the progress of the needle. Constant suction of the needle is maintained to identify vessels if encountered. The periosteum and the needle tract are anesthetized. The Craig needle biopsy is advanced in the same tract under C-arm fluoroscopic guidance. The cannulated, serrated biopsy needle is inserted to complete the procedure. In the event of excess bleeding, one can insert a piece of gelfoam into the biopsy site. One should attempt to obtain adequate amount of tissue. Following biopsy, the patient must be closely monitored

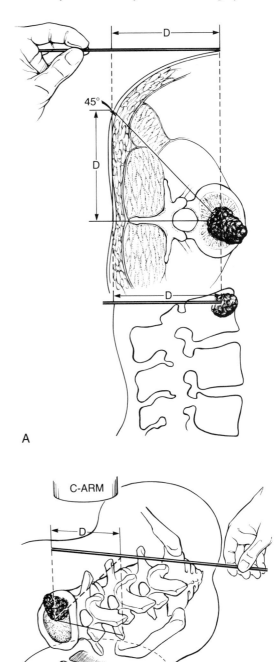

A

B

FIGURE 5–5. *(A)* A Steinmann pin is positioned so that its tip is at the center of the lesion with the patient in a lateral decubitus position. The entry point is selected at distance "D" from the spinous process, assuming that a 45-degree insertion angle would be used. *(B)* A three-dimensional illustration of this technique. (From Alexander, A. H.: Chymopapain chemonucleolysis, discography, and needle biopsy technique. In: Chapman, M. W. (ed.): *Operative Orthopaedics.* Philadelphia, J. B. Lippincott Company, 1988, p. 2134.)

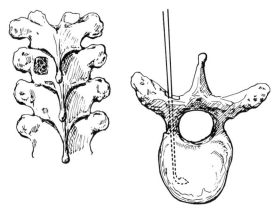

FIGURE 5–6. Illustration of transpedicular biopsy of the thoracic spine. (From Dunn, H. K.: Tumors of the thoracic and lumbar spine. In: Evarts, M. C. (ed.): *Surgery of the Musculoskeletal System.* New York, Churchill Livingstone, 1983, p. 4:191.)

for bleeding complications. Percutaneous needle biopsy is also possible in the cervical spine using a lateral approach.[71]

Computed tomography–guided needle biopsy has been reported to be more accurate and safer.[67] It allows a more precise passage of the needle without damaging vital structures. Bony lesions are more readily identified using computed tomography rather than fluoroscopy. Computed tomography allows better depiction of associated great vessels, nerves, and lungs as well as the lesion itself. For lesions in the cervical or thoracic spine, a CT-guided biopsy or open biopsy is safer and more effective than a fluoroscopic closed biopsy.[67] Biopsy of densely sclerotic and small lesions are also difficult with fluoroscopy-guided closed techniques. Although fluoroscopy-guided closed biopsy is considered safe up to T10 vertebra,[30] complications have been reported. These include neural injury, paraspinal hematoma, infection, pneumothorax, meningitis, and death.[3, 5, 20, 40, 51, 66]

Technique of open biopsy is simple for posteriorly located lesions. Routine anterior exposure is needed for anterior lesions of the cervical spine. Technique of open biopsy for anterior lesions located in the thoracic and lumbar spine frequently employs the transpedicular approaches[26] (Fig. 5–6). The precise localization of the thoracic and lumbar pedicles is important, and intraoperative imaging is of great help. Costotransversectomy and posterolateral approaches may also be used in selected cases of thoracic and lumbar lesions, respectively.

OPERATIVE TECHNIQUES OF EXPOSURE AND STABILIZATION

The goals of tumor surgery in the spine are to obtain a complete excision if possible, to preserve or restore normal neurological function, and to maintain spinal stability. Weinstein and McLain reported 82 cases of primary neoplasms of the spine, and prolonged survival was seen with complete excision of the malignant tumor as opposed to incomplete resection.[92] They also reported that giant cell tumors demonstrated an aggressive tendency to local recurrence if not completely resected initially.[92] Complete excision is not possible in metastatic lesions, but the goals should be to decompress the spinal cord and to stabilize the spine. O'Neil and coworkers reported 33 patients with tumorous conditions of the spine who were treated with anterior, posterior, or combined anterior and posterior surgical techniques.[68] They concluded that an aggressive surgical approach helps these patients to be pain free and to preserve spinal cord function.

Special considerations should be given to patients with neurological compromise. Therapeutic interventions include steroids, radiotherapy, decompressive laminectomy with or without stabilization, or anterior corpectomy and fusion. Steroids can be helpful in reducing edema of the spinal cord in the initial stage of treatment. Radiation therapy is the initial treatment of choice if neurological compromise is due to tumor infiltration rather than mechanical deformity or bony impingement. Young and associates compared 16 patients with spinal epidural metastases who received laminectomy plus radiotherapy with 13 patients who received radiotherapy alone.[96] No significant difference was found in the effectiveness of the two treatment methods in regard to pain relief, improved ambulation, or improved sphincter function.[96] A similar conclusion was reached by other authors.[27, 39] Certain tumors, such as lymphoma and multiple myeloma, are quite radiosensitive. Chordoma and chondrosarcoma are very radioresistant. Most metastatic tumors are moderately radiosensitive, and treatment with radiation may be effective in many situations. If radiotherapy is planned after surgery, it should be delayed at least two weeks to prevent wound complications.[4] Also, radiation above 1500 rad may adversely affect the incorporation of bone grafts.[4]

The precise method of surgical treatment depends on the nature, location, and extent of the tumor, the spinal level, and the patient's medical status, but most metastatic tumors should be decompressed anteriorly as the spinal cord is compressed from the anterior side.[56, 69, 82, 89] The indications for anterior decompression and stabilization are neural compromise after previous radiotherapy, neural deficit due to radioresistant tumors, neural deterioration during radiotherapy, and pathological fracture-dislocation with neural impairment. Siegal and associates documented an 85 per cent return of ambulation after 35 anterior decompressions and stabilizations and a 93 per cent retention of sphincter control after 41 procedures.[82] These results are superior to those obtained by radiation therapy alone or by radiation therapy combined with laminectomy.[82] If the spinal cord compression is due to a lesion located posteriorly, decompressive laminectomy and posterior stabilization is preferred. Laminectomy alone is not recommended because of the development of postsurgical kyphotic deformity. After the onset of neurological manifestations, surgery should be performed as soon as possible to obtain maximum neural recovery.[14] In metastatic disease of the spine, where neural impairment is not a problem but the patient has unrelenting pain despite radiotherapy and orthosis, palliative posterior stabilization alone may be appropriate.[18, 21, 73] Occasionally, debilitated patients with a limited life span who require surgery for neural decompression and spinal stabilization may be treated with posterior laminectomy and stabilization as a surgical means of palliation.[80] Posterior approach is less extensive compared with anterior decompression and fusion, and it improves the quality of the patient's remaining life.[80]

Spinal stabilization after excision of tumor is an important step in preventing postsurgical instability. Adequate stabilization is possible with various internal fixation devices, bone graft, or cement. Following anterior decompression, bone graft stabilization is preferred for long-term success. Methylmethacrylate and metal implants may also be used as augmentation.[47, 56] Methylmethacrylate provides only temporary stability and, therefore, should not be used in patients with a life expectancy of longer than one year.[64] Great caution should be exercised to avoid thermal and mechanical injuries to the spinal cord if methylmethacrylate is used.[22] Second-stage posterior stabilization is recommended for extensive lesions, particularly in the thoracolumbar region. A one-stage combined anterior and posterior approach may be considered in selected cases. The one-stage combined procedure requires prolonged operating time and results in more blood loss, but it provides better stabilization and rapid rehabilitation.[58]

Intraspinal neoplasms are classified according to their relation to the dura and the spinal cord. There are extradural, intradural-extramedullary, and intramedullary types. Extradural tumors are principally metastatic. Intradural tumors require microscopic dissection for removal. Most intradural tumors can be removed by laminectomy approach unless they are located anteriorly. Posterior stabilization is recommended if the spine becomes unstable following tumor excision. Postlaminectomy kyphosis is particularly common in younger patients and in regions of the cervical spine and cervicothoracic junction.[95]

UPPER CERVICAL SPINE

Stabilization of the upper cervical spine may be necessary after tumor excision. Many techniques of occipitocervical fusion have been described.[25, 43, 32, 93] Wertheim and Bohlman, using rigid wiring and iliac grafts[93] (Fig. 5–7), reported successful fusion in 13 patients. This technique seems to be safe and reliable.

Atlantoaxial stabilization and fusion can be accomplished with wires and iliac bone graft

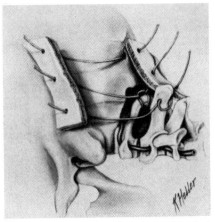

FIGURE 5–7. Illustration of occiput-C1-C2 fusion. (From Wertheim, S. B., and Bohlman, H. H.: Occipitocervical fusion. J. Bone Joint Surg. 69A:833, 1987.)

in the majority of cases (Fig. 5–8). The Halifax clamp may be used in selected cases where sublaminar wires would be difficult or dangerous to pass.[17] Magerl and associates described a transarticular screw technique for those who have deficient posterior arch of the atlas.[62] Roy-Camille and coworkers described plate fixation in the occipitocervical region.[77]

Complications associated with posterior occipitocervical fusion may be devastating. Care is required during passage of the wires or application of the screws to prevent injury to the brain stem or spinal cord. We recommend the use of somatosensory-evoked potential (SSEP) monitoring during these procedures. Dissection on the ring of the atlas must be done in a gentle manner as direct pressure may result in fracture or slippage of an instrument. One should dissect only laterally, approximately 1.5 cm., as the vertebral artery is at risk. One should avoid dissecting the foramen magnum from the inferior edge of the foramen to prevent uncontrollable venous bleeding. We recommend halo-vest immobilization after surgery to prevent failure of the surgical construct and to lessen the likelihood of pseudarthrosis.

Anterior approaches to the upper part of the cervical spine include dislocation of the temporomandibular joint,[74] osteotomy of the mandible,[46] transoral approach,[31] and anterior retropharyngeal approach.[19, 64, 94] Each procedure has advantages and disadvantages, and the surgeon should be thoroughly familiar with

the anatomy and potential complications associated with the particular procedure before undertaking this formidable task.

DeAndrade and MacNab described an anteromedial approach to the upper spine.[19] The neck is hyperextended, and the chin is turned to the opposite side. A skin incision is made along the anterior aspect of the sternocleidomastoid muscle and curved toward the mastoid process. Detach the sternocleidomastoid muscle from the mastoid process, and retract the carotid artery laterally. The superior thyroid artery and lingual vessels are ligated. The facial vein is identified at the upper portion of the incision, which helps to find the hypoglossal nerve. Careful retraction of this nerve is mandatory to avoid injury. Stripping of the longus colli muscle exposes the anterior aspect of the upper cervical spine.

The technique described by McAfee and associates is as follows[65] (Fig. 5–9A–E). A right-sided submandibular transverse incision and division of the platysma leads to the sternocleidomastoid muscle and its deep cervical fascia.[65] The mandibular branch of the facial nerve should be identified with the aid of a nerve stimulator, and the retromandibular vein is ligated during the initial stage of dissection. The anterior border of the sternocleidomastoid muscle is mobilized. The submandibular salivary gland and the jugular digastric lymph nodes are resected. Care should be taken to suture the salivary gland's duct to prevent a salivary fistula. The digastric tendon is divided

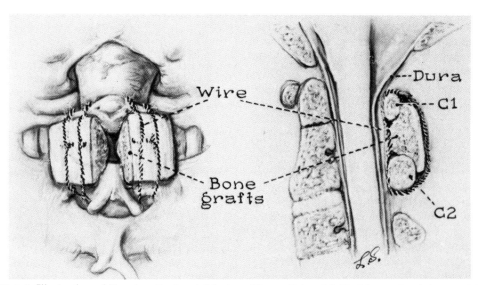

FIGURE 5–8. Illustration of Brooks atlantoaxial fusion. (From Griswold, D. M., et al.: Atlantoaxial fusion for instability. J. Bone Joint Surg. *60*A:285–292, 1978.)

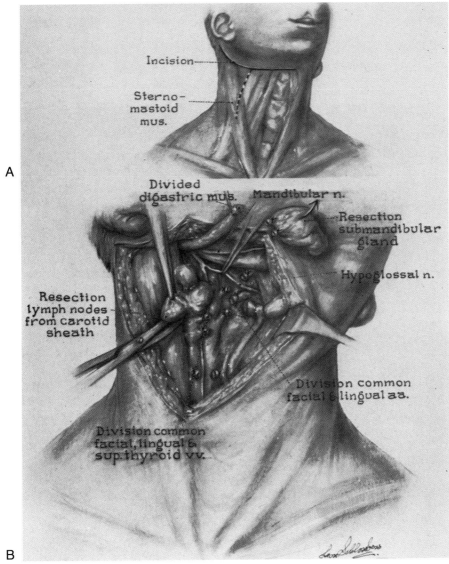

A

B

FIGURE 5–9. *(A–E)* Illustration of retropharyngeal anterior exposure of the upper cervical spine. (From McAfee, P. C., Bohlman, H. H., Riley, L. H., et al.: The anterior retropharyngeal approach to the upper part of the cervical spine. J. Bone Joint Surg. *69*A:1371, 1987.)

Illustration continued on following page

and tagged for later repair. The hypoglossal nerve is next identified and mobilized. In order to mobilize the carotid contents laterally, the carotid sheath is opened and arterial and venous branches are ligated. These include the superior thyroid artery and vein, lingual artery and vein, ascending pharyngeal artery and vein, and facial artery and vein, beginning inferiorly and progressing superiorly. The superior laryngeal nerve is also identified with the aid of a nerve stimulator and mobilized. The prevertebral fasciae are transected longitudinally to expose the longus colli muscles.

Tumor excision and bone graft stabilization can then be accomplished.

The lateral retropharyngeal approach described by Whitesides and Kelley provides exposure of both the upper and lower cervical areas[94] (Fig. 5–10). This involves dissection posterior to the carotid sheath. Dissection between the sternocleidomastoid muscle and anteriorly retracted carotid contents leads to the transverse processes of all the cervical vertebrae. In this manner, exposure is possible from the anterior ring of C1 to T1.

Anterior exposure from the occiput to C2 is

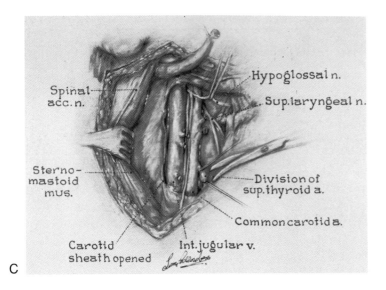

C

FIGURE 5-9 *Continued*

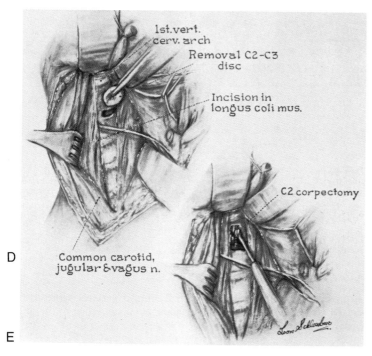

D

E

more directly and easily approached by the transoral route by splitting the soft palate and posterior pharyngeal wall, but it carries a high risk of infection.[31] Fang and Ong reported six patients who underwent anterior transoral approach to the upper cervical spine, and four had infections of the pharyngeal wall, including one patient who died of meningitis.[31] The vertebral artery is also at risk of injury during transoral approach. Potential complications associated with other anterior operations of the upper cervical spine can be numerous. Airway obstruction and difficulty with swallowing caused by retropharyngeal edema require prompt tracheostomy. Because dissection around the cranial nerves and vascular structures is involved, experience and thorough knowledge of the anatomy are required to prevent injuries to these structures. Proper positioning of the neck, fiberoptic nasotracheal awake intubation, and intraoperative monitoring of the spinal cord function are important measures to take in the prevention of spinal cord injury.

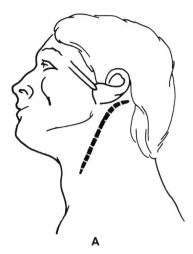

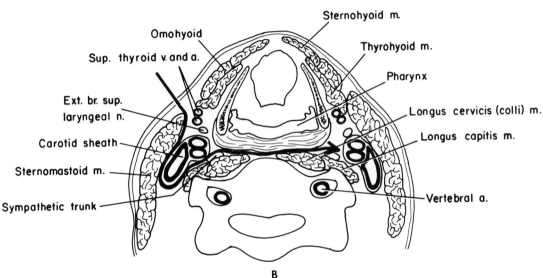

Sternohyoid m.

Omohyoid

Thyrohyoid m.

Sup. thyroid v. and a.

Pharynx

Ext. br. sup.
laryngeal n.

Longus cervicis (colli) m.

Carotid sheath

Longus capitis m.

Sternomastoid m.

Sympathetic trunk

Vertebral a.

B

FIGURE 5–10. Illustration of anterior exposure of the upper cervical spine with dissection lateral and posterior to the carotid sheath. (From Johnson, R. M., and Southwick, W. O.: Surgical approaches to the spine. In: Rothman, R. H., and Simeone, F. A. (eds.): *The Spine.* Philadelphia, W. B. Saunders Company, 1982, p. 111.)

LOWER CERVICAL SPINE

Tumor excision and stabilization in the lower cervical spine may be through anterior, posterior, or both routes depending on pathoanatomical processes of tumor. If the spinous processes and lamina are intact, a standard triple wiring and fusion with bone graft is performed.[9] If laminectomy is performed, a lateral facet wiring or lateral mass plating should be performed. Decompressive laminectomy for tumor excision is prone to progressive instability and late deformity, particularly in the younger individual.[95] Use of methylmethacrylate is possible, but only temporary benefit

may be expected.[24, 64] In general, methylmethacrylate should be used only as an adjunctive material in spinal stabilization.[13]

Exposure of the posterior elements of the lower cervical spine is simple, but stabilization after laminectomy is not easy. The techniques of cervical laminectomy were discussed under cervical disc disease. Facet fusion may be accomplished using the technique described by Callahan and associates[11] (Fig. 5–11A–D). The soft tissues and capsular ligaments are cleared from the facets and posterior pillars, and the facet joints are palpated using a small elevator. Drill holes are made in the inferior facets at a right angle to the plane of the facet joints.

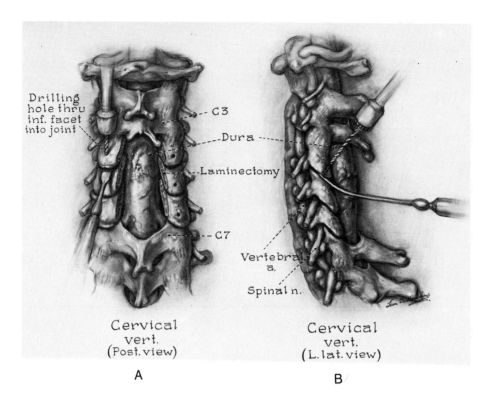

A

B

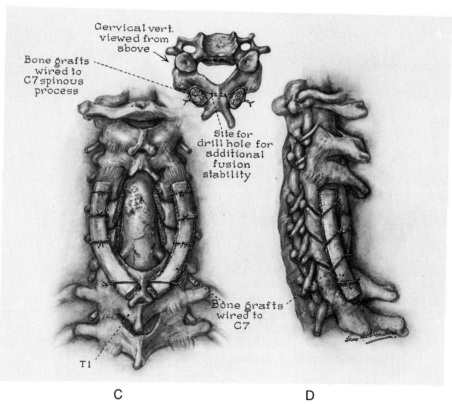

C

D

FIGURE 5–11. Illustration of facet wiring and bone grafting. (From Johnson, R. M., and Southwick W. O.: Surgical approaches to the spine. In: Rothman, R. H., and Simeone, F. A. (eds.): *The Spine*. Philadelphia, W. B. Saunders Company, 1982, pp. 138–139.)

Wires are inserted into each hole and tightened around the bone grafts.

Another method of facet fusion is posterior cervical plating, described by Roy-Camille.[28, 77] More rigid fixation is achievable with this technique. Bilateral exposure to the limits of the lateral masses is made. The center of the articular pillar is located and the cortex pierced with an awl (Fig. 5–12). The pillar is drilled with a 2- or 2.5-mm. bit and directed 15 to 20 degrees laterally for C3-C7 and straightforward for C2 vertebrae to avoid injuries to the vertebral artery. One should also aim the drill approximately 20 to 25 degrees in a cephalad direction to avoid the facet joint, particularly for the bottom screws. The opposite cortex is generally penetrated, using the drill with a stop guide. The drill hole is tapped with a 3.5-mm. tap, and a contoured Roy-Camille posterior cervical plate with a 3.5 mm. diameter is placed and secured with cortical screws 14 to 18 mm. long. Also, small pelvic reconstruction plates may be used instead of Roy-Camille plates. The posterior elements lateral to the plates are decorticated, and bone grafts are added.

Potential complications of posterior facet fusion after laminectomy include injuries to the vertebral artery and nerve roots and pseudarthrosis. Thorough familiarity with the articular pillar anatomy and surgical technique is important in the prevention of these complications. Another common complication after posterior cervical fusion is fusion extension. Exposure should be limited to the affected levels only to prevent this complication.

Anterior approach to the lower cervical spine has been described in the chapter on cervical disc disease. Anterior vertebral body resection and bone grafting is a curative procedure for benign lesions and a palliative one for metastatic lesions.[34, 73] A vertical incision parallel to the sternocleidomastoid muscle gives a more extensive exposure (Fig. 5–13). Corpectomy and the modified strut grafting method illustrated by Light and coworkers have been reliable in our hands.[60] The bone graft should span from the upper end-plate to the lower end-plate for greatest stability. A skeletal halo-vest should be fitted postoperatively in these patients. If adequate stability cannot be obtained after strut grafting, one should consider using an anterior plate with screws[91] or posterior fusion to provide additional stability.

Potential complications of anterior cervical spine exposure and bone graft stabilization have been discussed in the chapter on cervical disc disease. One of the common complications is dislodgement of the bone graft during application of the halo ring. In general, the halo ring should be applied at the beginning of surgery or before surgery. In this way, the surgery can be done with the patient in traction, and the vest can be applied right after surgery with less likelihood of bone graft dislodgement. Metal implants on the anterior aspects of the cervical spine should be avoided if possible. The mechanical strength of plated cervical spine with unicortical screws is inferior, and therefore, bicortical screws are recommended by most authors. Screw insertion to purchase posterior cortex of the vertebral body invites complications such as dural perforation and spinal cord injury. Prominence caused by the screw heads and the plate may also cause postoperative dysphagia or esophageal perforation. We prefer a second-stage posterior fusion over anterior plating if additional stability is required.

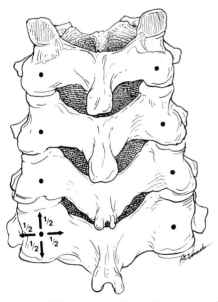

FIGURE 5–12. Illustration of lateral masses and the points of drill and screw entry for the lateral mass plating. (From Ebraheim, N. A., An, H. S., Jackson, W. T., et al.: Internal fixation of the unstable cervical spine using posterior Roy-Camille plates: Preliminary report. J. Orthop. Trauma 3:23, 1989.)

CERVICOTHORACIC JUNCTION

Lesions at upper thoracic vertebrae present a challenge to the spinal surgeon. Anterior

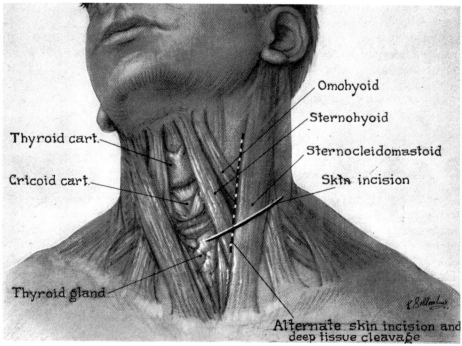

FIGURE 5–13. Illustration of skin incision of extensile anterior approach to the mid to lower cervical vertebrae. (From Southwick, W. O., and Robinson, R. A.: Surgical approaches to the vertebral bodies in the cervical and lumbar regions. J. Bone Joint Surg. *39*A:634, 1957.)

exposure of the upper thoracic vertebrae may be accomplished through supraclavicular approach, sternum splitting approach, or transthoracic approach. Supraclavicular approach entails a transverse incision above the clavicle and division of the clavicular head of the sternocleidomastoid and division of the scalenus anterior muscle.[54] After division of the sternocleidomastoid muscle, the fascia beneath is divided to release the omohyoid from its pulley. The internal jugular and subclavian veins as well as the carotid artery must be protected from injury during division of the sternocleidomastoid muscle. The subclavian artery and its branches, which include the thyrocervical trunk, suprascapular artery, and transcervical artery, must be identified. The suprascapular and transcervical arteries should be ligated as necessary. The dome of the lung and the phrenic nerve are in close proximity during division of the scalenus anterior muscle. The phrenic nerve should be identified and retracted before division of the scalenus anterior muscle. The brachial plexus and supraclavicular nerves are more superficial at the lateral border of the scalenus anterior muscle. Division of the scalenus anterior exposes the Sibson's fascia in the floor on the wound, which

covers the dome of the lung. Sibson's fascia is divided transversely using scissors, and the visceral pleura and lung should be retracted inferiorly. The trachea, the esophagus, and the recurrent laryngeal nerve must be protected during medial retraction. The recurrent laryngeal nerve should be identified and protected. The posterior thorax, stellate ganglion, and upper thoracic vertebral bodies are now visible, looking from above downward through the thoracic inlet. The inferior thyroid artery and vertebral artery should be identified. The thoracic duct should be identified if approached from the left. If damaged, the thoracic duct should be doubly ligated both proximally and distally to prevent chylothorax.

Sternum splitting approach provides better access to the cervicothoracic junction from C4 to T4, particularly in the obese patient[6] (Fig. 5–14A–C). The skin incision is made anterior to the left sternocleidomastoid muscle and extended along the midsternal area down to the xiphoid process. After division of the platysma muscle and superficial cervical fascia, blunt dissection is done between the laterally situated neurovascular bundle and medial visceral structures. The retrosternal adipose and thymus tissues are retracted from the manu-

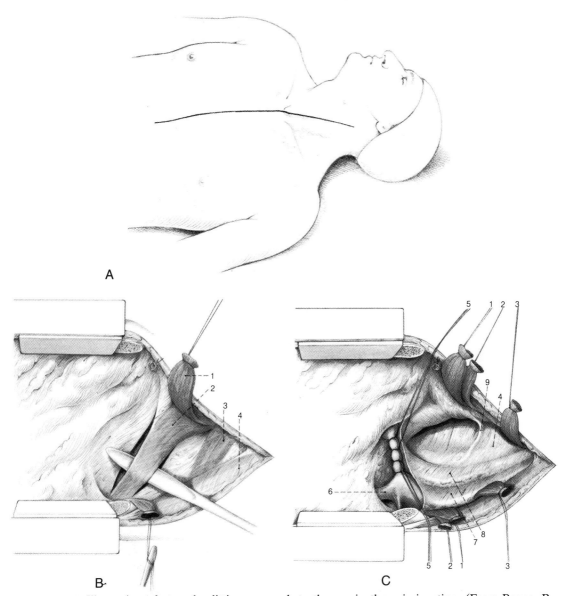

A

B

C

FIGURE 5–14. Illustration of sternal splitting approach to the cervicothoracic junction. (From Bauer, R., Kerschbaumer, F., and Poisel, S.: *Operative Approaches in Orthopaedic Surgery and Traumatology.* New York, Georg Thieme Verlag, 1987, p. 13.) *(A)* Skin incision is made on midline of sternum and anterior border of left sternomastoid. *(B)* Exposure and ligation of left brachicephalic vein if necessary. 1. Sternothyroid muscle; 2. Sternohyoid muscle; 3. Omohyoid muscle; 4. Cervical fascia, prevertebral layer. *(C)* Exposure of cervicothoracic junction from C6 to T3. 1. Left brachicephalic vein. 2. Left common carotid artery; 3. Left jugular vein; 4. Anterior longitudinal ligament; 5. Radiate ligament of head of rib; 6. Long muscle of the neck; 7. Inferior thyroid artery; 8. Omohyoid muscle; 9. Sternothyroid muscle.

brium. Median sternotomy should be performed carefully to prevent injury to the pleura. Sternohyoid, sternothyroid, and omohyoid muscles are identified and transected as necessary. The inferior thyroid artery is ligated

and transected. Blunt dissection is performed from the cranial toward the caudal portion until the left brachiocephalic vein is exposed. This vein may be ligated and transected if necessary, but postoperative edema of the left upper extremity may be a problem. Great caution should be exercised to avoid injuries to the sympathetic nerves, the cupola of the pleura at the level of T1, the great vessels, and the thoracic duct, which passes into the left venous angle between the subclavian artery and the common carotid artery.

Upper thoracic vertebrae may also be approached through a standard thoracotomy that enters the chest through the bed of the third rib, but access is greatly restricted by the scapula and remaining ribs. Recently, Turner and associates described a surgical approach to the upper thoracic spine from T1 to T3[90] (Fig. 5–15A,B). The right-sided approach is preferred to avoid the left subclavian artery, which is more curved than the right brachiocephalic artery. The incision is medial and inferior to the scapula. The scapula is retracted laterally by dividing the trapezius, latissimus dorsi, rhomboids, and levator scapulae muscles. The posterior 7 to 10 cm. of each of the second, third, fourth, and fifth ribs are removed. If T1 is involved, 2 to 3 cm. of the first rib are also excised. Exposure of the vertebrae is made with an L-shaped incision in the pleura and intercostal muscles. Potential

complications of this approach may be restriction of scapular movement and paralysis of intercostal muscles owing to the muscle-splitting aspects of this dissection. Turner and coworkers recommended use of this approach in older patients and perhaps in patients with malignant conditions.[90]

THORACIC SPINE AND THORACOLUMBAR JUNCTION

Exposure of the thoracic vertebral bodies is best accomplished by the anterior transthoracic approach. We prefer a right thoracotomy for exposure of the upper thoracic spine to avoid the subclavian and carotid arteries in the left superior mediastinum. In the lower thoracic spine, a left thoracotomy is preferred to avoid the liver. Because dissection is easier from above downward, the rib at the one or two upper levels should be removed, particularly if multiple levels are involved. Exposure of the thoracolumbar junction is best achieved by a thoracoabdominal approach, which entails circumferential incision in the muscular portion of the diaphragm adjacent to the costal margin. The technique and associated complications of

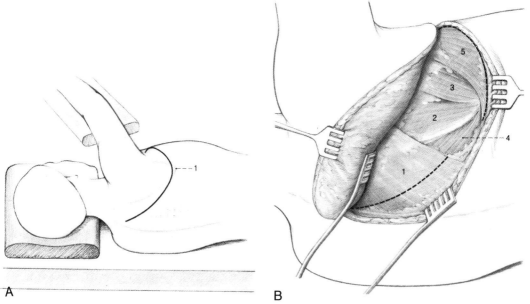

FIGURE 5–15. High thoracotomy for exposure of upper thoracic vertebrae. (From Bauer, R., Kerschbaumer, F., and Poisel, S.: *Operative Approaches in Orthopaedic Surgery and Traumatology.* New York, Georg Thieme Verlag, 1987, p. 33.) *(A)* Position and skin incision. 1. Inferior angle of scapula. *(B)* Exposure by division of muscles along the dashed line. 1. Trapezius muscle; 2. Infraspinous muscle; 3. Teres major muscle; 4. Greater rhomboid muscle; 5. Latissimus dorsi muscle.

anterior approach to the thoracic spine and thoracolumbar junction were discussed under scoliosis.

After tumor excision and decompression of the spinal cord, strut bone grafting should re-establish the stability of the spine (Fig. 5–16A–C). A trough is created in the involved verte-brae and the intervertebral disc tissue is re-moved. Rib or tricortical iliac crest grafts are inserted by countersinking the ends to prevent graft dislodgement.[15] It is important to place the bone graft against the end-plates to provide maximal stability. If sufficient stability is not achieved, augmentations with metal implants or methylmethacrylate may be considered, or posterior stabilization and fusion should be performed.[47, 63, 87] Metal implants should be used reluctantly around the anterior aspects of

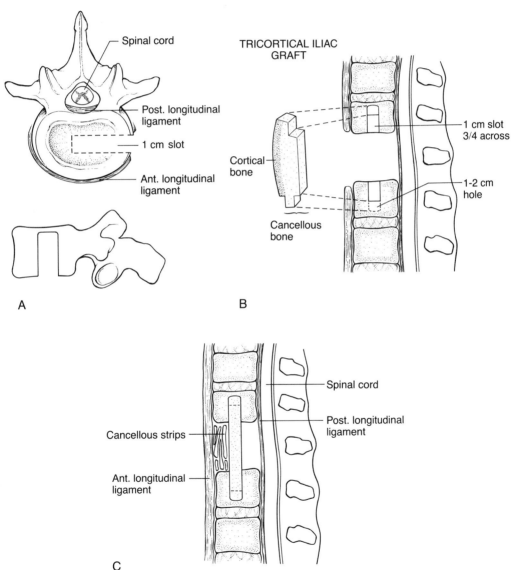

FIGURE 5–16. Strut bone grafting in the thoracic and lumbar region. *(A)* Sufficient bone with proximal and distal intervertebral disc is removed to decompress the neural canal, and tricortical iliac graft is fashioned. *(B)* Proximal and distal troughs are developed in the vertebral bodies adjacent to the junction of the anterior two-thirds and posterior one-third of the adjacent vertebral bodies. *(C)* The bone graft is secured from upper end-plate of the proximal vertebra and lower end-plate of distal vertebra. Additional cancellous bone is used to fill the defect.

the thoracolumbar spine, as any prominence caused by these implants may lead to devastating vascular erosion. One must be sure to place these implants away from great vessels or to place them within the vertebral column.

Another approach to the anterior and lateral aspect of the thoracic vertebrae is the posterolateral costotransversectomy technique (Fig. 5–17A,B). This approach is less extensive but may be preferred for lesions in the lateral aspect of the vertebral body, lesions that do not require a long strut graft, or patients who cannot tolerate a formal thoracotomy. The patient is placed half-way between a lateral decubitus and prone position with a pad in the axilla, and the upper arm is slightly extended and securely supported. A C-shape curved incision is made along the paraspinous muscles, spanning about four to five ribs. The middle part of the incision should be about 2.5 inches from the midline at the paraspinal depression. By undermining the skin and subcutaneous tissue, exposure of the paraspinous muscles and posterior elements of the spine is completed. The trapezius and latissimus dorsi muscles are divided either longitudinally or transversely. The rib and transverse process are resected at one to four levels depending on the extent of the lesion. The rib is exposed

subperiosteally and excised approximately 3.5 inches lateral to the vertebrae and disarticulated at the costovertebral junction. Careful retraction of the pleura will lead to the vertebrae. The pedicles, neural foramina, and spinal nerves should be identified. For neural decompression, the pedicles may be widened or excised to expose the dura. A strut bone graft may be applied if necessary.

Total spondylectomy through posterolateral approach has been described for lesions that require en bloc excision.[59, 78, 85, 86] This operation is a formidable procedure and should be performed by those with prior experience.

Operative complications associated with anterior or posterolateral approach of the thoracic spine may include spinal cord injury, dural tear, pneumothorax, bleeding, and bone graft problems. Again, SSEP monitoring is recommended if decompression of the spinal cord is planned. Power drill, curette, or rongeur should be used in a cautious manner, as neurovascular injury from use of these instruments may be devastating. Bone graft dislodgement is prevented by meticulous surgical technique. Stability of bone graft may be enhanced by use of metal or methylmethacrylate or posterior fusion if necessary.

Posterior approach to the thoracic spine is

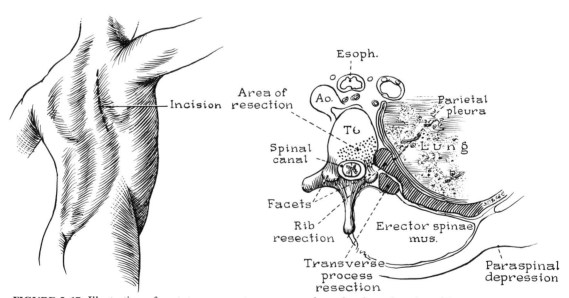

FIGURE 5–17. Illustration of costotransversectomy approach to the thoracic spine. (From Johnson, R. M., and Southwick, W. O.: Surgical approaches to the spine. In: Rothman, R. H., and Simeone, F. A. (eds.): *The Spine.* Philadelphia, W. B. Saunders Company, 1982, p. 166.) *(A)* A longitudinal or curvilinear incision is made lateral to the paraspinal muscle over the posterior angle of the ribs. *(B)* Cross-section of thoracic vertebrae with the hatched area to be removed.

straightforward. Almost all intraspinal tumors require laminectomy. Any lesion located in the posterior elements of the spine is approached posteriorly. Transpedicular approach is sometimes useful for biopsy of a lesion in the vertebral body or even for decompression of the spinal cord. Spinal stabilization with various types of instrumentation can be done posteriorly. Posterior spinal stablization should be considered when anterior corpectomy and bone grafting have not adequately restored spinal stability and when extensive laminectomy has been performed. There are too many instances in which laminectomy without stabilization resulted in kyphotic deformity and neurological deterioration.

Transpedicular biopsy or decompression requires a thorough knowledge of anatomy of the thoracic pedicle. The thoracic pedicle is located by crossing a horizontal line at the midportion of the transverse process and a vertical line at the junction between the lamina and transverse process ("the valleys"). A power burr is used to remove the outer cortex. A pin is placed to confirm the location of the pedicle with a roentgenogram. An angle-tipped curette can be used to remove tissues from the body. Decompression of the spinal cord can be done by excising the pedicle and by removing tissues from a posterolateral direction.

Posterior stabilization of the thoracic or thoracolumbar spine can be achieved by various instrumentations. We have been satisfied with Luque rods with sublaminar wires or Harrington distraction rods with sublaminar wires in the majority of cases[16, 35] (Fig. 5–18). It is important to achieve maximal stability for rapid rehabilitation, particularly in debilitated patients with cancer. The surgical construct usually consists of implants and bone grafts extending three levels above and three below. When anterior corpectomy and fusion is performed first, posterior stabilization is best accomplished by a compression construct. Care should be taken to prevent iatrogenic complications such as neural injury, laminar fracture, and implant failure. Recently, Cotrel-Dubousset and transpedicular instrumentations have been introduced. These instrumentations provide more rigid stabilization, but the surgical technique is more precise and difficult.

LUMBAR SPINE AND SACRUM

In the lower lumbar region, a standard retroperitoneal flank approach is used (Fig. 5–

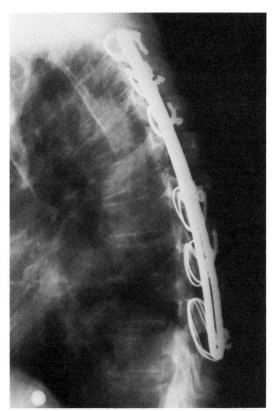

FIGURE 5–18. Lateral roentgenogram showing stabilization with boxed Luque rod and sublaminar wires in a 65-year-old male with metastatic melanoma to T7.

19A,B). The patient is placed in the right lateral decubitus position. The incision extends from the midaxillary line to the edge of the rectus sheath. The level of the incision varies according to the level of the spine approached. Dissection is through the external oblique, internal oblique, and transversus abdominis muscles. The retroperitoneal space is entered laterally by identifying the retroperitoneal fat, taking care to avoid penetration of the peritoneum just lateral to the rectus sheath. Blunt finger dissection anterior to the psoas muscle should lead to the spine. One should identify the genitofemoral nerve on the anterior surface of the psoas muscle and the sympathetic chains medial to the muscle. One should take extreme caution to avoid injuries to the ureter, which can be identified medially along the undersurface of the peritoneum, and the pulsating aorta, which is easily palpated. These structures are at risk with careless dissection. At the L4-L5 region, the iliolumbar vein should be identified and ligated to mobilize the great vessels.

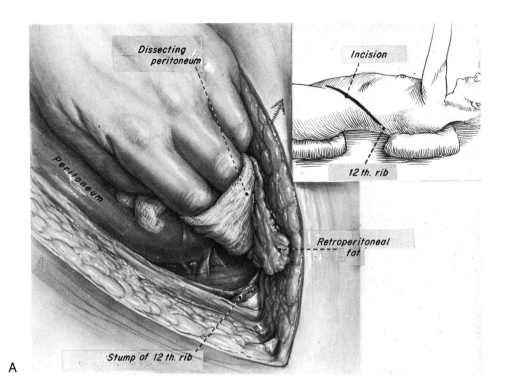

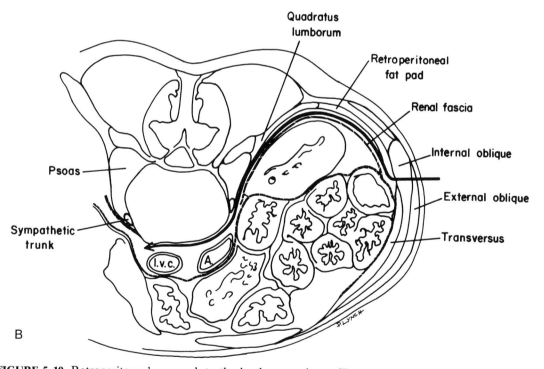

FIGURE 5–19. Retroperitoneal approach to the lumbar vertebrae. (From Johnson, R. M., and Southwick, W. O.: Surgical approaches to the spine. In: Rothman, R. H., and Simeone, F. A. (eds.): *The Spine.* Philadelphia, W. B. Saunders Company, p. 173.) *(A)* An oblique flank incision is made, and the peritoneum is separated from the retroperitoneal structures. *(B)* Transverse section through the midlumbar vertebrae illustrating the plane of dissection between the renal fascia anteriorly and the retrorenal fat pad, quadratus lumborum, and psoas muscles posteriorly.

Transperitoneal approach through a vertical or transverse incision in the lower abdomen provides the best exposure for the L5 and sacrum. The bowel contents are retracted, and the aortic bifurcation is palpated at the L4-L5 region. Infiltrate the tissue over the anterior surface of the sacral promontory to elevate the peritoneum off the vascular structures. Open the posterior peritoneum and identify the L5-S1 disc. The sacral artery runs down along the anterior aspect of the sacrum and is ligated as necessary. Great caution should be taken to protect the left iliac vein in the aortic bifurcation and preserve presacral plexus of parasympathetic nerves, which is important to sexual function. Exposure can be extended to the L4-L5 region by mobilizing the great vessels to the right after ligating the fourth and fifth lumbar vessels. Take care not to injure the left ureter, which crosses the left common iliac vessels over the sacroiliac joint.

Resection of chordoma arising from the sacrococcygeal area is usually done by a team consisting of a general surgeon and an orthopedic surgeon. Because of likely recurrence after intralesional or marginal resection, wide resection of chordoma should be performed whenever possible. Bony instability is not a problem after resection of the sacrum as long as the upper half of the body of S1 remains intact.[45] If the upper three sacral roots on one side and two sacral roots on the other side are preserved, close to normal sphincter function can be expected. If a nerve is involved by tumor, it should be resected rather than attempting to save it and leaving tumor tissues behind. High amputation of the sacrum is usually required for wide resection of this tumor. Through the anterior approach, the rectum is mobilized from tumor, and the internal iliac arteries and the lateral and medial sacral vessels are divided. The transection of the sacrum is carried out between S1 and S2 or through S1. S1 motor nerves should be preserved. Posterior approach follows immediately or is done simultaneously to complete the resection of the sacrum. Posterior sacral nerves can be resected without ill effects. Other primary tumors such as giant cell tumor and chondrosarcoma may also arise from the sacrum.[88]

Potential complications during anterior dissection along the lower lumbar spine and sacrum include hemorrhage from great vessel injury, retrograde ejaculation and sterility from superior hypogastric sympathetic plexus injury, ureteral injury, and bowel injury. Failure of penile erection is not anticipated after superior hypogastric sympathetic plexus injury, unless the patient has, in addition, advanced peripheral vascular disease.[53] Postoperative ileus or adhesion may occur as well.

Posterior approach of the lower lumbar spine and sacrum may be done through laminectomy or posterolateral or transpedicular routes, depending on the pathoanatomical process of the tumor. Techniques and potential complications of transpedicular instrumentation were discussed in the chapter on spondylolisthesis.

COMPLICATIONS

Aside from many complications related to various surgical approaches for tumor resection and stabilization, other problems may arise later in patients with spinal tumors. These include neurological deficit, postoperative leakage of spinal fluid, infection, hematoma, postsurgical instability, instrument failure, recurrence, and so forth.

NEUROLOGICAL DEFICIT

Although neurological improvements are often observed after tumor resection, patients who have advanced neurological deficit preoperatively may have worsening of their deficit postoperatively. This is particularly true after intradural intramedullary tumor resections. Recovery may be slow and incomplete in this group, especially among those in whom complete removal is not possible. Intradural extramedullary tumors, however, are less frequently associated with postoperative neurological deficit. Neurological improvement is expected after most extradural tumor resections provided that surgical trauma is avoided. Surgical trauma to the spinal cord is prevented by adequate exposure, careful surgical technique, and use of SSEP monitoring. The operating microscope, better dissection instruments, including lasers, and ultrasonic aspiration devices have reduced the risk of worsening neurological deficit in intraspinal surgery. As mentioned before, air-drill thinning of the lamina is recommended during laminectomy. Tumors located anteriorly should be approached anteriorly to avoid retraction of the spinal cord.

Spinal cord ischemia may be the etiology for

postoperative neurological deficit in some cases. Great attention was given in the past to the artery of Adamkiewicz, which is the largest of the feeders of the lumbar spinal cord. It occurs on the left side in 80 per cent of patients between T7 and L4, with the most common site being T9–T11.[23] It usually enters the spinal canal with at least one feeder. There is a "critical zone of the spinal cord" which extends from T4–T9.[23] It is rare in spinal tumor surgery for one to involve as many feeding arteries as one does in extensive scoliosis surgery. In fact, many individual intercostal or lumbar arteries are expendable, and no ischemic injury to the spinal cord results. Nonetheless, segmental arteries should be preserved in the thoracolumbar spine if possible. Embolization of vascular tumors such as renal cell carcinoma should also be done, preserving these feeding vessels to the spinal cord.

In some cases postoperative neurological deficit has been attributed to edema. There are certain patients who, in the postoperative period, remain remarkably steroid dependent, particularly patients with intramedullary tumors. The patient awakens with severe neurological deficit postoperatively, but as steroids are administered, the neurological deficit recedes. When steroids are tapered, neurological deterioration is again evident, which is again partially reversible by increasing the steroid medication. The beneficial effect has been attributed to their ability to reduce edema.

POSTOPERATIVE SPINAL FLUID LEAK

Postoperative spinal fluid leaks, or meningocele, paradoxically, are more likely to occur when there are small openings in the dura rather than when the dura is left wide open. Any dural rent should be closed meticulously, and the wound should be closed in a watertight manner with multiple running layers. Drains should be avoided in most cases. Because of the necessity of durotomy during resection of intradural tumors, postoperative leakage of spinal fluid is a definite risk in these cases. Spinal fluid leakage seems to occur more commonly in the upper thoracic region where wound dehiscence caused by stretching of the skin is also more frequent. A patient who has had previous radiation therapy is more prone to wound dehiscence and spinal fluid leakage. If skin dehiscence is present, skin closure may stop further leakage. Insertion of a lumbar subarachnoid or subcutaneous drain may lead to healing of the wound and ultimate closure of the fistulous tract. These bedside procedures are not predictable and are associated with bed confinement for several days, headaches, and the potential for infection. If prompt improvement is not observed, the surgeon is encouraged to reopen the incision and repair the dural leak. If the exact site of leakage is difficult to discover, a lumbar injection of 10 ml. of indigo carmine may help to identify the dural opening. Methylene blue should never be used because of its neurotoxicity. After the last dural stitch is made, the anesthesiologist is asked to increase intrathoracic pressure by Valsalva maneuver. This will distend the dura and reveal the site of potential leakage so that additional sutures may be placed.

POSTOPERATIVE INSTABILITY

Postoperative kyphosis or instability is frequent after laminectomy without stabilization. This is particularly common in the young patient. Several reports cite the high incidence of postlaminectomy deformities occurring in children.[36, 95] Yasuoka and coworkers reviewed laminectomies in patients under 25 years of age.[95] Twelve of 26 patients (46 per cent) under age 15 developed a deformity, and in 8 surgery was necessary to stabilize it. Patients between 15 and 25 years of age did not develop postoperative deformities, with the exception of two patients (6 per cent). These two patients developed mild deformities that did not progress after maturity and did not require further treatment. The site of laminectomy is also an important factor. The incidence of spinal deformities is high in cervical or cervicothoracic laminectomies, ranging between 80 to 100 per cent in young individuals.[36, 61, 95] The incidence of deformities after laminectomy is about 50 per cent in the thoracic region, 20 per cent in the thoracolumbar region, and very low in the lumbar region.[36] If the patient had preoperative kyphosis because of tumor, further deformity is surely expected after laminectomy. If unilateral or bilateral facet excision has been performed along with laminectomy, spinal deformity is more likely to ensue.[61] Acute angular kyphosis is prone to occur if the facets are removed compared with more gradual rounded kyphosis after laminectomies alone. Multilevel laminectomy probably has a worse prognosis than one-level laminectomy. Irradiation affects the growing cartilage cells in the growth plate of the vertebral bodies and may be attributed to the development of spinal deformities.

Prevention of postlaminectomy deformity is therefore important. Technique of laminectomy may be altered in some cases in order to lessen instability. Expansive open-door laminoplasty may be appropriate in some cases. Fusion at the time of the initial decompressive laminectomy may be appropriate in those patients at high risk for postoperative deformities. Close observation is essential for early recognition of spinal deformities. With children, roentgenograms should be taken every three months for the first year. Close follow-up visits are also important during the adolescent growth spurt.

The treatment of these postlaminectomy deformities is largely surgical since bracing is ineffective. The anterior approach is preferred in most cases as it is biomechanically more sound. A combined anterior and posterior procedure may be necessary in more severe cases to achieve a better correction and fusion.

INSTRUMENT PROBLEMS

Postoperative instabilities may also stem from inadequate stabilizations or failures of the surgical construct. Rigid stabilization is particularly important in older patients with metastatic tumors. One of the goals of surgery is to provide rigid stability so that the patient can move early without pain. If anterior reconstruction does not provide adequate stability, posterior stabilization should be performed without hesitation. Recent development of new instrumentations such as Luque rods, pedicular screws, and the Cotrel-Dubousset system helps the surgeon to choose appropriate instrumentation to provide maximal stability of the spine. Thorough knowledge and experience of the particular instrumentation system is required to avoid instrument problems such as hook dislodgement, rod or wire breakage, and recurrence of deformities. Other instrument-related problems such as neurological injury, pseudarthrosis, and loss of fixation were discussed under scoliosis. We prefer not to use anterior instrumentations in both cervical and thoracolumbar areas if possible. Complications such as dysphagia, vascular erosion, and death have been reported after insertion of hardware anteriorly.

RECURRENCE OF TUMOR

Recurrence of tumor is related to the biology of the primary tumor and the surgical margin achieved during the initial operation. More aggressive tumors, such as giant cell tumor and chordoma, are likely to recur if a complete excision is not done initially.[92] Every effort must be made to remove all tumor tissue unless it is very radiosensitive or metastatic. Frequently, a combined anterior and posterior procedure is necessary to eradicate the entire tumor. Repeat surgery for recurrence is not only difficult because of scar formation but also holds a worse prognosis for the patient. On the other hand, excision of the entire tumor is curative in many cases.

MISCELLANEOUS COMPLICATIONS

Other perioperative complications may relate to the general medical status of the patient. Older patients with metastatic tumors or multiple myeloma should have particular attention paid to their cardiovascular, pulmonary, and nutritional status. Careful fluid and electrolyte balance is needed to prevent pulmonary congestion, dehydration, and cardiac arrhythmia. Postoperative compression boots and early mobilization should be routine to prevent thrombosis and pulmonary embolism. Those who received chemotherapy or irradiation are more likely nutritionally depleted and prone to infection postoperatively. Nutritional or calorie support is vitally important for proper wound healing and postoperative recovery. Particular attention should be paid to those individuals who are receiving steroids, as they may die from stress gastrointestinal hemorrhage. These patients should receive prophylactic antacids. Patients with diffuse skeletal involvement may develop hypercalcemia with associated complications such as nausea, vomiting, abdominal pain, or cardiac symptoms.

REFERENCES

1. Akbarnia, B. A., and Rooholamini, S. A.: Scoliosis caused by benign osteoblastoma of the thoracic or lumbar spine. J. Bone Joint Surg. 63A:1146–1155, 1981.
2. Alexander, A. H.: Chymopapain chemonucleolysis, discography, and needle biopsy technique. In: Chapman, M. W. (ed.): *Operative Orthopaedics*. Philadelphia, J. B. Lippincott Company, 1988, pp. 2125–2135.
3. Amrose, G. B., Alpert, M., and Neer, C. S.: Vertebral osteomyelitis: A diagnostic problem. J.A.M.A. *197*:619–622, 1966.
4. Aprin, H.: Metastatic tumors of the spine. Spine: State of the Art Reviews 2:301–311, 1987.

5. Armstrong, P.: Needle aspiration, biopsy of the spine and suspected disc space infections. Br. J. Radiol. *51*:333–337, 1978.
6. Bauer, R., Kerschbaumer, F., and Poisel, S.: *Operative Approaches to Orthopaedic Surgery and Traumatology.* New York, Georg Thieme Verlag, 1987, pp. 13–16.
7. Beltran, J., Noto, A. M., Chakeres, D. W., et al.: Tumors of the osseous spine: Staging with MR imaging versus CT. Radiology *162*:565–569, 1987.
8. Bender, C. E., Berquist, T. H., and Wold, L. E.: Imaging-assisted percutaneous biopsy of the thoracic spine. Mayo Clin. Proc. *61*:942–950, 1986.
9. Bohlman, H. H., Sachs, B. L., Carter, J. R., et al.: Primary neoplasms of the cervical spine: Diagnosis and treatment of twenty-three patients. J. Bone Joint Surg. *68A*:483–494, 1986.
10. Boland, P. J., Lane, J. M., and Sundaresan, N.: Metastatic disease of the spine. Clin. Orthop. *169*:95–102, 1982.
11. Callahan, R. A., Johnson, R. M., Margolis, R. N., et al.: Cervical facet fusion for control of instability following laminectomy. J. Bone Joint Surg. *59A*:991–1002, 1977.
12. Capanna, R., Albisinni, U., Picci, P., et al.: Aneurysmal bone cyst of the spine. J. Bone Joint Surg. *67A*:527–531, 1985.
13. Clark, C. R., Keggi, K. J., and Panjabi, M. M.: Methylmethacrylate stabilization of the cervical spine. J. Bone Joint Surg. *66A*:40–46, 1984.
14. Constans, J. P., DeDivitiis, E., Donzelli, R., et al.: Spinal metastases with neurological manifestations. Review of 600 cases. J. Neurosurg. *59*:11–118, 1983.
15. Cotler, H. B., Cotler, J. M., Stoloff, A., et al.: The use of autograft for vertebral body replacement of the thoracic and lumbar spine. Spine *10*:748–756, 1985.
16. Cusick, J. F., Larson, S. J., Walsh, P. R., et al.: Distraction rod stabilization in the treatment of metastatic carcinoma. J. Neurosurg. *59*:861–866, 1983.
17. Cybulski, G. R., Stone, J. L., Crowell, R. M., et al.: Use of Halifax interlaminar clamps for posterior C1-2 arthrodesis. Neurosurgery *22*:429–31, 1988.
18. Danzig, L. A., Resnick, D., and Akeson, W. H.: The treatment of cervical spine metastasis from the prostate with a halo cast. Spine *5*:395–398, 1980.
19. DeAndrade, J. R., and MacNab, I.: Anterior occipitocervical fusion using an extra-pharyngeal exposure. J. Bone Joint Surg. *51A*:1621–1626, 1969.
20. Debnam, J. W., and Staple, T. W.: Needle biopsy of bone. Radiol. Clin North Am. *13*:157–164, 1975.
21. DeWald, R. L., Bridwell, K. H., Prodromas, C., et al.: Reconstructive spinal surgery as palliation for metastatic malignancies of the spine. Spine *10*:21–26, 1985.
22. Dolin, M. G.: Acute massive dural compression secondary to methylmethacrylate replacement of a tumorous lumbar vertebral body. Spine *14*:108–110, 1989.
23. Dommisse, G. F.: The blood supply of the spinal cord. J. Bone Joint Surg. *56B*:225, 1974.
24. Dunn, E. J., and Anas, P. P.: Tumors of the cervical spine. In: Evarts, M. C. (ed.): *Surgery of the Musculoskeletal System.* New York, Churchill Livingstone, 1983, pp. 4:175–189.
25. Dunn, E. J., and Anas, P. P.: The management of tumors of the upper cervical spine. Orthop. Clin. North Am. *9*:1065–1080, 1978.
26. Dunn, H. K.: Tumors of the thoracic and lumbar spine. In: Evarts, M. C. (ed.): *Surgery of the Musculoskeletal System.* New York, Churchill Livingstone, 1983, pp. 4:191–210.
27. Dunn, R. C., Jr., Kelley, W. A., Wohns, R. N., et al.: Spinal epidural neoplasia. A 15-year review of the results of surgical therapy. J. Neurosurg. *52*:47–51, 1980.
28. Ebraheim, N. A., An, H. S., Jackson, W. T., et al.: Internal fixation of the unstable cervical spine using posterior Roy-Camille plates: Preliminary report. J. Orthop. Trauma *3*:23–28, 1989.
29. Eismont, F. J., Green, B. A., Brown, M. D., et al.: Coexistent infection and tumor of the spine. A report of three cases. J. Bone Joint Surg. *69A*:452–458, 1987.
30. Evarts, C. M.: Diagnostic techniques: Closed biopsy of bone. Clin. Orthop. *107*:100–111, 1974.
31. Fang, H. S. Y., and Ong, G. B.: Direct anterior approach to the upper cervical spine. J. Bone Joint Surg. *44*:1588, 1962.
32. Fidler, M. W.: Pathological fractures of the cervical spine. J. Bone Joint Surg. *67B*:352–357, 1985.
33. Fielding, J. W., Pyle, R. N., and Fietti, V. G.: Anterior cervical vertebral body resection and bone grafting for benign and malignant tumors. J. Bone Joint Surg. *61A*:251–253, 1979.
34. Fielding, J. W., and Ratzan, S.: Osteochondroma of the cervical spine. J. Bone Joint Surg. *55A*:640–641, 1973.
35. Flatley, T. J., Anderson, M. H., and Anast, G. T.: Spinal instability due to malignant disease. J. Bone Joint Surg. *65A*:47–52, 1984.
36. Fraser, R. D., Paterson, D. C., and Simpson, D. A.: Orthopaedic aspects of spinal tumors in children. J. Bone Joint Surg. *59A*:143–151, 1977.
37. Friedlander, G. E., and Southwick, W. O.: Tumors of the spine. In: Rothman, R. H., and Simeone, F. A. (eds): *The Spine.* Philadelphia, W. B. Saunders Company, 1982, pp. 1022–1040.
38. Fyfe, I. S., Henry, A. P. J., and Mulholland, R. C.: Closed vertebral biopsy. J. Bone Joint Surg. *65B*:140–143, 1983.
39. Gilbert, R. W., Kim, J. H., and Posner, J. B.: Epidural spinal cord compression from metastatic tumor: Diagnosis and treatment. Ann. Neurol. *3*:40–51, 1978.
40. Gladstein, M. O., and Grantham, S. A.: Closed skeletal biopsy. Clin. Orthop. *103*:75–79, 1974.
41. Goyal, R. N., Russell, N. A., Benoit, B. G., et al.: Intraspinal cysts: A classification and literature review. Spine *12*:209–213, 1987.
42. Graham, J. J., and Yang, W. C.: Vertebral hemangioma with compression fracture and paraparesis treated with preoperative embolization and vertebral resection. Spine *9*:97–101, 1984.

43. Grantham, S. A., Dick, H. M., Thompson, R. C., et al.: Occipitocervical arthrodesis. Clin. Orthop. 65:118, 1969.

44. Gruszkiewicz, J., Doron, Y., Borovich, B., et al.: Spinal cord compression in Paget's disease of bone with reference to sacromatous degeneration and calcitonin treatment. Surg. Neurol. 27:117–125, 1987.

45. Gunterberg, B., Romanus, B., and Stener, B.: Pelvic strength after major amputation of the sacrum. An experimental study. Acta Orthop. Scand. 47:635, 1976.

46. Hall, J. E., Denis, F., and Murray, J.: Exposure of the upper cervical spine for spinal decompression. J. Bone Joint Surg. 59A:121–123, 1977.

47. Harrington, K. D.: The use of methylmethacrylate for vertebral body replacement and anterior stabilization of pathological fracture-dislocations of the spine due to metastatic malignant disease. J. Bone Joint Surg. 63A:36–46, 1981.

48. Hay, M. C., Paterson, D., and Taylor, T. K.: Aneurysmal bone cysts of the spine. J. Bone Joint Surg. 60B:406–411.

49. Hekster, R. E., Luyendijk, W., and Tan, T. I.: Spinal cord compression caused by vertebral hemangioma relieved by percutaneous catheter embolization. Neuroradiology 3:160–164, 1972.

50. Himmelfarb, Y. E., Sebes, J., and Rabinowitz, J.: Unusual roentgenographic presentations of multiple myeloma. J. Bone Joint Surg. 56A:1723–1728, 1974.

51. Hume, E. L., and Cotler, J. M.: Complications of needle biopsy of the spine. Jefferson Orthop. J. 9:66–69, 1980.

52. Ippolito, E., Farsetti, P., and Tudisco, C.: Vertebral plana. Long-term follow-up in five patients. J. Bone Joint Surg. 66A:1364–1368, 1984.

53. Johnson, R. M., and McGuire, E. J.: Urogenital complications of anterior approaches to the lumbar spine. Clin. Orthop 154:114–118, 1981.

54. Johnson, R. M., and Southwick, W. O.: Surgical approaches to the spine. In: Rothman, R. H., and Simeone, F. A. (eds.): The Spine. Philadelphia, W. B. Saunders Company, 1982, pp. 67–188.

55. Ker, N. B., and Jones, C. B.: Tumours of the cauda equina. J. Bone Joint Surg. 67B:358–362, 1985.

56. Kostuik, J. P., Errico, T. J., Gleason, T. F., et al.: Spinal stabilization of vertebral column tumors. Spine 13:250–256, 1988.

57. Laredo, J., and Bard, M.: Thoracic spine: Percutaneous trephine biopsy. Radiology 160:485–489, 1986.

58. Lee, C. K., Rosa, R., and Fernand, R.: Surgical treatment of tumors of the spine. Spine 11:201–208, 1986.

59. Lesoin, F., Rousseaux, M., Lozes, G., et al.: Posterolateral approach to tumours of the dorsolumbar spine. Acta Neurochir. (Wien) 81:40–44, 1986.

60. Light, T. R., Wagner, F. C., Johnson, R. M., et al.: Correction of spinal instability and recovery of neurologic loss following cervical vertebral body replacement. Spine 5:392–394, 1980.

61. Lonstein, J. E.: Spinal stability after tumor resection by laminectomy. Spine: State of the Art Reviews 2:363–373, 1987.

62. Magerl, F., Grob, D., and Seemann, P.: Stable dorsal fusion of the cervical spine (C2-T1) using hook plates. In: Kehr, P., and Weidner, A. (eds.): Cervical Spine I. New York, Springer Verlag, 1987, p. 217.

63. Manabe, S., Tateishi, A., Abe, M., et al.: Surgical treatment of metastatic tumors of the spine. Spine 14:41–47, 1989.

64. McAfee, P. C., Bohlman, H. H., Ducker, T., et al.: Failure of stabilization of the spine with methylmethacrylate: A retrospective analysis of twenty-four cases. J. Bone Joint Surg. 68A:1145–1157, 1986.

65. McAfee, P.C., Bohlman, H. H., Riley, L. H., et al.: The anterior retropharyngeal approach to the upper part of the cervical spine. J. Bone Joint Surg. 69A:1371–1383, 1987.

66. McLaughlin, R. E., Miller, W. R., and Miller, C. W.: Quadriparesis after needle aspiration of the cervical spine. J. Bone Joint Surg. 58A:1167–1168, 1976.

67. Mick, C. A., and Zinreich, J.: Percutaneous trephine bone biopsy of the thoracic spine. Spine 10:737–740, 1985.

68. O'Neil, J., Gardner, V., and Armstrong, G.: Treatment of tumors of the thoracic and lumbar spinal column. Clin. Orthop. 227:103–112, 1988.

69. Onimus, M., Schraub, S., Bosset, J. F., et al.: Surgical treatment of vertebral metastasis. Spine 11:883–891, 1986.

70. Ottolenghi, C. E., and Aires, B.: Aspiration biopsy of the spine. Technique for the thoracic spine and results of twenty-eight biopsies in this region and overall results of 1050 biopsies of other spinal segments. J. Bone Joint Surg. 51A:1531–1544, 1969.

71. Ottolenghi, C. E., Shajowicz, F., and DeSchant, F. A.: Aspiration biopsy of the cervical spine. Techniques and results in twenty-four cases. J. Bone Joint Surg. 46A:715–733, 1964.

72. Pettine, K. A., and Klassen, R. A.: Osteoid osteoma and osteoblastoma of the spine. J. Bone Joint Surg. 68A:354–361, 1986.

73. Raycroft, J. F., Hockman, R. P., and Southwick, W. O.: Metastatic tumors involving the cervical vertebrae: Surgical palliation. J. Bone Joint Surg. 60A:763–768, 1978.

74. Riley, L. H., Jr.: Surgical approaches to the anterior structures of the cervical spine. Clin. Orthop. 91:16–20, 1973.

75. Rodichok, L. D., Harper, G. R., Ruckdeschel, J. C., et al.: Early diagnosis of spinal epidural metastases. Am. J. Med. 70:1181–1188, 1981.

76. Roscoe, M. W., McBroom, R. J., St. Louis, E., et al.: Preoperative embolization in the treatment of osseous metastases from renal cell carcinoma. Clin. Orthop. 238:302–307, 1989.

77. Roy-Camille, R., Sailliant, G., and Mazel, C.: Internal fixation of the unstable cervical spine by a posterior osteosynthesis with plates and screws. In: Sherk, H. H., et al. (eds.): The Cervical Spine. Philadelphia, J. B. Lippincott Company, 1989, pp. 390–421.

78. Roy-Camille, R.: One stage posterior resection of thoracic tumors (personal communication).

79. Schaberg, J., and Gainor, B. J.: A profile of

metastatic carcinoma of the spine. Spine *10*:19–20, 1985.

80. Sherman, R. M. P., and Waddell, J. P.: Laminectomy for metastatic epidural spinal cord tumors. Clin. Orthop. *207*:55–63, 1986.

81. Shives, T. C., Dahlin, D. C., Sim, F. H., et al.: Osteosarcoma of the spine. J. Bone Joint Surg. *68A*:660–668, 1986.

82. Siegal, T., Tiqva, P., and Siegal, T.: Vertebral body resection for epidural compression by malignant tumors. J. Bone Joint Surg. *67A*:375–382, 1985.

83. Simeone, F. A., and Lawner, P. M.: Intraspinal neoplasms. In: Rothman, R. H., and Simeone, F. A. (eds): *The Spine.* Philadelphia, W. B. Saunders Company, 1982, pp. 1041–1054.

84. Simeone, F. A.: Intraspinal neoplasms: Complications of surgery for intraspinal neoplasms. In: Horwitz, N. H., and Rizzoli, H. V.: *Postoperative Complications of Extracranial Neurological Surgery.* Baltimore, Williams & Wilkins, 1987.

85. Stener, B.: Total spondylectomy in chondrosarcoma arising from the seventh thoracic vertebra. J. Bone Joint Surg. *53B*:288–295, 1971.

86. Stener, B., and Johnson, O. E.: Complete removal of three vertebrae for giant cell tumour. J. Bone Joint Surg. *53B*:278–287, 1971.

87. Sundaresan, N., Galicich, J. H., Lane, J. M., et al.: Treatment of neoplastic epidural cord compression by vertebral body resection and stabilization. J. Neurosurg. *63*:676–684, 1985.

88. Sung, H. W., Shu, W. P., Wang, H. M., et al.: Surgical treatment of primary tumors of the sacrum. Clin. Orthop. *215*:91–98, 1987.

89. Turner, P. L., and Webb, J. K.: A surgical approach to the upper thoracic spine. J. Bone Joint Surg. *69B*:542–544, 1987.

90. Turner, P. L., Prince, H. G., Webb, J. K., et al.: Surgery for malignant extradural tumours of the spine. J. Bone Joint Surg. *70B*:51–56, 1988.

91. Weidner, A.: Internal fixation with metal plates and screws. In: Sherk, H. H., et al. (eds.): *The Cervical Spine.* Philadelphia, J. B. Lippincott Company, 1989, pp. 404–421.

92. Weinstein, J. N., and McLain, R. F.: Primary tumors of the spine. Spine *12*:843–851, 1987.

93. Wertheim, S. B., and Bohlman, H. H.: Occipitocervical fusion. J. Bone Joint Surg. *69A*:833–836, 1987.

94. Whitesides, T. E., Jr., and Kelley, R. P.: Lateral approach to the upper cervical spine for anterior fusion. South. Med. J. *59*:879–883, 1966.

95. Yasuoka, S., Peterson, H. A., MacCarty, C. S.: Incidence of spinal column deformity after multilevel laminectomy in children and adults. J. Neurosurg. *57*:441–445, 1982.

96. Young, R. F., Post, E. M., and King, G. A.: Treatment of spinal epidural metastases. J. Neurosurg. *53*:741–748, 1980.

SIX

Complications in Cervical Spine Injury

Michael R. Piazza, M.D.

Jerome M. Cotler, M.D.

Richard A. Balderston, M.D.

"Whoever wishes to investigate medicine properly should consider the greater particular nature of disease and what effects each produces . . . so he will not be in doubt as to treatment . . . or commit mistakes, as is likely to be the case provided one has not considered these matters."

Hippocrates 400 BC

Cervical spine injuries range from mild muscular strains to catastrophic injuries that can result in quadriplegia and death. The incidence of cervical fractures and fracture-dislocations is approximately 32.2 per million per year, and approximately 12.7 per million people per year sustain spinal cord injury (SCI).[177, 245] These estimates are in all likelihood low owing to the fact that many fatal cervical spine injuries are not diagnosed. Alker[5] studied 200 auto fatalities and discovered that 25 per cent had occult cervical spine injuries. This finding is in agreement with Bucholz and Burkehead,[50] who found 26 cervical lesions in 112 consecutive multiple trauma victims.

Physicians who participate in the care of these patients need to have a thorough understanding of the potential complications and pitfalls that reside at every stage of treatment. Many of the these complications are inherent to the disease process, while others can be attributed to errors in judgment or errors in technique. Knowledge of these complications allows the treating physician to avoid repeating the mistakes of others and allows academicians

the raw material with which to design clinical and basic science studies.

The material presented in this chapter was obtained by a thorough review of the literature and also represents our experience at Thomas Jefferson University Hospital, the acute care facility of the Delaware Valley Regional Spinal Cord Injury Center. Since the inception of the center in 1979, a total of 1,089 newly injured persons with traumatic spinal cord injury were admitted. In addition, the center has admitted 268 persons with spinal injury only (no neurological deficit) in the past three years.

Although the information presented is categorized into different sections, the reader should recognize that these are artificial divisions and one should treat the patient on a continuum.

INITIAL EVALUATION

The treatment of cervical spine injuries has evolved throughout the twentieth century. Clinicians have begun to achieve the fundamental goals of treatment, which include protection of the neural elements, facilitation of neurological return, restoration of spinal alignment, and establishment of spinal stability, while maximizing rehabilitation efforts. The attainment of these goals depends on the early recognition and initiation of treatment in persons suspected of having cervical spine injuries. A high index of suspicion must be present in all health care and rescue personnel. Failure to diagnose a cervical injury is one of the most common and potentially catastrophic complications that can occur to this patient population.

Rogers[248] reported that 10 per cent of patients in his series developed spinal cord compression prior to diagnosis and the initiation of treatment. Geisler[124] reported a 3 per cent incidence of delayed cord injury secondary to failure to diagnose early. In a more recent series, Bohlman[32] reported on 300 patients with cervical spine injuries. One third of this group were not initially diagnosed as having a cervical injury. Eleven of these persons died or developed a paralysis after the initiation of care. The scenarios most commonly implicated in a missed diagnosis were multiple trauma, head injury, ethanol intoxication, and inadequate radiographs.

The upper cervical spine is a common location of the missed lesions. Injury at this level should be suspected in any patient with facial trauma or scalp laceration.[50] Other signs that should alert the physician to a possible upper cervical injury are the triad of hypotension, hypothermia, and bradycardia seen in patients with sympathetic disruption.[233]

ACCIDENT SITE

At the site of the accident, failure to recognize a potential cervical injury can lead to permanent neurological injury or even death. All personnel involved with the initial evaluation and the extrication must be familiar with techniques of cervical stabilization and splinting.[1] This should include the police and firemen in addition to the medical and paramedical personnel.

There is often confusion at an accident site initially. It is during this critical period of time that a well-meaning person may inappropriately extricate the victim. In general, the victim should remain in the motor vehicle or water, in cases of a diving accident, until adequate stabilization has been obtained and an adequate number of trained personnel are present to safely move the patient.

Initial evaluation of the ABCs (airway, breathing, and circulation) should begin immediately at the accident scene and appropriate cardiopulmonary resuscitation measures initiated. In the case of a drowning victim with a suspected cervical spine injury, CPR can be

initiated in the water while the head and neck are maintained in a neutral position.

Transport to the nearest hospital emergency department should be performed in a supine position. Ideally the patient should be strapped to a spine board and careful attention paid to the maintenance of a neutral cervical alignment. Care should be taken to avoid the placement of cushions or pillows beneath the victim's head, as this causes the cervical spine to assume a flexed position. This alignment should be avoided because the majority of injuries to the cervical spine are flexion injuries. The one notable exception to this rule is a patient with a known diagnosis of ankylosing spondylitis and a previous cervical kyphotic deformity. This patient should be transported in the position in which he or she was found at the accident scene. The appropriate cervical alignment can be determined only after appropriate radiographs are obtained.

If a cervical spine injury is suspected in a young child, one must pay particular attention to cervical alignment during transport. Herzenberg and associates[152] reported that the cervical spine in children would be placed into cervical kyphosis if the child is placed on a flat spine board in a supine position. This occurs because of the relatively large head in comparison with the remainder of the child's body (Fig. 6–1). These authors recommended using a specially designed spine board that contains a recess for the child's head or use of a double mattress under the child's shoulders to eliminate the cervical kyphosis.

The application of traction during the initial

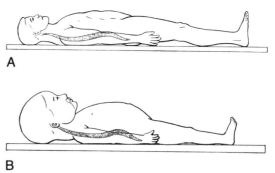

A

B

FIGURE 6–1. (A) Adult immobilized on a standard backboard. (B) Young child on a standard backboard. The relatively large head forces the neck into a kyphotic position. (From Herzenberg, J.E., Hensinger, R.N., Dedrick, D.K., and Phillips, W.A.: Emergency transport and positioning of young children who have an injury of the cervical spine. J. Bone Joint Surg. *71*A:1, 15–22, 1989.)

transport is a controversial topic. Although the majority of cervical injuries occur in flexion, it is impossible to determine the exact mechanism of injury or the severity of soft tissue disruption at the scene of the accident. If traction is used, small weights should be used owing to the possibility of overdistracting a cervical spine with severe three-column disruption.

At present, we instruct all referring physicians to discontinue cervical traction during transport to the Spinal Cord Injury Center. The only exception to this rule is a patient whose spinal alignment can only be maintained with longitudinal traction or a patient whose neurological status deteriorates out of traction. In these instances, traction should be maintained and the patient should be accompanied during the transport by a physician experienced in transport of the spinal cord–injured patient. If traction is required, consideration should be given to the use of an orthosis which can maintain longitudinal traction without the use of free-hanging weights.

INITIAL HOSPITAL EVALUATION

Any patient who comes to the accident ward with a head injury, neck injury, or multiple trauma should be evaluated and treated as having a potentially unstable cervical spine injury until proven otherwise. When a patient with a suspected cervical spine injury arrives at the Regional Spinal Cord Injury Center of the Delaware Valley, they are met by the team of treating physicians, which includes members of the orthopedic, neurosurgical, and physical medicine and rehabilitation departments. Careful evaluation to rule out thoracic or abdominal injuries must be done. Patients with cervical spine injuries are at particular risk of having these concurrent injuries missed owing to the presence of a neurological deficit or altered sensorium. The incidence of closed head injuries has been reported to be 15 to 49 per cent of patients with cervical injuries.[76] It is in these situations that peritoneal lavage or CT scan evaluation may be needed to rule out these serious, potentially life-threatening injuries.

Upon arrival at the emergency department, appropriate resuscitative measures (ABCs) and medications should be initiated. It should be remembered that appropriate cervical immobilization needs to be included in this initial treatment. Failure to suspect an unstable cervical spine lesion may result in a devastating neurological injury during maneuvers to protect the airway or during intubation. A stiff cervical collar such as a Philadelphia collar can be used initially. In cases with a defined neurological lesion, skeletal traction using light weight can be initiated after ruling out a skull fracture. This is accomplished in the emergency room by performing a careful physical exam. This includes palpation of the skull and otoscopic examination to rule out the presence of a hemotympanum. If there is evidence to suggest a skull fracture, the patient should be further evaluated with skull radiographs and computed tomography as necessary to rule out a fracture. Failure to rule out the presence of a skull fracture prior to placement of skeletal pins can lead to dural penetration, intracranial aneurysms, brain abscesses, and epidural hematomas.[32, 83, 157, 295]

Skeletal traction of the cervical spine in the acute trauma situation has been found to be safe and effective. In a review of his experience with cervical trauma, Rogers stated, "The cord is safe when the patient is in skull traction."[249] In a review of 300 patients hospitalized with acute injuries of the cervical spine, Bohlman reported that only one patient incurred a neurological worsening in traction.[32] This patient fell out of bed during an episode of ethanol withdrawal delirium.

Cervical traction must be initiated with light weights owing to the risk of overdistraction. The patient with an upper cervical injury is at particular risk for this complication if large weights are used. At the Spinal Cord Injury Center we usually begin traction with a weight of ten pounds. Lateral radiographs are obtained immediately after the initiation of traction, and further weight is added as deemed necessary. The goal of skeletal traction is realignment of the spine. Attaining proper alignment allows for immediate decompression and stabilization of the injured segment. The use of traction in the treatment of cervical injuries and its associated complications will be discussed in greater detail in the section dealing with nonoperative treatment.

INITIAL RADIOGRAPHIC EVALUATION

A lateral radiograph of the entire cervical spine, including the top of T1, should be obtained initially. Failure to visualize the cervicothoracic junction may result in a failure to diagnose a potentially catastrophic injury (Fig. 6–2). Obtaining a lateral film that includes the top of T1 may be difficult in large and heavily muscled patients. In this situation, a swimmer's view may allow visualization of the articulation between C6 and T1. Although longitudinal traction of the arms is often advocated, care should be taken because excessive longitudinal traction may be placed across a cervical fracture. If these techniques fail to adequately visualize down to T1, lateral tomograms may be used as described by Lauritzen.[182] Another option is to obtain a CT scan with lateral reconstructions. The lateral tomograms are useful for patients who are neurologically intact and when there is a low index of suspicion of injury. The CT scan, on the other hand, is useful in patients who have a neurological injury compatible with a lower cervical injury. The CT scan provides excellent definition of the skeletal injury and obviates the need to turn this high-risk patient to a lateral decubitus position to obtain the lateral tomograms.

An adequate lateral radiograph will reveal the vast majority of cervical spine injuries. If there is no apparent fracture, fracture-dislocation, subluxation, or significant soft tissue finding on the lateral film, one should proceed with the remainder of the cervical spine series.[233] This should include anteroposterior, open mouth, and oblique views. These views are helpful in defining injuries of the facet joints and of the upper cervical spine. As stated previously, upper cervical spine lesions can be difficult to diagnose and therefore represent a large number of the cervical injuries missed during initial evaluation.[32] The specific upper cervical injuries will be discussed in detail later.

If the plain radiographs fail to reveal an injury and a high index of suspicion remains, one should proceed with a stretch test.[319] Obvious indications for this type of thorough evaluation include a neurological deficit or specific point tenderness to palpation of the cervical spine. Flexion-extension radiographs should be used cautiously in the acute setting because of the risk of neurological injury.[91] If flexion-extension radiographs are used, the patient should flex and extend his neck actively, and the physician ordering the study should be present to ensure that the x-ray technologist and the patient fully understand these instructions.

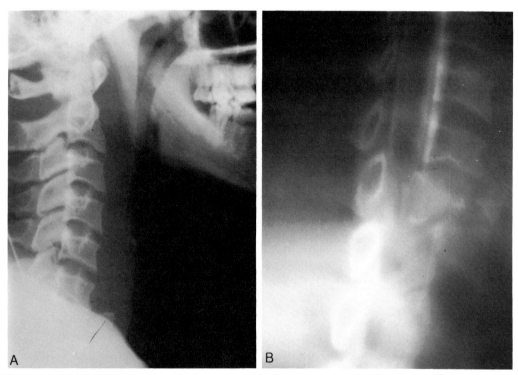

FIGURE 6–2. *(A)* Initial lateral cervical roentgenograph suggests bony pathology at the cervicothoracic junction. *(B)* Tomograms were necessary to further define the lesion.

The pediatric population is at significant risk for incurring a neurological injury without an obvious skeletal injury.[2, 15, 16, 51, 52, 128, 143, 172, 201, 207, 257, 299] This is especially true in children less than 10 years of age.[16, 207, 211] Quadriplegia has been reported to occur in children with negative radiographs and myelograms.[2, 299] Plain films may reveal only small fissures in the vertebral bodies or mildly widened intervertebral disc spaces.[16]

Prevertebral soft tissue swelling may be the only finding on plain radiographs that localizes the level of injury. This finding must be interpreted carefully because of the possibility of its being a false-positive finding. The measurement of the prevertebral soft tissue space may be enlarged if the child is either crying or speaking at the time when the film is taken. Wholly and coworkers[322] found that the average soft tissue space anterior to C2 is 3.5 mm., while Weir[311] recorded an average measurement of 5 mm. anterior to C3 in a pediatric population. An increase in the prevertebral soft tissue space may not be present in all cases of cervical injury in a child. Pepin and Hawkins[227] reported that 30 per cent of their pediatric population with cervical injury were without anterior soft tissue swelling that could be appreciated on plain radiographs.

Histological examination has revealed that most pediatric spinal cord injuries are associated with end-plate avulsions of the vertebral bodies.[16] This is analogous to a Salter I type of injury of the vertebral body. In general, these injuries heal well with immobilization. Intervertebral disc herniations are extremely rare in children with spinal cord injury.[16]

If a child has a neurological deficit and no evidence of injury is appreciated on the plain radiographs, one should proceed with further special studies. A cervical myelogram has been recommended in this situation.[172] CT scans as well as magnetic resonance imaging may also be used.[127, 160] Tomograms may be particularly useful in evaluating C1-C2 injuries, odontoid fractures, lateral mass fractures, and facet injuries. Bone scans can also be used to define the level of injury.

On the other end of the spectrum are children who are seen after significant injury and who are neurologically intact. If the plain radiographs are without significant findings, one must correlate this with the clinical examination of the neck. Further studies should then be obtained as deemed appropriate. As in the adult population, significant ligamentous injuries without obvious bone injury can occur in the pediatric group.[211] If the child is cooperative, lateral flexion and extension radiographs can be obtained at two to four weeks after injury to rule out persistent instability.

When evaluating the plain radiographs of a pediatric patient with a suspected cervical injury, one should take great care not to misinterpret the normal radiographic variants seen in the pediatric population. Knowledge of these normal variants avoids overtreatment.[19, 85, 158, 300] In general, the variants commonly misinterpreted include epiphyseal variations, unique vertebral architecture, incomplete ossification, and age-related increased laxity of the pediatric cervical spine.

The cervical spine attains an adult appearance at approximately age 8.[269] One of the more common variants seen on review of plain radiographs is pseudosubluxation of the vertebral bodies. This finding was first described in 1952[19, 300] and was further defined in ensuing reports.[60, 85, 289] This finding is most common at the C2-C3 interspace but can occur further caudad in the subaxial cervical spine. Pseudosubluxation of as much as 4 mm. may be normal on lateral radiographs when the spine is flexed.[19, 60, 305] Cattell and Filtzer studied 160 children who were without a history of trauma.[60] Nine per cent demonstrated marked pseudosubluxation, while an additional 15 per cent had moderate displacement. Of the subjects who were less than 8 years of age, 40 per cent demonstrated evidence of anterior displacement of C2 on C3. These areas of pseudosubluxation often are associated with evidence of hypermobility as demonstrated on flexion and extension radiographs. This hypermobility and hence the pseudosubluxation have been explained by the age-related ligamentous laxity, anterior wedging of the vertebral bodies, lack of development of the joints of Luschka, and the relatively horizontal plane of the articular processes of the upper cervical spine.[19, 60, 214, 236, 289]

A second common variant seen in the pediatric cervical spine is the absence of lordosis in a neutral position.[109, 167] When seen in the adult spine, this often is suggestive of a cervical injury and is attributed to paraspinal muscle spasm. In children, this is a relatively common variant found in 14 per cent of normal children.[60]

An additional variant is the absence of uniform angular changes between adjacent vertebrae.[60, 269] This finding may be seen at one or multiple levels and is more pronounced with flexion. Cattell and Filtzer found this variant in 25 (16 per cent) of 160 normal subjects.[60]

The radiographic appearance of the developing odontoid process can also be difficult to evaluate in a trauma setting.[55] The odontoid basilar synchondrosis can be easily mistaken for an undisplaced fracture at the base of the odontoid process or an os odontoideum. This synchrondrosis is present at birth and begins to close at 3 years of age.[19] Sullivan and associates reported that the synchondrosis is present in 100 per cent of children at age 3 and 50 per cent of children ages 4 and 5, and remains visible in a vestigial form in 50 per cent up to age 11.[60]

The apical odontoid epiphysis appears at age 2 and unites with the body of the odontoid at approximately age 12.[19] This epiphysis can be difficult to see on a lateral film. It was found in only 18 of 70 subjects between the ages of 5 and 11 years.[60] The apparent foreshortening of the odontoid process associated with the delayed appearance of this epiphysis can resemble a hypoplastic odontoid and can render the evaluation of C1-C2 stability difficult. When the epiphysis is not present, the arch of the atlas can appear to override the odontoid with extension. This is especially true if the odontoid is angulated posteriorly. Cattell found this apparent overriding in 20 per cent of his study group.[60] He found that the overriding decreased with growth and disappears at about 7 years of age.

Owing to the cartilaginous makeup of the ring of the atlas, congenital fusions of the atlas and axis can be difficult to appreciate in a young child. Also, owing to the thickened cartilage, the atlantodens interval (ADI) will appear widened. Approximately, 20 per cent of children less than 7 years of age will have an ADI greater than 3 mm.[60]

The final variant that has been described in the literature as causing confusion is the secondary centers of ossification of the spinous processes. These are said to resemble potential avulsion fractures.[265, 269] In his review of 160 subjects, Cattell found only one example of a secondary center of ossification that resembled an avulsion fracture.[60] This single example was seen in a 16-year-old male.

SYSTEMIC COMPLICATIONS

CARDIOVASCULAR

Patients who are exposed to cervical trauma are at risk for developing cardiovascular instability secondary to sympathetic disruption.[301] This is especially true in spinal cord injuries above the level of T5. Sympathetic disruption results in a significant decrease in systemic vascular resistance and marked blood vessel dilatation. This can result in marked bradycardia, hypotension, and the development of pulmonary edema. The pulmonary edema can be further exacerbated by cardiac arrhythmias and hypertension which can occur as spinal shock resolves.[3, 89, 97, 296] In a review of 83 consecutive patients with traumatic quadriplegia, Winslow and associates documented bradycardia in 22.[328] The bradycardia was found to be self-limiting and resolved three to five weeks after injury. No patient required permanent pacemaker therapy.

As spinal shock resolves, autonomic hyperreflexia can occur. This condition is potentially life-threatening owing to the development of severe hypertension. Other associated symptoms include diaphoresis, vasodilatation, nasal congestion, headaches, and bradycardia. Visceral stimulation, most commonly bladder distention, is the triggering agent. If this cause-and-effect relationship is not appreciated and immediate treatment instituted, the marked hypertension can result in myocardial infarction and subarachnoid and intracerebral hemorrhage.[125] Treatment includes removal of the visceral stimulation (bladder catheterization) and pharmacological agents that can block the sympathetic ganglia. Phentolamine and phenoxybenzamine (alpha-adrenergic blocking agents) have been found to be effective in the treatment of the life-threatening hypertension. Although the true incidence of this condition has not been delineated in cervical trauma, it has been documented in up to 70 per cent of patients with severe cord trauma above T7.[179]

Autonomic dysfunction can also result in poikilothermia. The spinal cord–injured patient may lose the ability to sweat or vasoconstrict, resulting in hyper- or hypothermia. Care must be taken to monitor the patient's temperature closely during the acute period after injury.

PULMONARY

Normal respiratory function depends on the normal functioning of the primary and accessory muscles of ventilation. The primary muscles include the diaphragm and the intercostal muscles. The diaphragm is innervated by the phrenic nerves which are made up of the nerve roots of C3-C5. The intercostal muscles are innervated by the intercostal nerves which arise from the thoracic nerve roots from T1 through T11. During normal breathing, inspiration is an active process mainly attributable to contraction of the diaphragm. Expiration, on the other hand, is a passive process which results from elastic recoil of the lung and chest wall. Exertional breathing requires the recruitment of the intercostal muscles and, when necessary, the accessory muscles of ventilation.

The accessory muscles include two groups, the cervical and the abdominal. The cervical group consists of the scalenes, sternocleidomastoid, pectoralis, and trapezius muscles. These muscles are innervated by the upper cervical roots and assist in exertional inspiration. The abdominal muscles include the external and internal obliques, rectus abdominis, and transversalis muscles. Innervation of this group is supplied via the nerve roots from T6-L1. These muscles become active during exertional breathing by increasing intra-abdominal pressure during active expiration. The intercostal muscles and these accessory muscles of respiration provide the great reserve of ventilatory function needed for exertional breathing.

Spinal cord injury in the cervical and thoracic regions can have significant detrimental effects on pulmonary function through denervation of these respiratory muscles. Fuglmeyer reported a decrease in total lung capacity to 69 per cent of predicted normal in patients with chronic lower cervical lesions.[116, 117] Vital capacity was found to be reduced to 42 per cent of normal. In the acute setting, even greater reductions in pulmonary function occur initially. Ohrey and associates found vital capacity to be 31 per cent of normal in the acute phase of treatment.[221] These values were found to increase to 40 per cent of predicted values within 6 months of injury. Other studies have documented decreases in vital capacity to 20 per cent of normal in acute injuries located at the C6 to C8 levels.[59, 285] After aggressive therapy, the vital capacities of these patients increased from 50 to 70 per cent of predicted normals. It appears that the greatest improvement in vital capacity occurs during the initial week after injury.[57] Aggressive physical therapy of the remaining respiratory musculature needs to be initiated early.[139, 183, 224] A plateau in respiratory function can be expected after 10 to 14 days of aggressive therapy.[57]

The level of cord injury correlates closely with the severity of pulmonary function compromise. Injuries at C5 or below usually retain normal diaphragm function and hence the ability to ventilate in nonstress situations. Careful evaluation of the spontaneously ventilating patient needs to be performed in the acute setting. At the Regional Spinal Cord Injury Center, immediate measurement of vital capacity (VC) is obtained on admission. A VC of less than 10 ml per kg or evidence of respiratory difficulty is considered a strong indication for intubation.[57, 125] The patient should also be carefully evaluated to rule out the presence of aspiration or pulmonary contusion. Initial chest radiograph and arterial blood gas should be obtained. Close observation of respiratory function must be performed during the critical first week after injury. Respiratory function deterioration can develop insidiously for up to four days after injury.[18] Daily pulmonary function testing should be included with the routine pulmonary therapy that these patients receive.

Lesions at the level of C3 and C4 will give evidence of severely compromised pulmonary function. Vital capacities range from 600 to 1000 ml (15 per cent of normal).[314] Careful inspection of these patients reveals recruitment of all accessory muscles that retain innervation. Early intubation of these patients is imperative before ventilatory muscle fatigue results in respiratory failure.

Pulmonary complications occur frequently in patients with spinal cord injury. These complications can be attributed to the effects of neurological injury on pulmonary function and the effects of immobilization. Difficulties with secretions and development of atelectasis universally affect all patients with cervical cord injury. Pneumonia is a frequent complication despite aggressive, modern respiratory care. Respiratory failure has been noted to occur in 15 to 40 per cent of patients with spinal cord injury and remains a common cause of death in the acute phase.[26, 64, 142, 198]

GASTROINTESTINAL

Spinal cord injury along with the disruption of the autonomic nervous system and immobilization all affect gastrointestinal (GI) function. There is a tendency to develop gastric stasis, intestinal atony, and increased gastric secretions in this patient population. These events all predispose patients with spinal cord injuries to gastrointestinal bleeding.[156, 312] This complication occurs frequently in spinal cord injured patients and usually manifests itself approximately 10 to 14 days after injury. The use of steroids during this acute phase increases the likelihood of developing gastrointestinal bleeding. In a review of patients with cervical spine trauma, Bohlman discovered a 40 per cent incidence of GI bleeding in those treated with steroids within 72 hours after injury.[34] This is compared with an incidence of 9 per cent in those patients who did not receive corticosteroids.

Prophylaxis must be initiated on admission for all patients with spinal cord injury. This should include nasogastric suction, an appropriate H2 antagonist, and antacids. Care should be taken to monitor the patient closely for occult GI bleeding. In quadriplegic patients, there may be no associated symptoms. Unexplained decrease in hemoglobin/hematocrit, tachycardia, or hypotension should alert the physician to this potential complication. Immediate placement of a nasogastric tube, Hemoccult testing of stools, and frequent blood count evaluations should be initiated.

THROMBOEMBOLIC

Deep venous thrombosis (DVT) and pulmonary embolism are serious, life-threatening complications frequently seen in spinal cord–injured patients. The incidence of deep venous thrombosis in acute spinal cord injury ranges from 10 to 100 per cent depending on the diagnostic tests used. When clinical examination is used alone, 10 to 64 per cent of subjects have been reported to develop DVT.[42, 209, 228, 308] Recognizing that clinical examination can result in a large number of false positives and negatives, studies that attempt to delineate the true incidence of DVT should use a venogram as an end-point of the study. Venography remains the most accurate method of documenting DVT.[161, 239] Using venography, Bors and associates reported an overall incidence of 60 per cent in SCI.[41] In a more recent report, Merli and associates discovered an incidence of DVT of 47 per cent using close surveillance with IPG and ^{125}I fibrinogen scans.[202] The end-point of this study was venography in all patients.

The severity of the spinal cord injury and its effect on the incidence of DVT have been studied. Bors and associates reported an incidence of 58 per cent in complete lesions and 59 per cent in incomplete cases.[41] Using ^{125}I fibrinogen scanning only, Myllynen and associates[209] reported an incidence of 100 per cent in complete lesions and 63 per cent in incomplete ones. Recent close surveillance of neuro-intact patients with spinal fracture at our Spinal Cord Injury Center has revealed

the development of DVT in 3 of 20 patients (15 per cent). No prophylaxis was used in any of these studies. These studies demonstrate that patients with SCI are at significant risk of developing DVT if prophylaxis is not used. The data also suggest that neuro-intact patients may benefit from prophylaxis. Further study of this patient population needs to be done.

Pulmonary embolism is the leading cause of death in acute SCI.[286, 298] In 1963, Tribe reported a 37 per cent incidence of fatal pulmonary embolism in acute SCI.[298] More recently, Stover[286] reported on the National Data Base for the second quarter of 1983 that the incidence of fatal pulmonary emboli was 14 per cent.

Most pulmonary emboli are assumed to originate from lower extremity deep vein thrombi.[216] Owing to the significant morbidity and mortality associated with this complication it would seem reasonable to undertake prophylaxis against the formation of deep vein thrombi. The NIH Consensus Conference on the prevention of venous thrombosis and pulmonary embolus has stated its opinion that prevention is far superior to treatment.[216]

The prophylaxis of DVT needs to be initiated as soon after injury as possible. This statement is based on the finding that 34 of 87 acute SCI patients were diagnosed as having DVT on admission to our Spinal Cord Injury Center.[202] All patients were admitted within two weeks of injury. Other studies have demonstrated that the first two weeks after injury is the highest risk period for the development of DVT.[42, 130]

Although there is little agreement in the literature on which type of prophylaxis is best, most authors agree that some type is warranted in this patient population. The high incidence of DVT in SCI has been attributed to increased coagulability and decreased venous return.[212, 250] Prophylaxis that addresses only one of these factors has shown variable results.[130, 209, 308] Subcutaneous low-dose heparin prophylaxis was found to have no significant effect on the incidence of DVT in our population.[202] In this prospective, randomized study, electrical stimulation of the calf musculature combined with low-dose heparin significantly reduced the incidence of DVT from 47 to 7 per cent. It is our opinion that all spinal cord–injured patients should be placed on prophylaxis for DVT. This should include an agent, such as heparin, which will counteract the increased coagulopathy and include a treatment for the decreased venous return. This could be accomplished with the addition of either electrical stimulation of the calf musculature or external pneumatic compression boots.

UROLOGICAL

Complications of the genitourinary tract are common in both the acute and chronic phases of treatment of spinal cord injury. In the acute phase, the majority of patients present with a neurogenic, or "shock," bladder. This hypotonic, areflexic, paresthetic bladder is usually a temporary phenomenon that lasts from 6 to 12 weeks.[184] The goal of therapy during this acute phase is prevention of urinary tract infection. This is best accomplished by the early institution of an intermittent catheterization program.[25, 38, 141, 287] Indwelling catheters should be used only in the immediate postinjury and postoperative periods, in females with decubiti, and in patients who are experiencing a rapid diuresis.[25] Although the goal is discontinuation of an indwelling catheter, it appears that a short period of catheter drainage does not adversely affect the long-term goals of being catheter-free or infection-free.[188]

Despite aggressive observation and treatment, urinary tract infection continues to be one of the most common complications seen in SCI.[287] Systemic prophylactic antibiotics have not proved to have long-term efficacy.[178, 205] Chronic urinary tract colonization and infection represent a significant risk to an SCI patient's well-being.

Renal calculi develop in approximately 8 per cent of spinal cord–injured patients.[11, 80] Ninety-eight per cent of these stones result from chronic urea-producing infections. If untreated, these stones can produce obstruction in the kidneys and lead to hydronephrosis, pyelonephritis, parenchymal abscesses, and potentially to septicemia and death.

Owing to the significant potential of developing renal complications, all spinal cord–injured patients should be closely followed by a nephrologist or urologist. This close follow-up must continue throughout the patient's life. Using modern treatment regimens, the mortality associated with renal failure has dramatically decreased in patients with spinal cord injury.[123, 144]

NEUROLOGICAL

The primary goal in the treatment of cervical injuries is prevention or limitation of a neurological deficit. Despite concerted efforts to protect patients, significant neural progression or ascension can occur. Although rare, this can occur at any time after injury.[22, 135] Early ascension of paralysis is usually related to central necrosis of the gray matter. Massive epidural hemorrhage may also produce neurological loss in the early period after injury.[135] This is especially true in patients with ankylosing spondylitis who incur spinal fractures.[32, 36]

Late loss of neurological function should alert the physician to an enlarging central syrinx of the spinal cord.[12, 219] The incidence of syrinx formation after SCI ranges from 0.3 to 2.3 per cent.[23] The clinical symptoms may surface a few months after injury or years later.[304] Although most common after thoracolumbar injuries, a syrinx may occur after cervical trauma.[12] Also, syrinx formation may occur in both complete and incomplete lesions.

Extensive research of spinal cord injury has provided great insight into the pathology and possible mechanisms of controlling and limiting cord injury. Within seconds after sustaining an injury, flame hemorrhages can be found in the gray matter and pia-arachnoid membranes.[7, 14, 112] A few minutes later, the hemorrhage spreads into the white matter while extravasation of blood and fluid from blood vessels begins.[81, 168] Significant cord edema can begin within hours after a severe injury and is usually present within 2 to 3 days after injury.[129, 187] Complete transection of the cord leads to cavitation and formation of microcysts.[170] Later these microcysts may rupture, forming larger cysts.[170]

Both clinical and basic science researchers have determined that the most significant factor in SCI is the amount of mechanical energy transferred to the cord at the time of impact.[35, 181, 190, 195, 292] There are also vascular mechanisms of injury involved. As in the traumatized brain, the spinal cord looses its autoregulation of arteriovenous blood flow patterns.[264] Significant occlusion of major veins and arteries of the cervical cord can also occur due to malalignment, fracture fragment impingement, or vascular spasm after injury.

In animal studies, the two factors that appear to determine the severity of SCI are the magnitude and duration of compression. Based on this finding, many authors have recommended early reduction as a mechanism of protecting the neural elements. Studies using somatosensory-evoked potential monitoring (SSEP) have documented the beneficial effects of early reduction.[231, 251] Our clinical impression is in agreement with this finding, and our present policy is to reduce all fractures with skeletal traction as soon as possible after radiographic delineation of the injury. An additional benefit obtained with traction is the immobilization it affords. Immobilization alone has been found in experimental studies to raise the threshold for SCI and is a critical factor in the initial treatment of these patients.

The use of steroids has been studied extensively in SCI. A large number of investigators have found steroids to be beneficial and have advocated their use in the early treatment of SCI.[10, 29, 47, 99, 145, 187] It has been suggested that the mechanism of action is restoration of blood pressure, stabilization of cell membranes, prevention of lysozomal enzymes, and inhibition of complement activation. Other investigators have documented no significant benefit with the use of steroids in SCI.[43, 77, 90, 151, 173] One multicenter, randomized clinical trial failed to demonstrate any difference between high- and low-dose steroids and also showed no difference in clinical improvement as compared with patients who did not receive steroids.[44]

The use of steroids in SCI has also been found to have detrimental effects. The risk of developing GI bleeding is increased when steroids are used in this patient population.[32, 34, 96] The infection rate has also been adversely affected with high-dose steroids.[68] Other potential risks are delayed wound healing and possible fluid and electrolyte aberrations.

Diuretics have also been advocated in the early treatment of SCI. Mannitol and dextran have been studied in the laboratory and found to have a beneficial effect.[151, 241, 266, 329] Reed and associates observed improved blood flow patterns in the white matter of the cord after treatment with mannitol.[241] Clinical studies documenting the efficacy of diuretics in the treatment of SCI are lacking at present.

Other forms of therapy currently under investigation include naloxone,[84] dimethyl sulfoxide (DMSO),[77, 78, 168] hyperbaric oxygen,[153, 332, 333] and local hypothermia.[2, 200, 320] Further research on these modalities needs to be completed prior to their clinical use.

SKIN

Measures to prevent decubitus ulcer must be instituted in all patients with cervical spine injuries. This should include frequent movement through the use of turning frames and Rotorest type beds, massage of pressure areas, avoidance of sepsis, and maintenance of proper nutrition.[125] A routine schedule of turn-

ing and daily skin examinations should be performed. If pressure sores are detected, aggressive treatment should be initiated to decrease the risk of sepsis.

Patients with complete neurological lesions are at particular risk of developing skin problems. These most commonly occur at bony prominences, such as the scapula, the sacrum, and the heels. Other common sites include the skin underlying casts and orthoses. In the treatment of complete lesions, consideration should be given to the use of removable orthoses which allow frequent skin checks.

HETEROTOPIC OSSIFICATION

Heterotopic ossification (HO) of the hip has been found to occur in 10 to 25 per cent of patients with SCI.[30, 159, 294, 315] In one third of those affected, there exists a significant loss of motion which limits their rehabilitation potential.[315] Problems associated with HO of the hip in SCI include a limitation in sitting, difficulty dressing, and an increased incidence of decubitus ulcers.[147, 294, 316]

Physical therapy does not appear to decrease the incidence of HO.[315] Diphosphonates have been of questionable value.[253, 288] Surgical resection of HO has been successful in some series and fraught with significant complication rates and high rates of recurrence in others.[72, 75, 122, 147, 159, 294] The complications that often occur with this surgical procedure include significant bleeding, hematoma formation, wound infection, osteomyelitis, and chronic pressure sores.

Criteria for successful resection have been defined. The surgery should be performed a minimum of 18 months after injury and only after the HO is considered mature as determined by serial radiographs, bone scans, and serum alkaline phosphatase.[294, 315] Patients should also demonstrate severe restriction of hip motion before being considered candidates for this procedure. Recent data reported by Garland and associates have questioned these criteria for a successful resection of HO.[122] In a review of 24 consecutive SCI patients who underwent resection of HO at Rancho Los Amigos, the authors found that normal bone scans, alkaline phosphatase levels, and a mature radiographic appearance of HO were poor predictors of success. The best predictor of success, improved hip motion, was preoperative range of motion. In this study, 92 per cent of hips experienced bony recurrence. Other complications included superficial wound infections in 33 per cent and osteomyelitis in 33 per cent. Complications other than HO recurrence were found in 79 percent of the hips operated on. These authors concluded that patients with severe restrictions in range of motion or ankylosis of the hip should be considered candidates for prophylaxis against recurrence. Although prophylaxis has not been studied extensively in this population, consideration should be given to the use of low-dose radiation or anti-inflammatory medication such as indomethacin.

MALNUTRITION

Quadriplegic patients frequently become malnourished owing to the increased metabolic demands associated with multiple trauma and the disruption of normal caloric intake.[225] Gastric stasis and intestinal atony often occur initially after injury, requiring nasogastric suctioning. Gastrointestinal injuries or complications such as GI bleeding can further delay the onset of enteric feedings. If sufficient caloric intake is not initiated early, malnutrition with its associated complications may result. These patients are more likely to develop wound infections or delayed wound healing.

Malnutrition should be prevented with early total parenteral nutrition (TPN) and initiation of enteral feedings as soon as gastric stasis and intestinal atony resolve. It has been our experience that this patient population responds quickly to aggressive nutritional support. The nutrition specialists at Thomas Jefferson University Hospital are important members of the SCI team.

COMPLICATIONS OF NONOPERATIVE TREATMENT

SKELETAL TRACTION

Cervical skeletal traction was first described by Crutchfield in 1933.[73] Since that time, this method of immobilization and reduction has become accepted as the standard of care for a patient with an unstable cervical spine injury. Bohlman has stated that all cervical SCI patients should be placed into traction even if no obvious bony injury is appreciated.[34] This allows for protection of the cervical spine while further evaluating for occult bone and soft tissue injury.

Cervical traction has been found to be an effective method of preventing neurological deterioration.[32, 258] Rogers believed that the cord is safe when the patient is in skull traction.[249] In a report of 300 patients with cervical spine injuries, only one experienced a neurological injury while in traction.[32]

Although infrequent, complications of cervical traction have been reported. In general, halter skin traction should be condemned owing to the large weights often needed to obtain reductions and maintain alignment. These large weights cause significant discomfort and result in patient restlessness, which can lead to further SCI.[248] Pressure sores beneath the skin straps can also develop if weights greater than 5 pounds are used.

The use of skeletal traction pins has been associated with multiple complications. In general, the risk of developing these complications is related to the length of time in traction.[32, 157] These complications include pin tract infections which can lead to osteomyelitis,[17, 83, 113] epidural abscess,[83] and brain abscess.[295] The traction pins can also penetrate the skull, resulting in a laceration of the meningeal vessels which can lead to epidural hematoma.[83]

A potentially catastrophic complication that can occur with traction is overdistraction of the injured segment (Fig. 6–3). This can result in increased neurological injury[34, 74] and death.[53, 115] Overdistraction can occur if all of the anterior and posterior ligamentous structures are torn. This is most commonly found in patients with severe rotational injuries and patients with ankylosing spondylitis and osteoarthritis. Overdistraction can also occur over a long period secondary to ligament attenuation. Prevention of this complication can be assured by carefully delineating the injury prior to the start of traction, ruling out occult injuries of the spine at secondary locations, beginning with low weights, and obtaining frequent radiographic and clinical evaluations.[203]

Other complications that have been attributed to long-term traction include decreased pulmonary function, increased incidence of pulmonary embolus, infection, decubitus ulcer, increased cost of hospitalization, and delay in rehabilitation. In addition, there is no assurance that instability and recurrent deformity will not be present after a lengthy course of traction.[32, 248]

ORTHOSIS

There exists a variety of orthoses manufactured for use in the cervical region. Their ability to immobilize the cervical region ranges

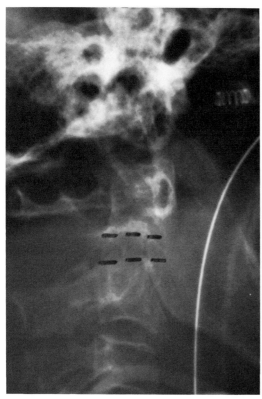

FIGURE 6–3. This odontoid fracture is overdistracted by 5 mm. with only 10 pounds of skeletal traction.

from a minimal effect with soft collars to the maximum ability to immobilize with a halo vest orthosis. Johnson and associates found that the halo vest orthosis allows only 4 per cent of normal flexion and extension.[165] These reports are in contrast to Koch and Nickel's report which documented an average of 31 per cent of normal motion in six patients who had incurred an unstable cervical injury.[174] They also noted that the halo was inadequate in controlling axial loading of the cervical spine. They documented an average variation in distraction force of 20 pounds in different positions. Despite these shortcomings, the halo vest orthosis remains the most rigid form of immobilization for the cervical spine.[165]

Complications that occur with the stiff collar orthoses and the cervical-thoracic orthoses include pressure sores and loss of spinal alignment. The pressure sores frequently occur in areas of a bony prominence and are most likely to develop on insensate skin. The "at risk" areas for these orthoses include the scapulae, clavicles, and the mandible. Patients with rheumatoid arthritis are particularly prone to skin breakdown under these orthoses.

The advantages of the halo vest orthosis include the rigid immobilization of the cervical spine, the ability to precisely control the position of the neck, and less interference with mandibular motion and eating.[69, 174, 215, 229, 230, 235, 238] Despite these advantages, there is a significant risk of complications associated with its use. Garfin and associates studied 179 patients who were treated with this orthosis.[119] They documented pin loosening in 36 per cent, pin infection in 20 per cent, pressure sores under vests in 11 per cent, nerve injury in 2 per cent, and a dural penetration risk of 1 per cent. In a follow-up series, increasing the insertion torque from 6 in-lb to 8 in-lb significantly decreased the risk of developing these complications. The infection rate dropped to 2 per cent, while the loosening rate decreased to 7 per cent. The higher insertion torque was not associated with an increased risk of dural penetration. Further design modifications of the halo pins and careful application of the halo and vest should decrease the incidence of these complications.[120, 121]

We have found that one must also pay particular attention to the vest to ensure adequate fit. Patients with neurological injury frequently require a vest change to a smaller size within a few weeks after injury owing to muscle atrophy. Also, it has been our experience that a natural sheepskin liner is more efficacious in preventing skin breakdown under the vest.

Another serious complication of the halo vest orthosis is failure to adequately immobilize. Glaser and Whitehall reported on a group of 101 patients treated with a halo vest orthosis.[126] Fourteen developed a loss of reduction, and four demonstrated a recurrent bilateral facet jump. Posterior ligament injury has been reported to be a predisposing factor in failure of immobilization with a halo.[321] Recognizing this limitation of the halo vest orthosis, it would appear prudent to consider operative stabilization in those patients with unstable injuries associated with posterior column disruption (Table 6–1).

Last, the rigid immobilization of the halo vest orthosis has been implicated in the development of facet joint degenerative arthritis.[297] In a review of 100 consecutive patients, 47 per cent demonstrated facet degenerative changes.[297] These changes were found to be associated with the patient's age and the length of time in the halo device.

UPPER CERVICAL SPINE

Diagnosis and treatment of injuries to the occipitocervical and atlantoaxial regions are

Table 6–1
Instability Found after Nonoperative Treatment of Flexion-Distraction and Flexion-Rotation Injuries

	# OF PTS	% LATE INSTABILITY
Ramadier et al. 1963	37	27%
Cheshire 1969	19	21%
Dorr et al. 1982	25	30%
O'Brien et al. 1982	28	17%
Cotler et al. 1989	14	64%

fraught with complications. As stated previously, the upper portion of the cervical spine is the most common location of a missed injury.[32] To prevent this potentially catastrophic complication, one must have a high index of suspicion. All patients with facial or scalp trauma or multiple trauma should have a cervical spine series of radiographs, including open mouth and oblique views. Of course, the lateral radiograph should be cleared of injury down to T1 prior to obtaining the remainder of the series. Computed axial tomography or tomographic radiographs should be obtained when a suspicious lesion exists.

Skeletal traction should not be used in suspected upper cervical injuries owing to the risk of overdistraction. This can occur with small weights and may result in upper cervical cord injury and vertebral artery injury.

OCCIPITOCERVICAL INJURIES

These injuries usually occur in motor vehicle accidents and other high velocity trauma. The mechanism of injury is a violent, rotational force that causes disruption of all the ligamentous connections between the occiput and the atlas. Although this injury is nearly always fatal, multiple case reports of survivors have been reported in the literature.[92, 98, 101, 302, 334]

Prevention of serious neurological injury should be given the highest priority when this injury is suspected. These patients should be immediately immobilized and radiographically evaluated to rule out this injury. Wiesel and Rothman have defined occipitoatlantal instability as translation of greater than 1 mm as measured from the basion to the tip of the odontoid.[323]

Traction should not be used when this injury is suspected owing to potential injury to the spinal cord and vertebral arteries. Owing to the marked soft tissue disruption, the treatment of choice for documented instability is posterior fusion. If deficiencies of the atlas posterior ring are present, the fusion will need to be extended to the axis.[323] Nonoperative treatment is not recommended because of the potential for postimmobilization instability and the risk of high neurological injury. The rate of nonunion for upper cervical fusions is low (Table 6–2).

Instability of the occipitocervical junction can also occur in the pediatric population. Evaluation and treatment should proceed as in the adult group. When instability is suspected at this level in children, careful review of radiographs should be performed to rule out congenital and developmental causes of instability. This is important in this age group because of the difficulty these patients have conveying accurate histories of injury or symptoms.

ATLAS FRACTURES

Fractures of the ring of C1 are uncommon injuries that account for 2 to 13 per cent of all cervical fractures.[248, 268] These injuries are generally considered benign lesions that are amenable to nonoperative treatment with immobilization.[155, 164, 268] Hinchley and Bickel[155] as well as Sherk and Nicholson[268] found that failure to achieve solid osseous union did not preclude a good clinical result and that this complication rarely resulted in any disability.

Segal and associates[262] in a study of 18 patients with a fractured atlas also found that a unilateral comminuted fracture predisposed to nonunion and a poor clinical result. This lesion is defined as one fracture that is anterior and one that is posterior to the lateral mass, along with an associated osteoperiosteal avulsion of the transverse ligament. This conclusion is supported by Bohlman, who found an increased risk of pain and loss of motion associated with fractures of the lateral mass with incongruity of the articular surface.[32, 38]

Nonunion of these fractures has been reported in the literature.[149, 154, 193, 204, 262] The incidence of this complication has varied with the technique of radiographic evaluation. Using computed axial tomography, Segal and associates found an incidence of 17 per cent in their series.[262] The one factor that has been widely implicated in the development of this complication is inadequate immobilization.[166, 174, 186, 280]

INSTABILITY OF C1-C2

In his classic laboratory study, Fielding defined the radiographic parameters for C1-C2

Table 6–2
Upper Cervical Spine Fusions

	# PTS	# NONUNIONS
Occiput-C1		
Fielding et al. 1976 AQ	11	2
C1–C2		
Fielding et al. 1976 AQ	46 Gallie	1 (2.2%)
Griswold et al. 1978 CU	10 Gallie	4 (40%)
	30 Brooks	1 (3.3%)
Brooks and Jenkins 1978 CT	15 Brooks	1 (6.6%)
	101	7 (7%)

instability.[105] The transverse ligament was found to tear when the atlanto-dens interval (ADI) was between 3 and 5 mm. This was found to be the major restraint which maintained the normal association between the atlas and the axis. The radiographic parameter of measuring the ADI on flexion and extension lateral radiographs is well accepted. The accepted upper limits of normal include 3 mm. in adults and 4 mm. in young children.[104, 108, 137, 162, 282]

Clinical studies have revealed that the majority of transverse ligament tears occur near its junction with the lateral mass.[262, 282] This finding differs with the cadaver study performed by Fielding and associates which noted 75 per cent midsubstance ruptures.[105] Late C1-C2 instability can occur in injuries of the transverse ligament which do not heal.[277] This instability carries a significant risk of subsequent neurological injury including death.[9, 13, 17, 136]

Careful evaluation with flexion and extension lateral radiographs should be performed at the completion of immobilization to rule out this potentially serious complication. Although the natural history of transverse ligament tears has not been fully delineated, it appears that the majority will heal spontaneously with immobilization. Segal and associates demonstrated a healing rate of more than 80 per cent of the documented osseous avulsions in their series.[262] Patients who demonstrate continued instability after a trial of immobilization should undergo appropriate operative fusion to prevent neurological injury.

Reduction of a C1-C2 subluxation or dislocation should be performed with the patient awake, using careful positioning and traction.[107, 118] The patient's neurological status should be closely monitored during this awake reduction process. Performing a reduction under general anesthesia has been associated with an increased risk of mortality and morbidity.[275, 306]

In the pediatric population, one must differentiate a traumatic C1-C2 instability from the more common Grisel's syndrome.[134, 192] Grisel's syndrome is a C1-C2 subluxation or dislocation which results from an inflammatory laxity of the transverse, apical, alar, and facet joint ligaments. Causes include pharyngitis, otitis, tonsillar abscess, and tuberculosis.[146] Most patients with Grisel's syndrome will respond to rest or light weight traction. Traumatic C1-C2 instability in this age group should be treated with rigid immobilization and surgical stabilization as in the adult population.

ODONTOID FRACTURES

The most common complication that occurs in the nonoperative treatment of odontoid fractures is nonunion. This has been reported with an incidence varying from 0 to 88 per cent.[17, 31, 113, 191, 246, 256, 260] The factors that have been found to be predictive of this outcome include Type II fractures of the Anderson and D'Alonzo classification,[9, 31, 255, 307] fracture displacement of 4 mm. or more,[13, 95, 254, 307] posterior dislocation,[8, 95, 256] fracture gaps,[17, 254, 256] lack of immobilization,[261] and older age.[13, 95, 256]

Nonoperative treatment of Types I and III odontoid fractures is uniformly successful. The union rate for these fractures has been reported at 100 per cent and 93 to 100 per cent, respectively.[9, 255, 307]

The treatment of Type II fractures remains controversial. Owing to the high risk of nonunion, many authors recommend surgical treatment acutely.[13, 95, 191, 254, 256, 284, 307] The relative indications for surgery of these fractures include injuries that cannot be held reduced in a halo, unreliable patients, multiple trauma, and older age.

In the pediatric population, odontoid fractures are one of the most common injuries of the cervical spine. In almost all reported cases, the fractures have occurred at the basilar synchondrosis.[9, 17, 28, 113, 133, 160, 210, 263, 324] These injuries are most commonly incurred in a short fall[263] and represent an epiphyseal separation of the basilar synchondrosis.[31] Forceps deliveries can also result in odontoid fractures when the head is rotated beyond 90 degrees.[48, 106, 272] Owing to the presence of the synchondrosis, nondisplaced fractures can be difficult to diagnose.[62] Open mouth radiographs are often useless in this age group.[133] Evaluation should be performed with a high-quality lateral film and lateral tomograms when necessary.

Displacement of the odontoid is almost always anterior.[28, 31, 133, 269] Rarely, the displacement may be posterior.[244] When anteriorly displaced, reduction can safely be achieved with gentle traction and cervical extension. The majority of these fractures heal nicely with nonoperative treatment. Treatment methods that have been used successfully include halo skeletal traction, halter traction, and immobilization with Minerva casts or halo vest orthoses.[28, 133, 244, 267] Surgical reduction or fusion is rarely indicated.[9, 17, 31, 133] No evidence of a growth disturbance of the odontoid has been demonstrated after the injury has healed.

Failure to diagnose an odontoid fracture in a child and the resulting failure to properly immobilize have resulted in the development of nonunion.[17, 102, 106, 113] Nonunion can cause resorption of the base of the odontoid and can lead to the radiographic picture of an os odontoideum.[102, 106, 113]

TRAUMATIC SPONDYLOLISTHESIS OF THE AXIS

Traumatic spondylolisthesis of the second cervical vertebra is a common cervical fracture which is also referred to as a hangman's fracture. This injury can result from a hyperextension-axial loading injury,[46, 88, 110, 293] or from a hyperextension-distraction injury as in a judicial hanging.[137, 150, 330, 331] The fracture line passes through the neural arch of the axis and may be associated with anterior displacement of C2 on C3.

The frequency of neurological injury associated with the traumatic variety of this fracture has varied from 6.5 to 73 per cent in the literature.[46, 70, 79, 88, 110, 326] Although the majority of patients present with mild, transient symptoms, the neurological injury can range from paresthesias to complete quadriplegia. This differs from a judicial hanging, which is fatal owing to the distraction force which causes complete disruption of the C2-C3 disc space. Traumatic injuries associated with a distraction force often result in severe neurological injury.[86, 326]

One must carefully evaluate the remainder of the cervical spine owing to the high number of fractures seen in association with traumatic spondylolisthesis of the axis. In a review of 52 patients, 13 (25 per cent) were noted to have associated injuries.[185] The majority of these were located in the upper cervical spine and included fractures of the atlas and the odontoid.

Treatment of this fracture includes reduction with skeletal traction followed by immobilization with a halo vest orthosis. This form of treatment is successful in obtaining union of this fracture as well as spontaneous fusion between C2 and C3 in a good percentage of cases.[110, 185] Francis and associates reviewed 123 patients[110] and reported a nonunion rate of 5.5 per cent and noted no correlation with initial displacement.

After the period of immobilization, lateral flexion and extension radiographs should be obtained to rule out persistent instability. If a fusion is considered necessary, an anterior fusion between C2 and C3 should be used.[110] This approach obviates the need to include C1 in the fusion as would be necessary in a posterior approach.

There exists a variant of this fracture which Levine and Edwards reported to be an indication for primary surgical reduction and fusion.[185] This injury includes both severe angulation and displacement with concomitant unilateral or bilateral facet dislocations at C2-C3. This injury complex was difficult to reduce with closed traction techniques and reductions often slipped while in halo vest immobilization.

A rare complication that has been reported in association with this injury is vertebral artery thrombosis.[88, 163, 226] Clinical signs and symptoms of vertebral artery insufficiency include difficulties moving the tongue or swallowing, diplopia, cortical blindness, and bilateral rotatory nystagmus. Death can also result from thrombosis of the vertebral arteries.[163, 259, 313, 327] Early reduction of severely displaced and angulated fractures should be performed to minimize the effects of kinking of the vertebral arteries.[226]

Traumatic spondylolisthesis of the axis has been noted in the pediatric population.[148, 236] Pizzutillo and associates reported the cases of five children who ranged in age from 6 months to 1 year.[236] Nonoperative treatment with mild extension and immobilization with either a Minerva jacket or halo cast appears to produce a high union rate. Instability following immobilization has been identified in this age group and needs to be ruled out at the completion of treatment. Care should be taken not to mistake a normal roentgenographic variant in this age group. Also, one should always maintain a high index of suspicion for child abuse in this age group.[196]

SUBAXIAL CERVICAL SPINE

Nonoperative treatment of lower cervical spine injuries is recommended by many authors as the preferred treatment.[24, 65, 111, 140] They cite the low incidence of late instability seen in patients treated nonoperatively. The incidence has been reported in the literature to be between 6 and 12 per cent.[24, 49, 53, 54, 65] Also, they have noted the frequent occurrence of spontaneous fusion after cervical trauma. This has been documented in up to 30 per cent of cases and is noted to appear 3 to 18 months after injury.[248] Others have argued that operative stabilization should be employed primarily.[20, 66, 67, 218, 233, 248] The allegations leveled at nonoperative treatment include increased risk of complications associated with prolonged immobilization, decreased neurological function due to inadequate decompression, delayed entrance into a formal rehabilitation program, and no assurance that late instability will not be present at the completion of the nonoperative treatment. In addition, Cotler and associates recently reported a significant cost savings in a group of flexion distraction injuries which were treated surgically as compared with a similar group treated nonoperatively[71] (see Table 6–1).

Patients with unstable cervical injuries are generally considered candidates for surgical stabilization. The graded checklist proposed by White and Panjabi offers an excellent method for evaluating instability.[317] In addition, surgical decompression should be considered in any patient with significant neural compression. The approach used to decompress should directly address the area of compression. Anterior compression by either bony fragments or disc material should be addressed with an anterior approach, while posterior compression from epidural hematomas or posterior bony element displacement should be decompressed by a posterior approach.

Although opinions remain diverse, there appears to have developed a swing away from nonoperative treatment of "potentially" unstable cervical injuries. Flexion distraction or flexion rotation injuries appear to be particularly prone to late instability. The incidence of late instability after nonoperative treatment of these injury patterns has been reported to be 21 to 64 per cent[65, 71, 82, 220, 240] (see Table 6–2).

A common error in the evaluation of subaxial cervical injuries is underestimation of ligamentous and disc pathology. Failure to diagnose posterior ligament injury in compression flexion injuries predisposes to late instability with late kyphosis formation[27, 66, 189, 194, 278, 310] (Fig. 6–4). Failure to diagnose disc herniations associated with cervical fractures may allow continued neural compression. In a series of 51 consecutive patients with cervical trauma admitted to the Regional Spinal Cord Injury Center, 43 per cent were noted to have significant disc injuries. The groups who appeared to be at particular risk of disc injury were those with anterior cord syndromes (100 per cent), central cord syndromes (60 per cent), and complete neurological injuries (40 per cent).

One must carefully review the routine radiographs to evaluate for widening of the interspinous ligaments and intervertebral subluxation. Further evaluation with computed axial tomography should be done to define bony injuries of the facet joints and pedicles. Magnetic resonance imaging (MRI) is particularly helpful in defining posterior ligament injury and injury of the intervertebral discs. An MRI should be obtained in any patient with suspected disc injury. This should include all patients with neurological injury, especially those with anterior cord syndromes.

Magnetic resonance imaging is also very helpful in defining epidural hemorrhages. This is a rare complication seen most frequently in patients with ankylosing spondylitis.[34] The epidural and prevertebral veins are fixed in scar tissue in this disease process and are easily torn with fracture displacement.[32, 36] As recently reported by Cotler and associates, spinal cord injury can be evaluated in the early post-injury period with MRI scanning. Careful radiological evaluation of patients with cervical trauma should identify or prevent the majority of complications associated with nonoperative treatment.

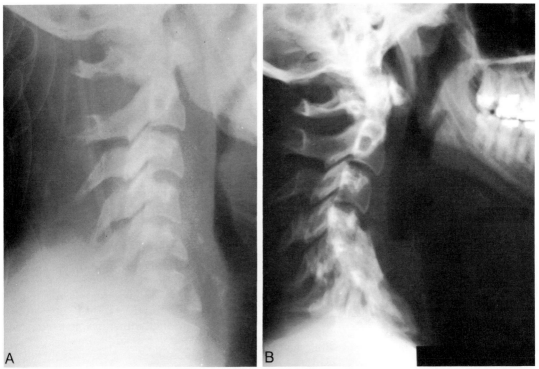

FIGURE 6-4. *(A)* Severe flexion-compression injury with multilevel involvement. Patient was treated with an anterior strut graft followed by halo immobilization for four months. *(B)* Kyphotic deformity demonstrating the halo vest's inability to control multicolumn failure. Posterior fusion with fixation should have been added at the time of anterior fusion.

Lower cervical spine injuries in children differ in that there is often a more profound neurological deficit than the bony injury would suggest.[290] It is not unusual for children with complete quadriplegic injuries to have normal radiographs and myelograms.[2] Often, the fractures occur at the vertebral end-plates and, if nondisplaced, can be difficult to identify.[16] In general, these fractures respond well to nonoperative treatment with closed reduction and immobilization. Surgical stabilization should be used only if instability is documented after a trial of immobilization or if reduction cannot be obtained with closed techniques.[160, 252] Adolescents with lower cervical fractures are less likely to develop spontaneous fusion and more often require surgical stabilization.[131] Remodeling of vertebral wedge fractures can be expected in children less than 10 years of age.

Spinal cord injuries in children often span multiple segments owing to damage by traction and rotational forces.[52] This pathological finding explains the disparity often seen between the neurological injury level and the level of bony injury. MRI can be used to rule out other causes for the disparity. These could include epidural hematoma formation or a missed second level of injury. Of note, intervertebral disc injury associated with cervical trauma is extremely rare in this age group.[16]

OPERATIVE COMPLICATIONS

Complications of surgical procedures in the treatment of cervical trauma include general complications that can occur with any surgical procedure on the spine and site-specific complications. Complications unique to cervical spine trauma patients will be included under these headings for completeness.

INTRAOPERATIVE COMPLICATIONS

Although rare, a large number of varied complications can occur during the surgical procedure. The majority of these can be attributed to poor preoperative planning and inadequate technique. Prevention of many of these complications can be attained by good preoperative planning, knowledge of anatomy, attention to detail, and gentle nontraumatic technique.

ANESTHETIC COMPLICATIONS

The risk of developing an anesthetic complication is increased in cervical trauma patients owing to the potentially unstable spine and the labile cardiovascular status. To prevent neurological injury during induction and intubation, an awake intubation using a blind nasotracheal or fiberoptic technique should be used. The patient may then be positioned and neurological function tested before being put to sleep. This system should be used in patients who are neurologically intact but have cervical instability, all patients with cervical myelopathy, and those with incomplete neurological lesions. Complete lesions may prove difficult to examine after positioning.

It is also important to remember that the cardiovascular system is lable owing to disruption of the sympathetic nervous system.[301] One must closely monitor the patient's vital signs during induction.

Succinylcholine is contraindicated in cases of SCI owing to a marked rise in serum potassium which has been noted in this clinical setting[21, 138] Paralyzed muscles can release large quantities of potassium in response to succinylcholine. Cardiorespiratory arrest can ensue.

VASCULAR COMPLICATIONS

Vascular injuries occur rarely in surgery of the traumatized cervical spine. Knowledge of vessel anatomy and common anatomical variations should help to prevent these complications.

The vertebral arteries are at particular risk as they traverse the posterior arch of the atlas. Dissection of the posterior arch of the atlas should be limited to 12 mm. lateral to the midline. Care should be taken to stop dissecting as soon as the sharp ridge of the outer margin of the vertebral groove is in view. Vertebral artery injury can also occur during transoral approaches to the upper cervical spine.[100] Injury to the vertebral arteries can result in symptoms of vertebral artery insufficiency as previously described.

Other vessels at risk include the subclavian vein during sternal splitting approaches to the cervicothoracic region and the retinal arteries, which can become thrombosed if circumferential pressure is placed on the eye. The latter complication can be prevented by using May-field tongs or a Gardener headrest. These head-holding devices are also critical to ensure adequate exposure and stability throughout the procedure.

NEUROLOGICAL COMPLICATIONS

Injury to the spinal cord with creation or aggravation of a neurological injury is a rare but major risk of cervical spine surgery. Breaches of technique that can result in neurologic injury include poorly controlled turning of the patient, improper positioning, and penetration of instruments into the spinal canal. Laminar fractures are particularly risky areas of canal penetration.

Spinal cord injury can also occur during anterior decompression of the lower cervical spine. The risk is increased if the canal is intentionally entered.[33, 36, 232] Preservation of the posterior longitudinal ligament appears to be protective against cord injury.[33, 40, 247]

Other potential nerve injuries include the hypoglossal nerve in upper cervical approaches, the superior thyroid nerve, the recurrent laryngeal nerve, and the cervical sympathetic chains. Prevention of these nerve injuries relies on the careful identification and protection of these structures.

CEREBROSPINAL FLUID (CSF) LEAKS

A CSF fistula may occur if a durotomy occurs and is left unrepaired. Eismont has reported that identification of the tear is the primary prerequisite for its successful management.[94] Repairs should use a 5-0 or 6-0 nonabsorbable suture on an atraumatic needle. The repair should be watertight, and this should be tested with multiple Valsalva maneuvers.

Dural tears that occur secondary to trauma are often anterior and very difficult to repair. The presence of such a tear is not an indication for surgical repair. Most of these tears will heal spontaneously.[184] If encountered during surgery, repair should be attempted when possible. An alternative, which is less than optimal, is placement of an Avitene or Gelfoam patch in the region of the tear. Antibiotics should be used in all cases of a dural tear as prophylaxis against meningitis. Other complications associated with dural tears include CSF fistulae, pseudomeningoceles, and subsequent neurological compromise.

ESOPHAGEAL PERFORATIONS

Esophageal perforations are rare complications associated with the use of sharp-tipped retractors or overaggressive retraction. Bohlman and Eismont noted one case in a series of 75 anterior cervical corpectomies.[39] Kewalramani and Riggins also noted one case in their series of 41 patients.[171] Injury to the esophagus can also result from anteriorly placed wires, screws, and methylmethacrylate.[34] Esophageal perforation has been noted to result in the formation of esophageal-cutaneous fistula and osteomyelitis of the cervical spine. These lesions should be suspected in any patient who develops a postoperative infection and should be diagnosed early with a barium swallow or endoscopic examination.

THORACIC DUCT INJURIES

Injury of the thoracic duct is a rare complication of the anterolateral approach to the cervical spine. Bohlman and Eismont reported one case in a series of 75 anterior cervical decompressions.[39] This single case was treated successfully with bedrest.

OPERATIVE LEVEL

The final intraoperative complication is surgery performed at the wrong level. This is a completely preventable complication. A lateral cervical radiograph should be obtained whenever one is not completely sure of the level. This is particularly true in the lower cervical spine. One must be careful to position the patient appropriately to obtain good quality films (Fig. 6–5).

POSTOPERATIVE COMPLICATIONS

All of the systemic complications described in the nonoperative section can also occur in the postoperative period. The team of physicians treating these patients should maintain a high index of suspicion and continue with prophylactic measures in the postoperative period.

INFECTION

Sepsis complicating cervical spine surgery is extremely rare in the treatment of traumatic lesions. It is reported to be less than 1 per cent in most series. The majority of infections reported are associated with other predisposing factors. These include esophageal perforations[34, 39] and the presence of a foreign material such as methylmethacrylate.[93, 223] A third predisposing factor is the placement of a tracheostomy within 3 days after an anterior cervical procedure.[217]

Abscess formation in the cervical region is a potentially catastrophic complication owing to the risk of airway obstruction and neural compression. Respiratory distress and death can ensue if this condition is not addressed quickly. Early drainage and debridement should be considered in anterior cervical spine infections to prevent these complications.

RESPIRATORY COMPLICATIONS

The immediate postoperative period is a particularly risky time for the development of pulmonary complications. Cardiorespiratory instability, respiratory obstruction, and death have all been reported.[32, 34, 37, 218, 232] The risk factors that have been identified with the development of these complications include complete high cervical lesions, chronic obstructive pulmonary disease, age greater than 60 years, and severe depression.[32, 37]

Airway obstruction can also occur because of a wound hematoma which forms after an anterior cervical procedure. This can present as an acute compromise which demands rapid tracheostomy. It is for this reason that these patients should be monitored closely in the postoperative period and consideration be given to placement of a tracheostomy set at the bedside. A surgical drain should also be used to decrease the risk of hematoma formation.

Last, intraoperative injury of the high cervical cord may result in sleep-induced apnea (Ondine's curse) or prolonged respiratory depression.[32, 91, 107, 108, 176] Passage of sublaminar wires has been reported to cause similar respiratory dysfunction.[108] Owing to the ratio of canal size to spinal cord size in the lower cervical region, sublaminar wires should not be passed below C3.

Prevention of respiratory complications during the postoperative period depends on a thorough understanding of the pathogenesis and careful monitoring of the patient's respiratory status. Preoperative pulmonary function testing and arterial blood gas analysis can identify patients at risk. This should be coupled with an aggressive postoperative respiratory therapy program. Early use of a tracheostomy

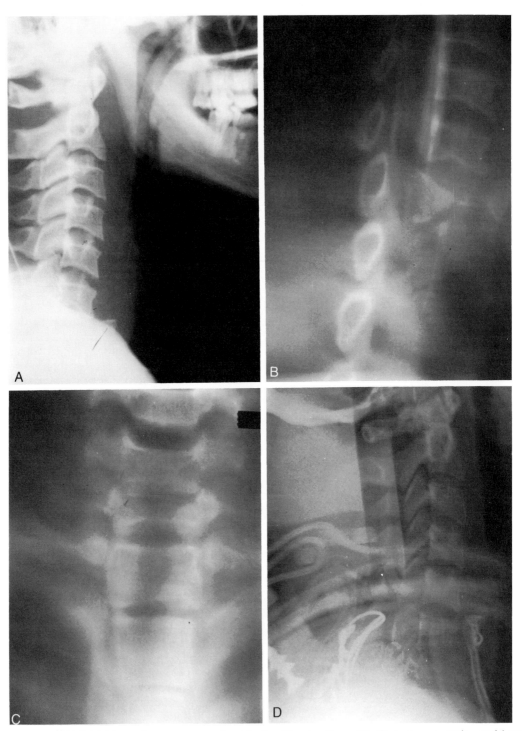

FIGURE 6–5. *(A)* Initial lateral roentgenograph with shoulder traction. *(B, C)* Anteroposterior and lateral tomography demonstrate a severe burst fracture of C7. *(D)* Crucial intraoperative roentgenograph after simultaneous anterior and posterior fusion demonstrating anterior graft subluxation.

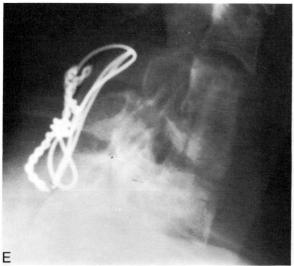
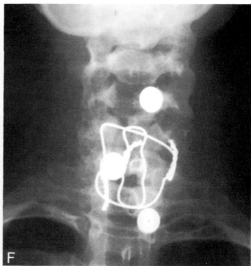

FIGURE 6–5 *Continued. (E, F)* After revision of the anterior graft, alignment of the anterior strut within the vertebral bodies has been achieved.

may reduce the mortality and morbidity in this patient population.[32, 37] Following an anterior cervical procedure, placement of a tracheostomy should be delayed to decrease the risk of infection.

COMPLICATIONS OF SURGICAL DECISION MAKING

The origin of a large number of postoperative complications can be traced to errors in surgical decision making which occurred prior to or during the procedure. Careful scrutiny of graft displacements and failures of internal fixation often reveals inappropriate use of a fixation device, failure to recognize and decipher the mechanisms of injury, and failure to adequately immobilize the patient until a solid fusion is achieved.

When choosing the appropriate surgical procedure, one must take into account the patient's bony and soft tissue injuries. Based upon these findings, the appropriate surgical procedures can be performed.

Surgical decompression is often necessary when compression of the neural elements is defined preoperatively. The route or approach used for the decompression should address the compressing bone and soft tissue directly. An anterior approach should be used for anterior bone and disc fragments, while the posterior approach should be reserved for epidural hematomas and other posterior compressing entities. This aggressive surgical attitude is supported by the excellent results obtained by late

anterior decompression in SCI.[39, 40, 180] Neurological improvement consisting of root return in complete lesions and improved distal function in incomplete lesions can occur if the decompression is done appropriately.

A fateful error is an attempt to decompress a spinal cord which is compressed anteriorly with a laminectomy. Not only is a laminectomy useless in relieving anterior compression,[6, 32, 36, 195, 206] but this procedure is also associated with a 22 to 30 per cent risk of further neurological injury.[32, 34, 36, 38, 206] This procedure has also been noted to increase the mortality rate in this patient population.[32, 33] In addition, laminectomy can result in significant instability which mandates internal stabilization.[56, 274, 281] If not appropriately stabilized, laminectomy can result in the development of cervical kyphosis with worsening of the anterior compression force upon the spinal cord.[20, 58, 270]

When one is considering an anterior decompression procedure, it is important to rule out injury to the posterior bony and ligamentous elements. Failure to recognize a posterior column disruption is one of the most common causes of anterior graft displacement in the postoperative period.[27, 66, 103, 234, 278] Cloward recognized the association and recommended using a posterior cervical wiring and fusion to prevent this.[66] Stauffer and Kelly found a high correlation between posterior column injury and the development of graft displacement or late kyphosis deformity.[278] These studies are further supported by a recent study performed at our Regional Spinal Cord Injury Center.[234]

We reviewed 138 patients who underwent anterior cervical vertebrectomy and reconstruction with an iliac crest autograft. Those patients with posterior column injury who were treated with a primary or simultaneous posterior cervical wiring and fusion experienced a significant decrease in graft complications as compared with those patients who were treated with primary anterior reconstruction (P <.005). It is important to point out that all patients in this study were treated postoperatively with a halo vest orthosis. This form of immobilization, although the most rigid today, cannot take the place of internal stabilization as demonstrated by the high graft complication rate in the group with three-column disruption and primary anterior reconstruction (see Fig. 6–4).

COMPLICATIONS OF SPECIFIC SITES

Lower Cervical Spine

Nonunion after posterior cervical wiring and fusion using the Rogers technique or the three-wire technique (Bohlman) appears to be a nonexistent problem. In a review of 72 patients, Bohlman and associates found no instances of nonunion.[32] This has been our experience at the Regional Spinal Cord Injury Center. When the spinous processes remain intact, this is the internal fixation technique of choice in the lower cervical spine.

One of the more common complications encountered in posterior fusions of the lower cervical spine is spontaneous extension of the fusion mass to involve levels above and below the area intended to be fused. Although children appear to be particularly prone to this, this complication can be found in all age groups. To prevent this, the surgeon must be careful to expose only the levels he intends to fuse surgically. Obtaining an early intraoperative lateral radiograph to confirm levels should facilitate this limited exposure.

UPPER CERVICAL SPINE

The occipitocervical and atlantoaxial regions of the spine are historically prone to the development of nonunions[114, 197, 213, 248, 256] (see Table 6–2). Use of different wire fixation techniques has improved the rate of fusion. In a review of 66 patients, Edmunds and associates documented 3 nonunions in 20 occipitocervical fusions and 18 nonunions in 44 C1-C2 fusions.[87] They found that nonunion correlated with the use of light wire, postoperative infection, and the use of only grafts without wire fixation. Fielding and coworkers reviewed their experience with 46 C1-C2 Gallie type of fusions and 11 occipitocervical fusions.[107] Only one of the Gallie fusions resulted in a nonunion, while 2 of the 11 occipitocervical fusions developed a nonunion. Griswold and associates reviewed their experience with 10 Gallie and 30 Brooks type of C1-C2 fusions.[136] Sixty per cent of the Gallie procedures were successful as compared with 96 percent of the Brooks type of fusions. These authors felt that the Brooks procedure offered superior immediate stability as compared with the Gallie technique. This concept is further substantiated by the laboratory work of White and associates, who demonstrated that the lateral position of the wires in a Brooks type fusion could control rotation as well as flexion and extension.[318]

Fusion of the pediatric upper cervical spine appears to have a higher success rate than that in the adult.[175] Koop and coworkers reviewed nine children who underwent posterior fusion of the upper cervical spine using a halo vest orthosis as the postoperative immobilization. Of this group, the eight patients who were fused with autograft went on to a solid fusion. The single patient in whom allograft was used developed a nonunion. Further evidence against the use of allograft in the pediatric cervical spine was reported by Stabler and associates.[279] Of the seven children who underwent posterior cervical wiring and fusion with allograft, all seven developed nonunions.

FAILURE OF INTERNAL FIXATION DEVICES

The individual devices will not be reviewed owing to the constant evolution and large number of internal fixation devices being used at present in the cervical region. This discussion is beyond the scope of a chapter dealing with the complications of cervical trauma. Instead the discussion will be centered on the common complications seen and the preventive measures.

Failure of internal fixation in the early postoperative period is an indication of inadequate immobilization. Despite the biomechanics laboratory studies that demonstrate excellent rigidity of the different systems, it is important to recognize that uncooperative patients, patients with poor bone quality, and less-than-perfect application of the internal fixation devices can markedly increase the risk of failure if the patient is not immobilized. We at the

Regional Spinal Cord Injury Center have a low threshold for the application of a halo vest orthosis. The risks of the temporary immobilization are considered minimal in comparison with the risk associated with the failure of an internal fixation device.

Failure of an internal fixation device in the late postoperative period is most often associated with the development of a pseudarthrosis. One must remember that no internal device can take the place of a solid fusion. Careful surgical technique to ensure an excellent fusion is the best method to prevent a late failure of internal fixation.

LATE COMPLICATIONS

Late Deformities

Late kyphotic deformity of the cervical spine can occur if posterior column disruption is not addressed,[32, 34, 56, 184, 208, 274] if a posterior cervical fusion is performed in burst injuries without consideration of an anterior reconstruction, and in cases where laminectomy is used for decompression.[20, 34, 56, 61, 271, 274, 281, 291] The development of the deformity can occur early after injury or as late as 25 years after.[20] If severe, significant anterior cord compression and nerve root tethering can result in neurological injury.[32, 56, 274]

In the pediatric population, the development of a kyphotic deformity tends to occur more rapidly and to be more severe.[20, 58, 61, 274] In addition to the above risk factors, complete neurological injuries predispose to the development of kyphotic deformity.[58, 274] Incomplete neurological lesions appear to be protective.[58] In addition, the growth potential of the pediatric spine may result in the production of further kyphosis.[61]

Along these lines scoliosis can develop after cervical trauma in the pediatric age group. Nearly 100 per cent of quadriplegic patients develop scoliosis of the thoracic and lumbar spine.

Late Syrinx Formation

A syrinx of the cervical cord can develop after a spinal cord injury.[12, 23, 132, 222, 303, 304, 309, 325] The incidence has been quoted to range from 0.3 to 2.3 per cent of spinal cord–injured patients.[23] This is an important clinical entity which must be placed into the differential diagnosis whenever a patient presents with a decrease in neurological function or a loss of the ability to perform activities of daily living. Physicians who participate in the long-term care of SCI patients should have a low threshold for obtaining a radiographic study to rule out the presence of a syrinx.

Neuropathic Arthropathy of the Spine

Neuropathic, or Charcot, changes of the spine can occur after SCI.[63, 169, 199, 237, 243, 276, 283] These changes can occur as late as 20 years after injury.[169] The differential diagnosis of this disease process is mainly an infectious process. Appropriate radiographic studies including bone scans, indium-111 scans, and computed axial tomography should be used to differentiate these disease processes.[45] Biopsy and cultures should be obtained when an infectious process is suspected. Late syrinx formation may also be a predisposing factor and therefore should be excluded when a neuropathic change is seen.[242]

REFERENCES

1. Advanced Trauma Life Support Course, Instructor's Manual. Committee on Trauma, American College of Surgeons, 1984.
2. Ahmann, P.A., Smith, S.A., et al.: Spinal cord infarction due to minor trauma in children. Neurology 25:301, 1975.
3. Albin, M.S., Bunegin, L., et al.: Brain and lungs at risk after cervical spinal cord transection. Surg. Neurol. 24:191, 1985.
4. Albin, M.S., White, R.J., and Acosta-Rua, G.: Study of functional recovery produced by delayed localized cooling after spinal cord injury in primates. J. Neurosurg. 29:113, 1968.
5. Alker, G.J., Oh, Y.S., and Leslie E.B.: High cervical spine and craniocervical junction injuries in fatal traffic accidents: A radiologic study. Orthop. Clin. North Am., 9(4):1003, 1978.
6. Allen, B.L., Tencer, A.F., and Ferguson, R.L.: The biomechanics of decompressive laminectomy. Spine 12:803, 1987.
7. Allen, W.E., D'Angelo, C.M., and Kier, E.L.: Correlation of microangiographic and electrophysiologic changes in experimental spinal cord trauma. Radiology 111:107, 1974.
8. Altoff, B., and Bardholm, P.: Fractures of the odontoid process: A clinical and radiographic study. Acta Orthop. Scand. 177:61, 1979.
9. Anderson, L.D., and D'Alonzo, R.T.: Fractures of the odontoid process of the axis. J. Bone Joint Surg. 15A:1663, 1974.
10. Anderson, D.K., Means, E.D., Waters, T.R., et al.: Microvascular perfusion and metabolism in injured spinal cord after methylprednisolone treatment. J. Neurosurg. 56:106, 1982.
11. Anderson, R.U.: Urinary tract infections in spinal cord injury patients. In: Walsh, P.C., Gittes, R.E., Perlmutter, A.D., and Stamey, T.A. (eds.): Campbell's Urology, 5th ed. Philadelphia, W.B. Saunders Company, 1986, 888–899.

12. Anton, H.A., and Schweigel, J.F.: Postraumatic syringomyelia: The British Columbia experience. Spine *11*:865, 1986.

13. Apuzzo, M.L.J., Heiden, J.S., et al.: Acute fractures of the odontoid process. J. Neurosurg. 48:85, 1978.

14. Assenmacher, R.R., and Ducker, T.D.: Experimental traumatic paraplegia. J. Bone Joint Surg. 53A:671, 1971.

15. Audic, B., and Maury, J.: Secondary vertebral deformities in childhood and adolescence. Paraplegia 7:10, 1969.

16. Aufdermaur, M.: Spinal injuries in juveniles. Necroscopy findings in twelve cases. J. Bone Joint Surg. 56B:513, 1974.

17. Aymes, E.W., and Anderson, F.M.: Fracture of the odontoid process. Arch. Surg. 72:377, 1956.

18. Babinski, M.F., Gilbert, T.J., and Holmstrom, F.: Early pulmonary assessment in acute spinal cord trauma. Proceedings Eighth World Conference of Anesthesia, Manila, 1984.

19. Bailey, D.K.: The normal cervical spine in infants and children. Radiology 59:712, 1952.

20. Bailey, R.W., and Badgely, C.E.: Stabilization of the cervical spine by anterior fusion. J. Bone Joint Surg. 42A:565, 1960.

21. Baker, B.B., Wagner, J.A., and Hemenway, W.G.: Succinylcholine-induced hyperkalemia and cardiac arrest. Arch. Otolaryngol. 96:464, 1972.

22. Barnett, H.J.M., Botterell, A.T., et al.: Progressive myelopathy as a sequel to traumatic paraplegia. Brain 89:159, 1966.

23. Barnett, H.J.M., Foster, J.B., and Hudgson, P.: Syringomyelia. In: *Major Problems in Neurology*, Vol. 1. Philadelphia, WB Saunders Company, 1973, pp. 129–153.

24. Bedbrook, G.M.: Stability of spinal fractures and fracture dislocations. Paraplegia 9:23, 1971.

25. Bedbrook, G.M.: *The Care and Management of Spinal Cord Injuries*. New York, Springer Verlag, 1981.

26. Bellamy, R., Pitts, F.W., and Stauffer, E.S.: Respiratory complications in traumatic quadriplegia: Analysis of twenty years experience. J. Neurosurg. 39:596, 1973.

27. Bell, G.D., and Bailey, S.I.: Anterior cervical fusion for trauma. Clin. Orthop. *128*:155, 1977.

28. Bhattacharyya, S.K.: Fracture and displacement of the odontoid process in a child. J. Bone Joint Surg. 56A:1071, 1974.

29. Black, P., and Markowitz, R.S.: Experimental spinal cord injury in monkeys: Comparison of steroids and local hypothermia. Surg. Forum 22:409, 1971.

30. Blane, C.E., and Perkasn, I.: True heterotopic bone in the paralyzed patient. Skeletal Radiol. 7:21, 1981.

31. Blockley, N.J., and Purser, D.W.: Fractures of the odontoid process of the axis. J. Bone Joint Surg. 38B:794, 1956.

32. Bohlman, H.H.: Acute fractures and dislocations of the cervical spine. An analysis of three hundred hospitalized patients and review of the literature. J. Bone Joint Surg. 61A:1119–1142, 1979.

33. Bohlman, H.H.: Cervical spondylosis with moderate to severe myelopathy: A report of seventeen cases treated by Robinson anterior cervical discectomy and fusion. Spine 2:151, 1977.

34. Bohlman, H.H.: Complications of treatment of fractures and dislocations of the cervical spine. In: Epps, C.H. Jr. (ed.): *Complications in Orthopaedic Surgery.* Philadelphia, J.B. Lippincott Company, 1978, pp. 611–641.

35. Bohlman, H.H: Late, progressive paralysis and pain following fractures of the thoracolumbar spine. J. Bone Joint Surg. 58A:728, 1976.

36. Bohlman, H.H.: The pathology and current treatment concepts of cervical spine injuries. Instr Course Lectures 21:108, 1972.

37. Bohlman, H.H.: Upper thoracic spine fractures with paralysis: A study of 180 cases. J. Bone Joint Surg. 56A: 1299, 1974.

38. Bohlman, H.H., Ducker, T.B., and Lucas, J.T.: Spine and spinal cord injuries. In: Rothman, R.H., and Simeone, F.A. (eds.): *The Spine.* Philadelphia, W.B. Saunders Company, 1982.

39. Bohlman, H.H., and Eismont, F.J.: Surgical techniques of anterior decompression and fusion for spinal cord injuries. Clin. Orthop. *154*:57, 1981.

40. Bohlman, H.H., Freehafer, A.A., and Dejak, J.J.: Late anterior decompression of spinal cord injuries: A report of thirty-six cases. J. Bone Joint Surg. 57A:1025, 1975.

41. Bors, E., Conrad, C.A., and Massell, T.B.: Venous occlusion of lower extremities in paraplegic patients. Surg. Gynecol. Obstet. 99:451, 1954.

42. Brach, B.B., Moser, K.M., et al.: Venous thrombosis in acute spinal cord paralysis. J. Trauma 17:289, 1977.

43. Bracken, M.B., Collins, W.F., et al.: Efficacy of methylprednisolone in acute spinal cord injury. J.A.M.A. 251:45, 1984.

44. Bracken, M.B., Shepard, M.J., et al.: Methylprednisolone and neurological function 1 year after spinal cord injury: Results of the National Acute Spinal Cord Injury Study. J. Neurosurg. 63:704, 1985.

45. Brandt-Zwadzki, M., Burke, V.D., and Jeffrey, R.B.: CT in the evaluation of spine infection. Spine 8:358, 1983.

46. Brashear, H.R., Venters, G.C., and Preston, E.T.: Fractures of the neural arch of the axis. A report of twenty-nine cases. J. Bone Joint Surg. 57A:879, 1975.

47. Braughler, J.M., and Hall, E.D.: Effects of multidose methylprednisolone sodium succinate administration on injured cat spinal cord neurofilament degradation and energy metabolism. J. Neurosurg. 61:290, 1984.

48. Bresnan, M.J., and Abroms, I.F.: Neonatal spinal cord transection secondary to intrauterine hyperextension of the neck in breech presentation. J. Pediatr. 84:734, 1974.

49. Brookes, T.P.: Dislocations of the cervical spine: Their complications and treatment. Surg. Gynecol. Obstet. 57:772, 1933.

50. Bucholz, R.W., and Burkehead, W.Z.: The pathological anatomy of fatal atlanto-occipital dislocation. J. Bone Joint Surg. 59A:991–1002, 1977.

51. Burke, D.C.: Spinal cord trauma in children. Paraplegia. 9:1, 1971.

52. Burke, D.C.: Traumatic spinal deformities in children. Paraplegia *11*:268, 1973–1974.
53. Burke, D.C., and Berryman, D.: The place of closed manipulation in the management of flexion-rotation dislocations of the cervical spine. J. Bone Joint Surg. *53B*:165, 1971.
54. Burke, D.C., and Tiong, T.S.: Stability of the cervical spine after conservative treatment. Paraplegia, *13*:191, 1975.
55. Caffey, J.: *Pediatric X-Ray Diagnosis. A Textbook for Students and Practitioners of Pediatrics, Surgery, and Radiology.* Chicago, Year Book Publishers, 1961, pp. 205–212, 1182–1194.
56. Callahan, R.A., Johnson, K., et al.: Cervical facet fusion for control of instability following laminectomy. J. Bone Joint Surg. *59A*:991, 1977.
57. Cane, R.D., and Shapiro, B.A.: Pulmonary effects of acute spinal cord injury: Assessment and management. Surgery of Spine Trauma.
58. Capen, D.A., Nelson, R.W., et al.: Decompressive laminectomy in cervical spine trauma: A review of early and late complications. Contemp. Orthop. *17*:21, 1988.
59. Carter, R.E.: Medical management of pulmonary complications of spinal cord injury. Adv. Neurol. *22*:261, 1979.
60. Cattell, H.S., and Filtzer, D.L.: Pseudosubluxation and other normal variations of the cervical spine in children. J. Bone Joint Surg., *47A*:1295, 1965.
61. Cattell, H.S., and Clark, A.L.: Cervical kyphosis and instability following multiple laminectomies in children. J. Bone Joint Surg. *49A*:713, 1967.
62. Cattell, H.S., and Filtzer, D.L: Pseudosubluxation and other normal variations in the cervical spine in children. J. Bone Joint Surg. *47A*:1295, 1965.
63. Charcot, J.M.: Sur quelques arthopathies qui paraissent dependre d'une lesion du cerveau ou de la moelle epiniere. Arch. Physiol. Norm Pathol. *1*:161, 1868.
64. Cheshire, D.J.E.: Respiratory management in acute traumatic tetraplegia. Paraplegia *1*:252, 1964.
65. Cheshire, D.J.E.: The stability of the cervical spine following the conservative treatment of fractures and fracture-dislocations. Paraplegia 7:193, 1969.
66. Cloward, R.B.: Treatment of acute fractures and fracture dislocation of the cervical spine by vertebral body fusion: A report of eleven cases. J. Neurosurg. *18*:201, 1961.
67. Cloward, R.B.: Treatment of spinal cord injury. J.A.M.A. *228*:1096, 1974.
68. Collins, W.F.: A review and update of experiment and clinical studies of spinal cord injury. Paraplegia *21*:204, 1983.
69. Cooper, P.R., Maravilla, K.R., et al.: Halo immobilization of cervical spine fractures. Indications and results. J. Neurosurg. *50*:603, 1979.
70. Cornish, B.L.: Traumatic spondylolisthesis of the axis. J. Bone Joint Surg. *50B*:31, 1968.
71. Cotler, H.B., Cotler, J.M., et al.: The medical and economic impact of closed unstable cervical spine dislocations. Presented at the American Academy of Orthopaedic Surgeons Meeting, Las Vegas, 1989.

72. Couvee, L.M.J.: Heterotopic ossification in the surgical treatment of serious contractures. Paraplegia *19*:89, 1981.
73. Crutchfield, W.G.: Skeletal traction in treatment of injuries to the cervical spine. Report of a case. South. Surg. 2:156, 1933.
74. Crutchfield, W.G.: Skeletal traction in treatment of injuries to the cervical spine. J.A.M.A. *155*:29, 1954.
75. Damanski, M.: Heterotopic ossification in paraplegia. J. Bone Joint Surg. *43B*:286, 1961.
76. Davidoff, G., Thomas, P., Johnson, M., et al.: Closed head injury in acute traumatic spinal cord injury: Incidence and risk factors. Arch. Phys. Med. Rehabil. 69:869, 1988.
77. de la Torre, J.C., Johnson, C.M., Goode, D.J., et al.: Pharmacologic treatment and evaluation of permanent experimental spinal cord trauma. Neurology *25*:508, 1975.
78. de la Torre, J.C., Kajihara, K., et al.: Modification of experimental head and spinal cord injuries using dimethyl sulfoxide. Trans. Am. Neurol. Assoc. 97:230, 1972.
79. Delorme, T.L.: Axis-pedicle fractures. J. Bone Joint Surg. *49A*:1472, 1967.
80. Devivo, M.J., Fine, P.R., et al.: Risk of renal calculi in spinal cord injury patients. J. Urol. *131*:857, 1984.
81. Dohrman, G.J., Wagner, F.C., and Bucy, P.C.: The microvasculature in transitory traumatic paraplegia. An electron microscopic study in the monkey. J. Neurosurg. *35*:263, 1971.
82. Dorr, L.D., Harvey, J.P., and Nickel, V.L.: Clinical review of the early stability of spine injuries. Spine 7:545, 1982.
83. Drake, C.G.: Cervical spinal cord injury. J. Neurosurg. *19*:487, 1962.
84. Ducker, T.B., and Assenmacher, D.R.: Microvascular response to experimental spinal cord trauma. Surg. Forum *20*:428, 1969.
85. Dunlap, J.P., Morris, M., and Thompson, R.G.: Cervical spine injuries in children. J. Bone Joint Surg. *40A*:681, 1958.
86. Edgar, M.A., Fisher, T.R., et al.: Tetraplegia from hangman's fracture: Report of a case with recovery. Injury 3:199, 1972.
87. Edmunds, J.O., Goldner, J.L., et al.: Arthrodesis of the unstable upper cervical spine for instability with and without myelopathy. J. Bone Joint Surgery. *57A*:1025, 1975.
88. Effendi, B., Roy, D., et al.: Fractures of the ring of the axis. A classification based on the analysis of 131 cases. J. Bone Joint Surg. *63B*:319, 1981.
89. Eidelberg, E.E.: Cardiovascular response to experimental spinal cord compression. J. Neurosurg. 38:326, 1973.
90. Eidelberg, E.E., Staten, E., et al.: Treatment of experimental spinal cord injury in ferrets. Surg. Neurol. 6:243, 1976.
91. Eismont, F.J., and Bohlman, H.H.: Atlanto-occipital dislocation with survival. J. Bone Joint Surg. *60A*:397, 1978.
92. Eismont, F.J., and Bohlman, H.H.: Posterior atlanto-occipital dislocation with fractures of the odontoid process: Report of care with survival. J. Bone Joint Surg. *60A*:397, 1978.
93. Eismont, F.J., and Bohlman, H.H.: Posterior methylmethacrylate fixation for cervical trauma. Spine 6:347, 1981.

94. Eismont, F.J., Wieser, S.W., et al.: Treatment of dural tears associated with spinal surgery. J. Bone Joint Surg. 63A:1132, 1981.

95. Ekong, C.E.U., Schwartz, M.L., et al.: Odontoid fracture: Management with early mobilization using the halo device. J. Neurosurg. 9:631, 1981.

96. Epstein, E., Hood, D.C., and Ransohoff, J.: Gastrointestinal bleeding in patients with spinal cord injury. J. Neurosurg. 54:16, 1981.

97. Evans, D.E., Kobrine, A.L., and Rizzoli, H.V.: Cardiac arrhythmias accompanying acute compression of the spinal cord. J. Neurosurg. 52:52, 1980.

98. Evarts, C.M.: Traumatic occipito-atlantal dislocation. J. Bone Joint Surg. 52A:1653, 1970.

99. Faden, A.I., Jacobs, T.P., et al.: Megadose corticosteroid therapy following experimental traumatic spinal injury. J. Neurosurg. 60:712, 1984.

100. Fang, H.S.Y., and Ong, G.B.: Direct anterior approach to the upper cervical spine. J. Bone Joint Surg. 44A:1588, 1962.

101. Farthing, J.W.: Atlantocranial dislocation with survival: A case report. North Carolina Med. J. 9:34, 1948.

102. Fielding, J.W.: Disappearance of the central portion of the odontoid process. A case report. J. Bone Joint Surg. 47A:1228, 1965.

103. Fielding, J.W.: The status of arthrodesis of the cervical spine. A current concepts review. J. Bone Joint Surg. 70A:1571, 1988.

104. Fielding, J.W.: Selected observations on the cervical spine in the child. Curr. Pract. Orthop. Surg. 5:31, 1973.

105. Fielding, J.W., Cochran, G.V.B., et al.: Tears of the transverse ligament of the atlas. A clinical and biomechanical study. J. Bone Joint Surg. 56A:1683, 1974.

106. Fielding, J.W., and Griffin, P.P.: Os odontoideum: An acquired lesion. J. Bone Joint Surg. 56A:187, 1974.

107. Fielding, J.W., Hawkins, R.J., and Ratzan, S.A.: Spine fusion for atlanto-axial instability. J. Bone Joint Surg. 58A:400, 1976.

108. Fielding, J.W., Tuul, A., and Hawkins, R.J.: "Ondine's curse." A complication of upper cervical spine surgery. J. Bone Joint Surg. 57A:1000, 1975.

109. Fineman, S., Borrelli, F.J., et al.: The Cervical spine: transformation of the normal lordotic pattern into a linear pattern in the neutral posture. J. Bone Joint Surg. 45A:1179, 1963.

110. Francis, W.R., Feilding, J.W., et al.: Traumatic spondylolisthesis of the axis. J. Bone Joint Surg. 63B:313, 1981.

111. Frankel, H.L., Hancock, D.O., et al.: The value of postural reduction in the initial management of closed injuries of the spine with paraplegia and tetraplegia. Paraplegia 7:179, 1969.

112. Freeman, L.W., and Wright, T.W.: Experimental observations of concussion and contusion of the spinal cord. Ann. Surg. 137:433, 1953.

113. Freiberger, R.H., Wilson, P.D., and Nicholas, J.A.: Acquired absence of the odontoid process. A case report. J. Bone Joint Surg. 47A:1231, 1965.

114. Fried, L.C.: Atlanto-axial fracture dislocations. Failure of posterior C1 to C2 fusion. J. Bone Joint Surg. 55B:490, 1973.

115. Fried, L.C.: Cervical spinal cord injury during skeletal traction. J.A.M.A. 229:181, 1974.

116. Fuglmeyer, A.R.: Effects of respiratory muscle paralysis in tetraplegic and paraplegic patients. Scand. J. Rehabil. Med. 3:141, 1971.

117. Fuglmeyer, A.R.: Ventilatory function in tetraplegic patients. Scand. J. Rehabil. Med. 3:151, 1971.

118. Garber, J.N.: Abnormalities of the atlas and axis vertebrae: Congenital and traumatic. J. Bone Joint Surg. 46A:1782, 1964.

119. Garfin, S.R., Botte, M.J., et al.: Complications in the use of the halo fixation device. J. Bone Joint Surg. 68A:320, 1986.

120. Garfin, S.R., Botte, M.J., et al.: Osteology of the skull as it affects halo pin placement. Spine 10:696, 1985.

121. Garfin, S.R., Lee, T.Q., et al.: Structural behavior of the halo orthosis pin-bone interface: Biomechanical evaluation of standard and newly designed stainless steel halo fixation pins. Spine 11:977, 1986.

122. Garland, D.E., and Orwin, J.F.: Resection of heterotopic ossification in patients with spinal cord injuries. Clin. Orthop. 242:169, 1989.

123. Geisler, W.O., Jousse, A., et al.: Survival in traumatic spinal cord injury. Paraplegia, 21:364, 1983.

124. Geisler, W.O., Wynne-Jones, M., and Jousse, A.T.: Early management of patients with trauma to the spinal cord. Med. Serv. J. Can. 22:512–523, 1966.

125. Gilbert, J.: Critical care management of the patient with acute spinal cord injury. Crit. Care Clin. 3:549, 1987.

126. Glaser, J.A., and Whitehall, R.: Complications with use of the halo vest. Proceedings of the 13th Annual Meeting of the Cervical Spine Research Society, Cambridge, MA, 1978.

127. Glausser, F.E., and Cares, H.L.: Biomechanical features of traumatic paraplegia in infancy. J. Trauma 13:166, 1973.

128. Glausser, F.E., and Cares, H.L.: Traumatic paraplegia in infancy. J.A.M.A. 219:38, 1972.

129. Goodman, J.H., Bingham, W.G., and Hunt, W.E.: Ultrastructural blood-brain barrier alterations and edema formation in acute spinal cord trauma. J. Neurosurg. 44:418, 1976.

130. Green, D., Rossi, E.C., et al: Deep vein thrombosis in spinal cord injury: Effect of prophylaxis with calf compression, aspirin, and dipyridamole. Paraplegia 20:227, 1982.

131. Griffiths, E.R.: Growth problems in cervical injuries. Paraplegia 11:277, 1973.

132. Griffiths, E.R., and McCormick, C.C.: Posttraumatic syringomyelia. Paraplegia, 19:81–88, 1981.

133. Griffiths, S.C.: Fracture of the odontoid process in children. J. Pediatr. Surg. 7:680, 1972.

134. Grisel, P.: Enucleation de l'atlas et torticollis nasopharyngren. Presse Med. 38, 1930.

135. Grisolia, A., Bell, R.L., and Pletier, L.F.: Fractures and dislocations of the spine complicating ankylosing spondylitis: A report of six cases. J. Bone Joint Surg. 49A:339, 1967.

136. Griswold, D.M., Albright, J.A., et al.: Atlanto-axial fusion for instability. J. Bone Joint Surg. 60A:285, 1978.

137. Grogono, B.J.S.: Injuries of the atlas and axis. J. Bone Joint Surg. 36B:397, 1954.

138. Gronert, B.A., and Theye, R.A.: Effect of succinylcholine on skeletal muscle with immobilization atrophy. Anesthesia 40:268, 1974.

139. Gross, D., Ladd, H.W., et al.: The effect of training on strength and endurance of the diaphragm in quadriplegia. Am. J. Med. 68:27, 1980.

140. Guttmann, L.: Spinal deformities in traumatic paraplegics and tetraplegics following surgical procedures. Paraplegia 7:38, 1969.

141. Guttman, L., and Frankel, H.: Value of intermittent catheterization in early management of traumatic paraplegia and tetraplegia. Paraplegia 4:63, 1966.

142. Hachen, H.J.: Idealized care of the acutely injured spinal cord in Switzerland. J. Trauma 17:931, 1977.

143. Hachen, H.J.: Spinal cord injury in children and adolescents: Diagnostic pitfalls and therapeutic considerations in the acute stage. Paraplegia 15:55, 1977.

144. Hackler, R.H.: A 25-year prospective mortality study in spinal cord injured patient: Comparison with long term living paraplegic. J. Urol. 117:486, 1977.

145. Hall, E.D., Wolf, D.L., and Braughler, J.M.: Effects of a single large dose of methylprednisolone sodium succinate on experimental posttraumatic spinal cord ischemia. J. Neurosurg. 61:124, 1984.

146. Hanson, T.A., Kraft, J.P., and Adcock, D.W.: Subluxation of the cervical vertebrae due to pharyngitis. South. Med. J. 66:427, 1973.

147. Hardy, A.G., and Dickson, J.W.: Pathological ossification in traumatic paraplegia. J. Bone Joint Surg. 45B:76, 1963.

148. Hasue, M., Hoshino, R., et al.: Cervical spine injuries in children. Fukushima J. Med. Sci. 20:115, 1974.

149. Hatchette, S.: Isolated fracture of the atlas. Radiology 36:233, 1941.

150. Haughton, S.: On hanging, considered from a mechanical and physiologic point of view. London, Edinburgh and Dublin Philos. Mag. J. Sci. 32:23, 1866.

151. Hedeman, L.S., Shellenberger, M.K., and Gordon, J.H.: Studies in experimental spinal cord trauma. J. Neurosurg. 40:44, 1974.

152. Herzenberg, J.E., Hensinger, R.N., Dedrick, D.K., et al.: Emergency transport and positioning of young children who have an injury of the cervical pine. J. Bone Joint Surg. 71A:15, 1989.

153. Higgins, A.C., Pearlstein, R.D., et al.: Effects of hyperbaric oxygen therapy on long tract neuronal conduction in the acute phase of spinal cord injury. J. Neurosurg. 55:501, 1981.

154. Highland, T.R., and Salciccioli, G.G.: Is immobilization adequate treatment of unstable burst fractures of the atlas? A case report with long term follow-up evaluation. Clin. Orthop. 201:196, 1985.

155. Hinchley, J.J., and Bickel, W.H.: Fractures of the atlas. Review and presentation of data on eight cases. Ann. Surg. 121:826, 1945.

156. Hinchley, J.E., Hreno, A., et al.: The stress ulcer syndrome. In: Welch, C. (ed.): Advances in Surgery. Chicago, Year Book Medical Publishers, 1970, p. 325.

157. Hirsh, L.F.: Intracranial aneurysm and hemorrhage following skull caliper traction. A review of skull tractions complications. Spine 4:206, 1979.

158. Holmes, J.C., and Hall, J.E.: Fusion for instability and potential instability of the cervical spine in children and adolescents. Orthop. Clin. North Am. 9:923, 1978.

159. Hsu, J.D., Sakimura, I., and Stauffer, E.S.: Heterotopic ossification around the hip joint in spinal cord injured patients. Clin. Orthop. 112:165, 1975.

160. Hubbard, D.D.: Injuries of the spine in children and adolescents. Clin. Orthop. 100:56, 1974.

161. Hull, R., Hirsh, J., et al.: Clinical validity of negative venogram in patients with clinically suspected venous thrombosis. Circulation 64:622, 1981.

162. Jackson, H.: Diagnosis of minimal atlantoaxial subluxation. Br. J. Radiol. 23:672, 1950.

163. Jeanneret, B., Magerl, F., and Stanisic, M.: Thrombosis of the vertebral artery. Spine 11:179, 1986.

164. Jefferson, G.: Fracture of the atlas vertebrae. Report of four cases and a review of those previously recorded. Br. J. Surg. 7:407, 1920.

165. Johnson, R.M., Hart, D.L., et al.: Cervical orthoses. A study comparing their effectiveness in restricting cervical motion in normal subjects. J. Bone Joint Surg. 59A:332, 1977.

166. Johnson, R.M., Owen, J.R., et al.: Cervical orthoses. A guide to their selection and use. Clin. Orthop. 154:34, 1981.

167. Juhl, J.H., Miller, S.M., and Roberts, G.W.: Roentgenographic variations in the normal cervical spine. Radiology 78:591, 1962.

168. Kajihara, K., Kawanaga, H.M., et al.: Dimethyl sulfoxide in the treatment of experimental acute spinal cord injury. Surg. Neurol. 1:16, 1973.

169. Kalen, V., Isono, S.S., et al.: Charcot arthropathy of the spine in longstanding paraplegia. Spine 12:42, 1987.

170. Kao, C.C., Chang, L.W., and Bloodworth, M.B., Jr.: The mechanism of spinal cord cavitation following spinal cord transection. J. Neurosurg. 46:745, 1977.

171. Kewalramani, L.S., and Riggins, R.S.: Complications of anterior spondylodesis for traumatic lesions of the cervical spine. Spine 2:25, 1977.

172. Kewalramani, L.S., and Tori, J.A.: Spinal cord trauma in children. Neurologic patterns, radiologic features, and pathomechanics of injury. Spine 5:11, 1980.

173. Kobrine, A.I.: The question of steroids in neurotrauma. Editorial. J.A.M.A. 251:68, 1984.

174. Koch, R.A., and Nickel, V.L.: The halo vest. An evaluation of motion and forces across the neck. Spine 3:103, 1978.

175. Koop, S.E., Winter, R.B., and Lonstein, J.E.: The surgical treatment of instability of the upper part of the cervical spine in children and adolescents. J. Bone Joint Surg. 66A:403, 1984.

176. Kopits, S.E., Perovic, M.N., et al.: Congenital atlantoaxial dislocations in various forms of dwarfism. J. Bone Joint Surg. 54A:1349, 1972.

177. Kraus, J.F., Franti, C.E., Riggins, R.S., et al.: Incidence of traumatic spinal cord lesions. J. Chronic Dis. 28:471–492, 1975.

178. Kuhlemeir, K.V., Stover, S.L., and Lloyd, L.K.: Prophylactic antibacterial therapy for preventing urinary tract infections in spinal cord injury patients. J. Urol. 134:514, 1985.

179. Kurnick, N.B.: Autonomic hyperreflexia and its control in patients with spinal cord lesions. Ann. Intern. Med. 44:678, 1956.

180. Larson, S.J., Holst, R.A., et al.: Lateral extra-cavity approach to traumatic lesions of the thoracic and lumbar spine. J. Neurosurg. 45:628, 1976.

181. Larson, S.J., Walsh, P.R., et al.: Evoked potentials in experimental myelopathy. Spine 5:299, 1980.

182. Lauritzen, J.: Diagnostic difficulties in lower cervical spine dislocations. Acta Orthop. Scand. 39:439, 1968.

183. Leigh, D.E., and Bradley, M.: Ventilatory muscle strength and endurance training. J. Appl. Physiol. 41:508, 1976.

184. Levine, A.M., and Edwards, C.C.: Complications in the treatment of acute spinal injury. Orthop. Clin. North Am. 17:183, 1986.

185. Levine, A.M., and Edwards, C.C.: The management of traumatic spondylolisthesis of the axis. J. Bone Joint Surg. 67A:217, 1985.

186. Levine, A.M., and Edwards, C.C.: Treatment of injuries in the C1-C2 complex. Orthop. Clin. North Am. 17:31, 1986.

187. Lewin, M.G., Hansebout, R.R., and Pappius, H.M.: Chemical characteristics of spinal cord edema in cats: Effects of steroids on potassium depletion. J. Neurosurg. 40:65, 1974.

188. Lloyd, L.K., Kuhlemeier, K.V., et al.: Initial bladder management in spinal cord injury: Does it make a difference? J. Urol. 135:523, 1986.

189. Macnab, I.: Complications of anterior cervical fusion. Orthop. Rev. 1:29, 1973.

190. Maiman, D.J., Larson, S.J., and Benzel, E.C.: Neurological improvement associated with late decompression of the thoracolumbar spinal cord. Neurosurgery 14:302, 1984.

191. Maiman, D.J., and Larson, S.J.: Management of odontoid fractures. J. Neurosurg. 11:471, 1982.

192. Marar, B.C., and Balachandran, N.: Non-traumatic atlanto-axial dislocation in children. Clin. Orthop. 92:220, 1973.

193. Marlin, A.E., Williams, G.R., and Lee, J.F.: Jefferson fractures in children. Case report. J. Neurosurg. 58:277, 1983.

194. Mazur, J.M., and Stauffer, E.S.: Unrecognized spinal instability associated with seemingly "simple" cervical compression fractures. Spine 8:287, 1983.

195. McAfee, P.C., Bohlman, H.H., and Yuan, H.A.: Anterior decompression of traumatic thoracolumbar fractures with incomplete neurologic deficit using a retroperitoneal approach. J. Bone Joint Surg. 67A:89, 1985.

196. McGrory, B.E., and Fenichel, G.M.: Hangman's fracture subsequent to shaking an infant. Ann. Neurol. 2:82, 1977.

197. Mclaurin, R.L., Vernal, R., and Salmon, J.H.: Treatment of fractures of the atlas and axis by wiring without fusion. J. Neurosurg. 36:773, 1972.

198. McMichan, J.C., Michel, L., and Westbrook, P.R.: Pulmonary dysfunction following traumatic quadriplegia. J.A.M.A. 243:528, 1980.

199. McNeel, D.P. and Ehni, G.: Charcot joints of the lumbar spine. J. Neurosurg. 30:55, 1969.

200. Meacham, W.F., and McPherson, W.F.: Local hypothermia in the treatment of acute injuries in the spinal cord. South. Med. J. 66:95, 1973.

201. Melzak, J.: Paraplegia among children. Lancet 2:40, 1969.

202. Merli, G.J., Herbison, G.J., et al.: Deep vein thrombosis: Prophylaxis in acute spinal cord injured patients. Arch. Phys. Med. Rehabil. 69:661, 1988.

203. Miller, L.S., Cotler, H.B., et al.: Biomechanical analysis of cervical distraction. Spine 12:831, 1987.

204. Milward, F.J.: An unusual case of fracture of the atlas. Br. Med. J. 1:458, 1933.

205. Mohler, J.L., Cowen, D.L., and Flanigan, R.C.: Suppression and treatment of urinary tract infection in patients with intermittently catheterized neurogenic bladder. J. Urol. 138:336, 1987.

206. Morgan, T.H., Wharton, G.W., and Austin, G.N.: The results of laminectomy in patients with incomplete spinal cord injuries. Paraplegia 9:14, 1971.

207. Murphy, M.J., and Ogden, J.A.: Cervical spine injuries in the child. Contemp. Orthop. 3:615, 1981.

208. Murphy, M.J., Ogden, J.A., and Southwick, W.O.: Spinal stabilization in acute spinal injuries. Surg. Clin. North Am. 60:1035–1047, 1980.

209. Myllynen, P., Kammonen, M., et al.: Deep venous thrombosis and pulmonary embolism in patients with acute spinal cord injury: Comparison with non-paralyzed patients immobilized due to spinal fractures. J. Trauma 25:541, 1985.

210. Nachemson, A.: Fracture of the odontoid process of the axis. A clinical study based on 26 cases. Acta Orthop. Scand. 29:185, 1960.

211. Nash, C.L.: Acute cervical soft tissue injury and late deformity. J. Bone Joint Surg. 61A:305, 1979.

212. Naso, F.: Pulmonary embolism in acute spinal cord injury. Arch. Phys. Med. Rehabil. 55:275, 1974.

213. Newman, P., and Sweernam, R.: Occipto-cervical fusion. J. Bone Joint Surg. 51B:423, 1969.

214. Nicholson, J.T.: Aspects radiologiques chez l'enfant. Rev. Chir. Orthop. 50:715, 1964.

215. Nickel, V.L., Perry, J., et al.: The halo. A spinal traction fixation device. J. Bone Joint Surg. 50A:1400, 1968.

216. NIH Consensus Development Conference Prevention of venous thrombosis and pulmonary embolism. J.A.M.A. 256:744, 1986.

217. Norrell, H.: Fractures and dislocations of the spine. In: Rothman, R.H., and Simeone, F.A. (eds.): The Spine, vol 2. Philadelphia, W.B. Saunders Company, 1975, pp. 529–566.

218. Norrell, H., and Wilson, C.B.: Early anterior fusion for injuries of the cervical portion of the spine. J.A.M.A. 214:525, 1970.

219. Nurick, S., Russell, J.A., and Deck, M.D.F.: Cystic degeneration of the spinal cord following spinal cord injury. Brain 93:211, 1970.

220. O'Brien, P.J., Schweigel, J.F., and Thompson, W.J.: Dislocations of the lower cervical spine. J. Trauma 8:710, 1982.

221. Ohry, A., Molho, M., and Rozin, R.: Alterations of pulmonary function in spinal cord injured patients. Paraplegia 13:101, 1975.
222. Padilla, C.: Syringomyelia after spinal cord injury. Am. Fam. Physician 26:145, 1982.
223. Panjabi, M.M., Hopper, W., et al.: Posterior spine stabilization with methylmethacrylate. Biomechanical testing of a surgical specimen. Spine 7:241, 1977.
224. Pardy, R.L., and Leigh, D.E.: Ventilatory muscle training. Respir. Care 29:278, 1984.
225. Peiffer, S.C., Blust, P., and Leyson, J.F.: Nutritional assessment of the spinal cord injured patient. J. Am. Diet Assoc. 78:501, 1981.
226. Pelker, R.R., and Dorfman, G.S.: Fracture of the axis associated with vertebral artery injury. Spine 11:622, 1986.
227. Pepin, J.W., and Hawkins, R.J.: Traumatic spondylolisthesis of the axis. Hangman's fracture. Clin. Orthop. 157:133, 1981.
228. Perkash, A., Prakash, V., and Perkash, I.: Experience with management of thromboembolism in patients with spinal cord injury. Part 1. Incidence, diagnosis and role of some risk factors. Paraplegia 16:322, 1978–1979.
229. Perry, J.: The halo in spinal abnormalities. Orthop. Clin. North Am. 3:69, 1972.
230. Perry, J., and Nickel, V.L.: Total cervical spine fusion for neck paralysis. J. Bone Joint Surg. 41A:37, 1959.
231. Perot, P.L., Jr.: The clinical use of somatosensory evoked potentials in spinal cord injury. Clin. Neurosurg. 20:367, 1973.
232. Perret, G., and Greene, J.: Anterior interbody fusion in the treatment of cervical fracture dislocations. Arch. Surg. 96:530, 1968.
233. Petrie, G.J.: Flexion injuries of the cervical spine. J. Bone Joint Surg. 46A:1800, 1964.
234. Piazza, M.R., and Cotler, J.M.: Graft complications in anterior cervical spine reconstructions. Presented at the Federation of Spine Associations Meeting, Feb. 12, 1989, Las Vegas.
235. Pieron, A.P., and Welply, W.R.: Halo traction. J. Bone Joint Surg. 52B:119, 1970.
236. Pizzutillo, P.D., Rocha, E.F., et al.: Bilateral fracture of the pedicle of the second cervical vertebrae in the young child. J. Bone Joint Surg. 68A:892, 1986.
237. Potts, W.J.: The pathology of Charcot joints. Ann. Surg. 86:596, 1927.
238. Prolo, D.J., Runnels, J.B., and Jameson, R.M.: The injured cervical spine. Immediate and long term immobilization with the halo. J.A.M.A. 224:591, 1973.
239. Rabinov, K., and Paulin, S.: Roentgen diagnosis of venous thrombosis in leg. Arch. Surg. 104:134, 1972.
240. Ramadier, J.O., and Bombart, M.: Traitement sanglant et non sanglant des lesions traumatiques du rachis cervical sans lesions nerveuses. Proceedings of the IXth Congress of the International Society of Orthopaedic Surgery and Traumatology, Vienna, 1963.
241. Reed, J.E., Allen, W.E. III, and Dohrman, G.J.: Effect of mannitol on the traumatized spinal cord. Spine 4:319, 1979.
242. Rhoades, C.E., Neff, J.R., et al.: Diagnosis of post-traumatic syringomyelia presenting as neuropathic joints. Clin. Orthop. 180:182, 1983.
243. Ridlon, J., and Berkheiser, E.J.: Neuropathic arthopathies. Charcot spine. J.A.M.A. 79:1467, 1922.
244. Ries, M.D., and Ray, S.: Posterior displacement of an odontoid fracture in a child. Spine 11:1043, 1986.
245. Riggins, R.S., and Kraus, J.F.: The risk of neurologic damage with fractures of the vertebrae. J. Trauma 17:126–133, 1977.
246. Roberts, A., and Wickstrom, J.: Prognosis of odontoid fractures. Proceedings of the American Academy of Orthopaedic Surgeons. J. Bone Joint Surg. 54A:1353, 1972.
247. Robinson, R.A., and Southwick, W.O.: Surgical approaches to the cervical spine. Instructional Course Lectures 17:229, 1960.
248. Rogers, W.A.: Fractures and dislocations of the cervical spine. An end-result study. J. Bone Joint Surg. 39A:341–376, 1957.
249. Rogers, W.A.: Treatment of fracture-dislocation of the cervical spine. J. Bone Joint Surg. 24:245, 1942.
250. Rossi, E.C., Green, D., et al.: Sequential changes in factor VIII and platelets preceding deep vein thrombosis in patients with spinal cord injury. Br. J. Haematol. 45:143, 1980.
251. Rowed, D.W., McLean, J.A., and Tator, C.H.: Somatosensory evoked potentials in acute spinal cord injury: Prognostic value. Surg. Neurol. 9:203, 1978.
252. Roy, L., and Gibson, D.A.: Cervical spine fusions in children. Clin. Orthop. 73:151, 1970.
253. Russell, R.G.G., and Smith, R.: Diphosphonates. Experimental and clinical aspects. J. Bone Joint Surg. 55B:66, 1973.
254. Ryan, M.: Odontoid fractures. A rational approach to treatment. J. Bone Joint Surg. 64B:416, 1982.
255. Ryan, M.D., and Taylor, T.K.F.: Odontoid fractures. J. Bone Joint Surg. 64B:416, 1982.
256. Schatzker, J., Rorabeck, C.H., and Waddell, J.P.: Fracture of the dens. An analysis of thirty-seven cases. J. Bone Joint Surg. 53B:392, 1971.
257. Scher, A.T.: Trauma of the spinal cord in children. South Afr. Med. J. 50:2023, 1976.
258. Schneider, R.C., Cherry, G., and Pautek, H.: The syndrome of acute central cervical cord injury with special reference to the mechanism involved in hyperextension injuries of the cervical spine. J. Neurosurg. 11:546, 1954.
259. Schneider, R.C., and Schemm, G.W.: Vertebral artery insufficiency in acute and chronic spinal trauma. J. Neurosurg. 18:348, 1961.
260. Schweigel, J.S.: Halo-thoracic brace management of the odontoid process. Spine 4:192, 1979.
261. Schweigel, J.S.: Management of the odontoid fracture with halo-thoracic bracing. Spine 12:838, 1987.
262. Segal, L.S., Grimm, J.O., and Stauffer, E.S.: Non-union of fractures of the atlas. J. Bone Joint Surg. 69A:1423, 1987.
263. Seimon, L.P.: Fracture of the odontoid process in young children. J. Bone Joint Surg. 59A:943, 1977.
264. Senter, H.J., and Venes, J.L.: Loss of autoregulation and posttraumatic ischemia following experimental spinal cord trauma. J. Neurosurg. 50:198, 1979.

265. Shanks, S.C., and Kerley, P.: *A Textbook of X-Ray Diagnosis.* Philadelphia, W.B. Saunders Company, 1959.

266. Shenkin, H.A.: The use of mannitol for the reduction of intracranial surgery. J. Neurosurg. *19*:897, 1962.

267. Sherk, H.H., Nicholson, J.T., and Chung, S.M.: Fractures of the odontoid process in young children. J. Bone Joint Surg. *60A*:921, 1978.

268. Sherk, H.H., and Nicholson, J.T.: Fractures of the atlas. J. Bone Joint Surg. *52A*:1017, 1970.

269. Sherk, H.H., Schut, L., and Lane, J.M.: Fractures and dislocations of the cervical spine in children. Orthop. Clin. North Am. *7*:593, 1976.

270. Siegal, T., Petah, T., and Siegal, T.: Vertebral body resection for epidural compression by malignant tumors. J. Bone Joint Surg. *67A*:375, 1985.

271. Shields, C.L., and Stauffer, E.S.: Late instability in cervical spine fractures secondary to laminectomy. Clin. Orthop. *119*:144, 1976.

272. Shulman, S.T., Madden, J.D., et al.: Transection of spinal cord. A rare obstetrical complication of cephalic delivery. Arch. Dis. Child. *46*:291, 1971.

273. Silver, J.R., and Gibbon, N.O.K.: Prognosis in tetraplegia. Br. Med. J. *4*:79, 1968.

274. Sim, F.H., Svien, H.J., et al: Swan neck deformity following extensive cervical laminectomy. A review of twenty-one cases. J. Bone Joint Surg. *56A*:564, 1974.

275. Sinh, G., and Pandya, S.K.: Treatment of congenital atlantoaxial dislocations. Proc. Aust. Assoc. Neurol. *5*:507, 1968.

276. Slabaugh, P.B., and Smith, T.K.: Neuropathic spine after spinal cord injury: A case report. J. Bone Joint Surg. *60A*:605, 1978.

277. Spence, K.F., Decker, S., and Sell, K.W.: Bursting atlantal fracture associated with rupture of the transverse ligament. J. Bone Joint Surg. *52A*:543, 1970.

278. Stauffer, E.S., and Kelly, E.G.: Fracture-dislocation of the cervical spine. Instability and recurrent deformity following treatment by anterior interbody fusion. J. Bone Joint Surg. *59A*:45, 1977.

279. Stabler, C.L., Eismont, F.J., et al.: Failure of posterior cervical fusions using cadaveric bone graft in children. J. Bone Joint Surg. *67A*:370, 1985.

280. Stauffer, E.S.: Fractures and dislocations of the spine. Part 1: The cervical spine. In: Rockwood, C.R., and Green, D.P. (eds.): *Fractures in Adults.* Philadelphia, J.B. Lippincott Company, 1984.

281. Stauffer, E.S., Wood, R.W., et al.: Gunshot wounds of the spine: The effects of laminectomy. J. Bone Joint Surg. *61A*:389, 1979.

282. Steel, H.H.: Anatomical and mechanical considerations of the atlanto-axial articulations. Proceedings of the American Orthopaedic Association. J. Bone Joint Surg. *50A*:1481, 1968.

283. Soto-Hall, R., and Haldeman, K.O.: The diagnosis of neuropathic joint disease: An analysis of 40 cases. J.A.M.A. *114*:2076, 1940.

284. Southwick, W.O.: Management of fractures of the dens: Current concept review. J. Bone Joint Surg. *62A*:482, 1980.

285. Stone, D.J., and Keltz, H.: The effect of respiratory muscle dysfunction on pulmonary function. Am. Rev. Respir. Dis. *88*:621, 1963.

286. Stover, S.L., Fine, P.R., et al.: University of Alabama in Birmingham Spinal Cord Injury Data Management Service. Quarterly Report for the Period March 1, 1983, through June 30, 1983, pp. 21, 22.

287. Stover, S.L., Lloyd, K., et al.: Urinary tract infection in spinal cord injury. Arch. Phys. Med. Rehabil. *70*:47, 1989.

288. Stover, S.L., Niemann, K.M.W., and Miller, J.M. II: Disodium etidronate in the prevention of postoperative recurrence of heterotopic ossification in spinal cord injured patients. J. Bone Joint Surg. *58A*:683, 1976.

289. Sullivan, C.R., Bruwer, A.J., and Harris, L.E.: Hypermobility of the cervical spine in children. A pitfall in the diagnosis of cervical dislocation. Am. J. Surg. *95*:636, 1958.

290. Swischuk, L.E.: Spine and spinal cord trauma in the battered child syndrome. Radiology *92*:733, 1969.

291. Tachdijian, M.O., and Matson, D.D.: Orthopaedic aspects of intraspinal tumors in infants and children. J. Bone Joint Surg. *47A*:223, 1965.

292. Tarlov, I.M.: Acute spinal cord compression paralysis. J. Neurosurg. *36*:10, 1972.

293. Termansen, N.B.: Hangman's fracture. Acta Orthop. Scand. *45*:529, 1974.

294. Tibone, J., Sakimura, I., et al.: Heterotopic ossification around the hip in spinal cord injured patients. J. Bone Joint Surg. *60A*:769, 1978.

295. Tindall, G.T., Flanagan, J.F., and Nashold, B.S., Jr.: Brain abscess and osteomyelitis following skull traction. Arch. Surg. *79*:638, 1959.

296. Theodore, J., and Robin, E.D.: Speculations on neurogenic pulmonary edema. Am. Rev. Respir. Dis. *113*:405, 1976.

297. Tredwell, S.J., and O'Brien, J.P.: Apophyseal joint degeneration in the cervical spine following halo-pelvic distraction. Spine *5*:497, 1980.

298. Tribe, C.R.: Causes of death in early and late stages of paraplegia. Paraplegia *1*:19, 1963.

299. Towbin, A.: Spinal injury related to the syndrome of sudden death in infants. Am. J. Clin. Pathol. *49*:562, 1968.

300. Townsend, F.H. Jr., Rowe, M.L.: Mobility of the upper cervical spine in health and disease. Pediatrics *10*:567, 1952.

301. Troll, G.F., and Dohrmann, G.J.: Anaesthesia of the spinal cord injured patient. Cardiovascular problems and their management. Paraplegia *13*:162, 1975.

302. Van Den Bout, A.H., and Dommisse, G.F.: Traumatic atlantooccipital dislocation. Spine *11*:174, 1986.

303. Vernon, J.D., et al.: Post-traumatic syringomyelia: The results of surgery. Paraplegia *21*:37, 1983.

304. Vernon, J.D., Silver, J.R., and Ohry, A.: Post-traumatic syringomyelia. Paraplegia *20*:339, 1982.

305. Vigoroux, R.P., Baurance, C., Choux, M., et al.: Injuries of the cervical spine in children. Neurochir. *14*:689, 1968.

306. Wadia, N.H.: Myelopathy complicating congenital atlanto-axial dislcoation. Brain 90:449, 1967.

307. Wang, G.J., Mabie, K.N., et al.: The non-surgical management of odontoid fractures in adults. Spine 9:229, 1984.

308. Watson, N.: Anti-coagulant therapy in prevention of venous thrombosis and pulmonary embolism in spinal cord injury. Paraplegia 16:265, 1978–1979.

309. Watson, N.: Ascending cystic degeneration of the cord after spinal cord injury. Paraplegia 19:89, 1981.

310. Webb, J.K., Broughton, B.K., et al.: Hidden flexion injury of the cervical spine. J. Bone Joint Surg. 58B:322, 1976.

311. Weir, D.C.: Roentgenographic signs of cervical injury. Clin. Orthop. 109:9, 1975.

312. Welch, C.E.: Abdominal surgery. N. Engl. J. Med. 284:424, 1971.

313. Werne, S.: Studies in spontaneous atlas dislocation. Acta Orthop. Scand. 23, 1957.

314. Wetzel, J.: Spinal cord injury. Clin. Phys. Ther. 6:75–98, 1985.

315. Wharton, G.W.: Heterotopic ossification. Clin. Orthop. 112:142, 1975.

316. Wharton, G.W., and Morgan, T.H.: Ankylosis in the paralyzed patient. J. Bone Joint Surg. 52A:105, 1970.

317. White, A.A., and Panjabi, M.M.: *Clinical Biomechanics of the Spine*. Philadelphia, J.B. Lippincott Company, 1978, p. 225.

318. White, A.A. III, Southwick, W.O., et al.: Practical biomechanics of the spine for the orthopaedic surgeon. In Instructional Course Lectures. St. Louis, C.V. Mosby, 23:62, 1974.

319. White, A.A., Southwick, W.O., and Panjabi, M.M.: Clinical instability in the lower cervical spine. Spine 1:15, 1976.

320. White, R.J.: Current status of spinal cord cooling. Clin. Neurosurg. 20:400, 1973.

321. Whitehall, R., Richman, J.A., and Glaser, J.A.: Failure of immobilization of the cervical spine by the halo vest. J. Bone Joint Surg. 68A:326, 1986.

322. Wholey, M.H., Bruwer, A.J., and Baker, H.L., Jr.: The lateral roentgenogram of the neck. Radiology 71:350, 1958.

323. Wiesel, S.W., and Rothman, R.H.: Occipitoatlantal hypermobility. Spine 4:187, 1979.

324. Willard, D.P., and Nicholson, J.T.: Dislocation of the first cervical vertebra. Ann. Surg. 113:464, 1941.

325. Williams, B., Terry, A., et al.: Syringomyelia as a sequel to traumatic paraplegia. Paraplegia 19:67, 1981.

326. Williams, T.G.: Hangman's fracture. J. Bone Joint Surg. 57B:82, 1975.

327. Wilson, M.J., Michele, A.A., and Jacobson, E.W.: Spontaneous dislocation of the atlanto-axial articulation. J. Bone Joint Surg. 22:698, 1940.

328. Winslow, E.B.J., Lesch, M., et al.: Spinal cord injuries associated with cardiopulmonary complications. Spine 11:809, 1986.

329. Wise, B.L., and Chater, N.: The value of hypertonic mannitol solution in decreasing brain mass and lowering cerebrospinal fluid pressure. J. Neurosurg. 19:1038, 1962.

330. Wood Jones, F.: The examination of the bodies of 100 men executed in Nubia in Roman times. Br. Med. J. 1:736, 1908.

331. Wood Jones, F.: The ideal lesion produced by judical hanging. Lancet 1:53, 1913.

332. Yeo, J.D., Lowry, C., and McKenzie, B.: Preliminary report on ten patients with spinal cord injuries treated with hyperbaric oxygen. Med. J. Aust. 2:572, 1978.

333. Yeo, J.D., Stabback, S., and McKenzie, B.: A study of the effects of hyperbaric oxygen on the experimental spinal cord injury. Med. J. Aust. 2:145, 1977.

334. Zigler, J.E., Waters, R.L., et al.: Occipito-cervico-thoracic spine fusion in a patient with occipto-cervical dislocation and survival. Spine 11:645, 1986.

SEVEN

Complications of Treatment of Fractures and Dislocations of the Thoracolumbar Spine

Howard S. An, M.D.

Jerome M. Cotler, M.D.

Richard A. Balderston, M.D.

The treatment of unstable fractures and fracture-dislocations of the thoracolumbar and lumbar spine remains a controversial topic despite numerous publications advocating various treatment modalities.[7, 8, 19, 23, 27, 47, 97, 113, 126, 130, 136] A sound understanding of the anatomy of the thoracic and lumbar vertebrae, the concept of stability, pathomechanics of injury, and pathoanatomy of neural structures is vitally important in the proper management of these injuries.

Anatomically, the thoracic spine has a smaller canal diameter, which accounts for a high percentage of associated neurological deficits in this region. Because the thoracic spine is inherently stable owing to its attachment to the ribs, it takes a significantly high-energy trauma to produce a fracture-dislocation at the thoracic level.[13, 137] On the other hand, the thoracolumbar junction is relatively more susceptible to injury owing to its inherent junctional instability and stress concentration. It is important to appreciate that neurological deficits incurred at the thoracolumbar junction may be due to damage to the conus medullaris or injuries of the nerve roots or the cauda equina.[64] Unstable fractures of the low lumbar spine represent an uncommon injury.[3, 3a, 48] The lumbar spine has a larger mass and greater spinal canal diameter, which account for infrequently associated neural impairment. The cauda equina in the lumbar spine is also more resistant to extrinsic pressure than the conus

medullaris at the thoracolumbar region.[61] In addition, normal lordotic configuration of the lumbar spine decreases the tendency for the vertebrae to assume a kyphotic configuration.

The anatomical distinction between the thoracic and lumbar vertebrae is also important in terms of associated injuries. Hemothorax, pneumothorax, ruptured diaphragm, fractured ribs, cardiac tamponade, and injury to the great vessels are typical injuries associated with a thoracic fracture.[102, 106, 107] Abdominal visceral injuries are more frequently associated with lumbar fractures, particularly with seat-belt injuries. Careful assessment of associated injuries is obviously important.

Spinal stability is a difficult concept to comprehend, but its understanding has been expanded over the last two decades.[25, 64, 99, 137] The concept of a burst fracture was first described by Holdsworth in 1970 and was thought to represent a stable injury with intact anterior and posterior ligamentous complexes.[64] However, in 1983 Denis described such injuries of the thoracolumbar junction as unstable with structural damage to two of the three spinal columns.[25] Similarly, McAfee and associates expounded on the concept of the unstable burst fracture.[99] The criteria for instability included vertebral height loss greater than 50 per cent kyphosis progressing beyond 20 degrees, the disruption of the posterior column, and the presence of a neurological deficit.[99] Ferguson and Allen's mechanistic classification provided a better understanding of the mechanism of injury, which is important in the selection of appropriate treatment.[41]

The treatment of unstable thoracolumbar fractures depends greatly on the patient's neurological status. Most authors agree that decompression and stabilization are necessary in patients with partial neurological deficits.[9, 16, 37, 44, 51, 119] Also, there is little controversy about the necessity of early stabilization and rehabilitation for patients with complete neurological deficits.[13, 14, 127] Most authors agree that surgery to decompress a complete injury is not indicated in the thoracolumbar region, as decompression does not alter the course of neurological outcomes in these patients.[13, 15, 113]

However, it is not clear whether decompression or stabilization is beneficial in the absence of neurological deficit. Numerous reports cite relatively good long-term outcomes after conservative treatment.[62, 71, 81, 136] Conservative treatment is particularly appropriate in patients with low lumbar burst fractures unless there is a need to mobilize the patient early.[3, 3a, 24, 48] However, there seems to be a recent trend toward early stabilization without direct decompression for patients with unstable thoracolumbar fractures and intact neurological status.[27, 33, 140] Denis and associates reported 52 patients with acute thoracolumbar burst fractures in the absence of neurological deficit, comparing operative (13 patients) and nonoperative (39 patients) treatment.[27] Of the patients in the nonoperative group, 17 per cent developed neurological problems, and 25 per cent were unable to return to work. On the other hand, operative patients fared significantly better in terms of neurological stability, return to work, and deformity.[27] The treatment of these patients by early open reduction, fusion, and instrumentation also reduces the period of immobilization and hospitalization.[140] Recently, Edwards followed 15 patients with a canal compromise documented by CT scan and concluded that residual retropulsed fragments gradually resorb if posterior instrumentation provides spine realignment and solid fusion.[35] It is our view that direct decompression is not necessary unless the retropulsed fragment is causing neurological symptoms.

There have been other reports on early stabilization and fusion for patients with unstable fractures with or without neurological deficits.[9, 16, 27, 63, 65, 140] The advantages of operative reduction and stabilization of thoracolumbar fractures have been well substantiated.[31, 32, 65,] [66, 113] Operative treatment allows earlier ambulation and anatomical fracture reduction and, at times, improves neurological outcome. These advantages are especially important in the patient with neurological compromise or in the patient with an unstable fracture with complete three-column disruption. It has generally become accepted in the recent literature that operative intervention in the form of stabilization with or without decompression is the treatment of choice in many of these injuries.

The exact methods of decompression and stabilization are different from one author to another. Controversy prevails on the issue of anterior versus posterior approach for patients with an incomplete spinal cord injury.[9, 12, 13, 23, 33, 56, 84, 97, 119] We prefer to perform a posterior distraction instrumentation first and to consider posterolateral or anterior decompression if necessary. The quality of reduction following distraction instrumentation may be assessed by laminotomy,[44, 51] myelogram,[33] intraoperative ultrasound,[9, 36, 101, 103, 116, 135] or postoperative CT scans.[51]

The decision as to whether operative intervention is necessary also depends on many other factors. Patients who have a loss of vertebral height of more than 50 per cent usually have an unacceptable outcome from conservative treatment.[62, 100] Also, those patients with a failure of the posterior column in tension tend to have an unsatisfactory result from nonoperative care. Subluxations and dislocations that are purely ligamentous also have a poor treatment outcome without surgery. Conservative treatment by reduction and casting is appropriate for flexion-distraction injuries that involve the bone and for flexion-compression injuries without significant middle-column disruption. Conservative treatment may also be appropriate in the low lumbar region even with middle-column disruption as long as lumbar lordosis and neurological protection can be maintained with recumbency and casting.[3, 3a, 24, 48] Translational injuries and three-column disruptions require fusion. Patients who require rapid mobilization, such as multiple trauma victims and older patients, should be stabilized early to prevent complications associated with prolonged bedrest.

In this chapter, pitfalls and complications related to the management of patients with thoracolumbar fractures will be discussed. General complications associated with spinal cord injury have been discussed under cervical spine injuries.

PREOPERATIVE PLANNING

Proper preoperative management is important in decreasing the overall morbidity of patients with unstable thoracolumbar fractures. Acute complications associated with thoracolumbar fractures can be neurological, orthopedic, or medical in nature.

Neurological deterioration following hospitalization for spinal cord injury is relatively uncommon. Marshall and coworkers reported 14 out of 283 patients, or 4.9 per cent, with spinal cord injury who deteriorated neurologically during acute hospital management.[94] Five of these patients had a tho columbar fracture. In 12 of the 14 patients, the decline in neurological function was associated with a specific management event such as application of halo-vest, skeletal traction, or Stryker frame rotation.[94] This underscores the importance of meticulous repeated documentations of the neurological status and careful moving and transporting of the patient.

Neurological deterioration may also be due to ascending myelopathy.[107] Although the exact pathogenesis of this phenomenon is unknown, it may involve spinal cord ischemia owing to the disruption of the artery of Adamkiewicz, which is most frequently found at T10 on the left side.[107] Slower progressive neurological deterioration may be due to the extension of cord edema. Use of corticosteriods and mannitol may be justified in these cases.[107]

Occult conus injury may be easily overlooked, as many patients have a urinary catheter prior to complete assessment of sphincter function. Postvoiding urinary volumes should be recorded in all cases. Preoperative urodynamic studies are helpful in doubtful cases. Failure to accurately document the neurological status may result in a distressing legal conflict.

Herniated disc material, spinal epidural hematoma,[46, 52, 58] pseudomeningocele,[72] or infection[90] causing neurological deterioration is rare, but these entities must be suspected and diagnosed if the cause of neurological deterioration is not clear. Magnetic resonance imaging can be helpful in diagnosing epidural hematoma, herniated disc, or extent of spinal cord hemorrhage or edema.[22]

Neurological deterioration may be related to the lack of proper orthopedic management of patients with thoracolumbar fractures. A fracture may be totally missed, particularly in a patient with multiple injuries, intoxication, decreased level of consciousness, ankylosing spondylitis, and osteoporosis.[4, 117, 131, 134] Multiple noncontiguous injuries of the spine are common and are easily overlooked.[4, 87, 131] Vertebral malalignment should be reduced as soon as possible with halo-femoral traction. Acute medical complications may be of pulmonary, cardiovascular, gastrointestinal, genitourinary, cutaneous, or metabolic origins (Table 7–1). A team of physicians and nurses in a spinal cord injury center is of great value in taking care of these complicated problems.

OPERATIVE TECHNIQUES

The exact methods of decompression and stabilization vary among different authors. Understanding the mechanism of injury is the key to the proper selection of a specific treatment

---

Table 7–1
Acute Medical Complications in Patients with Thoracolumbar Fractures

PULMONARY COMPLICATIONS
Atelectasis
Pneumonia
Pulmonary embolism
Pleural effusion
Hemothorax
Pulmonary edema

CARDIOVASCULAR COMPLICATIONS
Cardiac arrhythmia
Myocardial infarction
Cardiac tamponade
Deep vein thrombosis
Aortic dissection or dilatation
Autonomic dysreflexia

GENITOURINARY COMPLICATIONS
Urinary tract infection
Renal calculus

GASTROINTESTINAL COMPLICATIONS
Stress ulcer
Paralytic ileus
Abdominal obstruction
Pancreatitis

CUTANEOUS COMPLICATIONS
Pressure sores
Cellulitis

ENDOCRINE-METABOLIC-NUTRITIONAL COMPLICATIONS
Calcium and phosphate imbalance
Sodium and potassium imbalance
Acid-base imbalance
Hypoalbuminemia

method.[23, 41] Compression-flexion injuries are best treated with distraction instrumentation as the nature of the problem is failure of the anterior and middle columns in compression. Compression-flexion injuries typically produce loss of vertebral heights and localized kyphosis (Fig. 7–1A). The retropulsed fragment is almost always situated at the level of the pedicles (Fig. 7–1B). The distal half of the vertebra is usually split sagittally (Fig. 7–1C). The distraction flexion injuries with failure of the middle column in tension leave the middle column resistant to compression, and thus the use of compression instrumentation for these fractures is appropriate.[53, 57] Occasionally, distraction-flexion injuries may produce an incomplete cord injury from canal impingement by bone or disc material.[53, 86] In these cases, dis-

traction instrumentation that imparts significant extension is recommended instead of compression instrumentation for fear of producing neurological deterioration.[53, 86] Lateral flexion injuries are treated best with distraction instrumentation as are vertical compression injuries, should surgery be required. Translational injuries and torsional flexion injuries are extremely unstable, and overdistraction must be avoided. Segmentally wired Luque instrumentation is quite appropriate for these injuries.[91]

Stabilization of low lumbar burst fractures deserves special consideration as instrumentation and fusion in this region carry an increased risk of back pain or flat back syndrome.[3, 60, 82] To circumvent problems of back pain associated with long fusion masses in the lumbar spine, pedicular screw systems are now receiv-

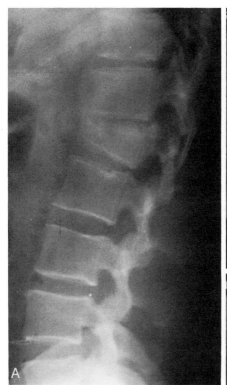

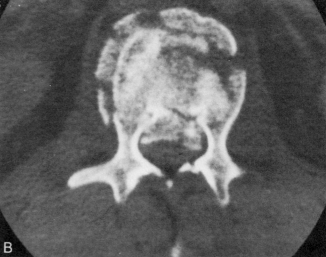

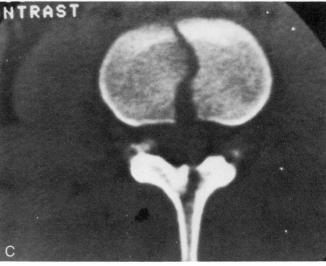

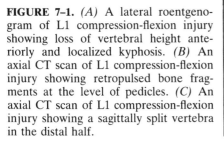

FIGURE 7–1. *(A)* A lateral roentgenogram of L1 compression-flexion injury showing loss of vertebral height anteriorly and localized kyphosis. *(B)* An axial CT scan of L1 compression-flexion injury showing retropulsed bone fragments at the level of pedicles. *(C)* An axial CT scan of L1 compression-flexion injury showing a sagittally split vertebra in the distal half.

ing much attention. Systems developed by Roy-Camille,[78, 123, 124] Steffee,[3, 128] and others have been demonstrated to provide rigid fixation of the lumbar spine. These systems, however, have minimal reduction capacity and depend more on postural reduction of the fracture. The modular spine system developed by Edwards, Cotrel-Dubousset instrumentation, and the fixateur interne by Dick are attractive since both distraction and extension moments can be applied, reducing the fracture, and restoring height and sagittal contours.[1, 10, 30, 34, 40, 74] All pedicular systems have been shown to provide rigid fixation. Generally, single motion segment immobilization and fusion above and below the injured vertebrae are adequate, provided that postoperative cast or brace support is used. We would like to emphasize the importance of postoperative external immobilization with cast or orthosis, as the potential problems from the absence of external immobilization significantly outweigh any possible ill effects from wearing an orthosis, except in those patients with decreased sensation.

Primary anterior decompression and fusion with or without anterior instrumentation may be valid in cases where a large midline retropulsed fragment is found in a patient with incomplete spinal cord injury.[11, 75, 80, 97] A secondary posterior procedure is recommended if ligamentous disruption is evident posteriorly.

POSTERIOR INSTRUMENTATIONS

The technique of Harrington distraction instrumentation has been discussed in the chapter on scoliosis. We will mention pertinent points that are relevant to thoracolumbar fractures.

Positioning is done on the four-poster or Relton-Hall frame. Postural reduction of the kyphotic deformity is aided by slightly raising the heights of the inferior posters and extending the legs. Gentle technique and care must be exercised during exposure of the posterior elements to prevent mechanical injury to the spinal cord. If laminar fractures were identified preoperatively by CT scans, added caution should be exercised during the subperiosteal exposure. Laminar fractures are frequently associated with traumatic dural tears or pseudomeningocele.[20, 72] Sublaminar wires are used to enhance the overall stability, particularly if the posterior column is disrupted.[17, 50, 98, 105, 129] Sublaminar wires should not be placed around the injured segment, as cord swelling leaves less

space for safe wire passage.[34] Interspinous wires with Wisconsin buttons may be used instead of sublaminar wires, recognizing that they provide less stability. The instrumentation is applied three segments above and two segments below the injured level. Purcell and associates tested 13 cadaver spinal segments and recommended the use of Harrington distraction rods by stabilizing three laminae above and two laminae below the point of instability. This construct provides additional stability against flexion mode by reducing the tendency for the upper hooks to back out during vertebral tilting.[115] We favor using square-ended Moe rods with Edwards' anatomical hooks or bifid pedicle hooks, since the plain, round-ended rods with plain or ribbed hooks provide less stability[28, 33, 49] (Fig. 7–2). Overdistraction must be avoided, particularly in cases where

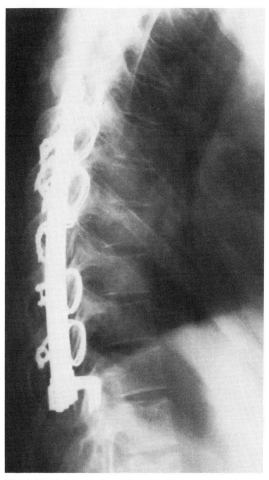

FIGURE 7–2. Postoperative roentgenogram of a patient with T8 burst fracture who underwent Moe rodding and fusion with Edwards' anatomical hooks and sublaminar wires.

the anterior longitudinal ligament is torn. Translational displacement or rotational injury is usually accompanied by disruption of the anterior longitudinal ligament. Magnetic resonance imaging is also helpful in defining the status of the anterior longitudinal ligament. In doubtful cases, two parallel K-wires may be inserted onto the spinous processes during surgery. If the anterior longitudinal ligament is torn, the wires will move apart in parallel planes rather than divergently during distraction maneuver.[5] A wire may be looped around the spinous processes prior to distraction if a potential problem of overdistraction is anticipated.[45] The rod should be bent to restore lumbar lordosis.[2, 29] The top of the rod should be contoured into a slight kyphosis to prevent dislodgement of the upper hook. Since the rod-ratchet junction is vulnerable to fatigue failure, the rod should be applied so that only two or three ratchets should be showing. C-washers are applied routinely. Furthermore, stabilizing transverse traction devices may be used.[40] A double transverse wire, Cotrel-Dubousset transverse device, or other cross-linking systems are known to significantly enhance the overall stability of surgical construct. Fusion with meticulous decortication and autogenous bone grafting is performed along the entire length of the instrumentation. The rods are not routinely removed.

The concept of "rod long and fuse short" was introduced by Jacobs, who believed that more stable constructs can be obtained by longer rods and spinal motion can be restored by short fusion and removing the rods later.[65, 66] There are potential problems with this approach. First, the facet joints undergo degeneration after prolonged immobilization, and arthritic pain and spinal stiffness may ensue.[60, 73] Also, early implant failures may occur as a result of motion at the nonfused segments. Osti and associates noted 48 per cent implant problems in patients with thoracolumbar fractures who had Harrington instrumentation without fusion.[114] Recurrence of deformity may also result after the hardware is removed.[60, 69, 108, 140] Furthermore, a second surgery to remove the rods may bring about additional morbidity to the patient.

Other modified distraction systems include the locking hook with contoured rod,[67, 68] Edwards' rod-sleeve,[33] and the Cotrel-Dubousset system. Early clinical results are encouraging using these systems. Edwards' rod-sleeve stabilization is particularly impressive in its ability to restore the spinal canal diameter and to

maintain correction.[33] When using the Cotrel-Dubousset instrumentation for axial instability, at least two segments above and two segments below should be stabilized, while stabilization of only one segment above and below the site of instability is adequate for rotational instability.[40] Combined use of pedicle screws and hooks is possible with the Cotrel-Dubousset and Edwards' universal systems, and a minimum number of segments can undergo instrumentation and fusion.

Compression instrumentation may be used in flexion-distraction injuries as mentioned before.[53] Also, in cases where primary anterior decompression and strut grafting have been performed, compression instrumentation can provide an effective posterior stabilization, fusing only one level above and below the injury. In addition, compression instrumentation following anterior procedure enhances the stability of the anterior strut graft. Harrington compression rods, Wisconsin compression system,[76] Edwards' reverse ratchet rods, Edwards' universal rods, or Cotrel-Dubousset rods can be used as compression devices. One must avoid the use of sublaminar wires along with compression devices, as the hooks may migrate anteriorly with wire tightening.[122]

Luque rods with sublaminar wires should be reserved for fracture/dislocations or translational injuries, as these rods and segmental wires do not provide resistance to axial forces. Late settling of burst fractures is a frequent complication with Luque rod fixation. These rods provide a stiff construct for very unstable fracture/dislocations or translational injuries.[91] We prefer using rectangular Luque rods over the original L-rods, which are slightly more cumbersome to insert and less stable.[43] The neural canal of the thoracic vertebrae is narrow, and great care must be exercised when passing sublaminar wires. Doubled Luque wires of 16 gauge are passed at each level, spanning three segments above and three segments below the site of instability. Sagittal contouring of the rods is obviously important.

The technique of transpedicular instrumentation has been discussed in the chapter on spondylolisthesis.[30, 39, 123, 128] The major advantage of pedicular instrumentation systems is fusing a minimum number of segments in the lumbar region. Recently, transpedicular instrumentation has been applied in the thoracolumbar junction as well[30, 39, 123] (Fig. 7–3A,B). Thorough knowledge of pedicular anatomy and identification of pedicular landmarks are important in the prevention of complications

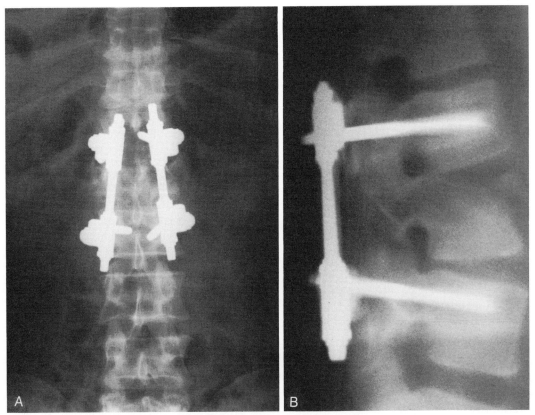

FIGURE 7–3. *(A)* Anteroposterior roentgenogram of a patient with L1 burst fracture who underwent AO fixateur interne instrumentation and fusion. *(B)* Lateral tomogram of this patient revealing the restoration of vertebral height and lordosis.

such as neural injury, pedicle fracture, and loss of fixation.[138]

NEURAL DECOMPRESSION

Restoration of spinal canal diameter is the most important part of the surgical procedure in the patient with an incomplete cord injury. Frequently, the distraction-hyperextension maneuver by spinal instrumentation will indirectly restore the spinal canal diameter.[33, 63, 133] Options for direct decompression include posterolateral decompression,[12, 84] transpedicular decompression,[44, 51] or anterior decompression.[97, 119, 139] Gertzbein and coworkers studied 60 consecutive patients and found no apparent difference between the degree of body encroachment of the spinal canal and the initial Frankel grade, nor was there a significant difference between those patients undergoing anterior versus posterior surgery.[55] Herndon and Galloway reported on 24 patients with incomplete spinal cord injuries and concluded that there was no correlation between neuro-

logical improvement and the amount of spinal canal encroachment.[63] Edwards and Levine believe that the presence of residual bone filling up to one-third of the canal has no effect on neural recovery, as long as vertebral height and lordosis are restored by posterior instrumentation.[34]

On the other hand, neural recovery has been observed in many patients following direct decompression even in chronic cases.[92, 93, 97] Hashimoto and associates studied the relationship between the traumatic spinal canal stenosis and neurological deficits in 112 consecutive patients and concluded that there is a definite relationship between the degree of stenosis and neurological deficit.[61] Furthermore, the relationship between the percentage of canal compromise and the presence of neurological deficit varies depending on the level of the fracture. Burst fractures having the following amounts of canal compromise were at significant risk of neurological involvement; at T11-T12, 35 per cent or more; at L1, 45 per cent or more; and at L2 and below, 55 per cent or more.[61] We are of the opinion that direct decompression is not justified in patients with normal neurological function, particularly if the canal compromise is less than 35 per cent at T11–L1 and less than 50 per cent at L2 and below. Remodeling of the spinal canal has been observed in patients who had initial canal compromise with thoracolumbar fractures.[42, 81] However, we believe that the canal diameter should be restored to near normal in patients with incomplete spinal cord injuries in order to provide the environment for maximal spinal cord recovery.

Laminectomy is contraindicated in most cases of thoracolumbar fractures in that it destabilizes the spine further without added benefits.[16, 19, 104, 132] Tencer and associates studied cadaveric spines that were prepared with a transducer device pushed into the canal to simulate the compressive effect of retropulsed bone on the spinal cord.[132] It was found that laminectomy has no decompressive effect on the spinal cord with up to 35 per cent occlusion of the spinal canal.[132] There have been numerous clinical cases that demonstrated the negative effects of laminectomy. If a laminectomy has been performed for an unusual reason, posterior instrumentation and fusion must accompany it to prevent the development of a kyphotic deformity.

Transpedicular or posterolateral decompression is relatively safe and effective in the lumbar region below the conus medullaris level. The anatomy of the retropulsed fragment must be carefully studied preoperatively.[77] A large midline retropulsed fragment often requires a bilateral transpedicular approach to adequately restore the spinal canal diameter.

Anterior retroperitoneal approach is the preferred method of decompression if a large midline retropulsed fragment is persistent after posterior instrumentation. If the retropulsed fragment is lodged to one side adjacent to the pedicle, a transpedicular or posterolateral approach is preferred.

Transpedicular or posterolateral decompression has been described in the literature.[37, 44, 51] A laminotomy is made at the level of the pedicle by taking down the inferior lamina of the vertebra above and superior lamina below. The retropulsed bone is almost always at the level of the pedicle. The pedicle and the transverse process are taken down with a burr. A reversed angle curette or a special impactor is placed lateral and anterior to the dura to allow safe tamping of the retropulsed fragment.[51, 112]

Prior to tamping, the vertebral body should be burred from a posterolateral direction in order to create a space for the retropulsed fragment to be pushed back. Bilateral approach may be necessary in selected cases. The cauda equina or roots may be gently retracted, but the spinal cord should never be retracted during this procedure.

Primary anterior decompression is preferred if the retropulsed fragment is large and located in the midline in a patient with incomplete neurological deficit or if the fracture is more than two weeks old.[14, 70, 97, 107] Secondary anterior decompression should also be done if there is persistent canal compromise following posterior instrumentation in a patient with an incomplete cord syndrome.[9, 16, 119] The patient is placed in the right lateral decubitus position, with the twelfth rib centered over the hinged portion of the operating table[97] (Fig. 7–4A). The skin incision is make along the twelfth rib from the costotransverse junction to 6 inches anterior to the tip of the twelfth rib. Divide muscle layers with electrocautery to the surface of the twelfth rib. Take care to protect the subcostal nerve and vessels. Disarticulate the rib at the costotransverse attachment, leaving it attached anteriorly. Attached to the tip of the twelfth rib is the diaphragm superiorly and the transverse abdominis musculature and fascia inferiorly. While removing the rib, split the cartilaginous tissue on the tip of the twelfth rib, and retract the diaphragmatic insertion cephalad and the abdominal musculature caudad. Identify the foamy fat of the retroperitoneal space. The retroperitoneal space is then bluntly dissected by sweeping the peritoneum from the undersurface of the abdominal wall and sweeping the pleura proximally. This maneuver exposes the left crus of the diaphragm and the psoas muscle. The disc spaces are prominent, whereas the vertebral bodies are shallow where the segmental vessels cross. The segmental vessels at the affected levels are carefully identified and tied in the midportion of the vertebral bodies. Follow the twelfth intercostal nerve toward the thecal sac, and remove the pedicle to expose the lateral wall of the thecal sac in case of L1 decompression (Fig. 7–4B). The disc material above and below the fractured level is removed, followed by removal of the retropulsed fragment. Epidural bleeding can be controlled by bipolar cautery. A headlight, magnification loupe, and power burr are essential equipment during decompression.

Strut fusion technique is performed by mak-

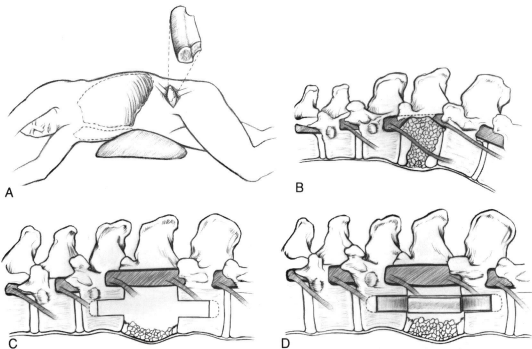

FIGURE 7–4. *(A)* The retroperitoneal approach to the first lumbar vertebra from the left through an incision overlying the twelfth rib. *(B)* Tracing the intercostal nerve leads to the dural sac. Removal of the pedicle exposes the retropulsed fragment in the anterior aspect of the spinal canal. *(C)* Using a high-speed burr, the retropulsed fragment is thinned and removed away from the spinal cord. *(D)* An iliac crest tricortical strut graft is placed from the upper end-plate of superior vertebra and inferior end-plate of inferior vertebra. (Modified from McAfee, P. C., Bohlman, H. H., and Yuan, H. A.: Anterior decompression of traumatic thoracolumbar fractures with incomplete neurological deficit using retroperitoneal approach. J. Bone Joint Surg. *67A:89*, 1985.)

ing a trough in the body of the T12 vertebra up to the upper end-plate and in the body of the L2 vertebra to the lower end-plate[21] (Fig. 7–4C). The iliac strut graft should extend from the upper end-plate of the T12 vertebrae to the lower end-plate of the L2 vertebra for maximum stability (Fig. 7–4D). After insertion of the tricortical graft, the operating table is flexed back to the neutral position in order to lock the graft in place.

POSTOPERATIVE COMPLICATIONS

Despite careful preoperative planning and meticulous surgery, complications do occur postoperatively (Table 7–2). Early recognition of such problems and prompt treatment are important to decrease the overall morbidity.

NEURAL INJURY

The incidence of neurological deterioration following surgery is about 1 per cent but such deterioration poses a significant problem if it occurs.[34] This problem may occur following either a posterior or an anterior procedure. McAfee and Bohlman reported five patients who had neurological deterioration following posterior Harrington instrumentation for fractures of the thoracolumbar spine.[96] One of these patients had laminectomy for decompression along with distraction rods, which resulted in an ascending paraplegia, loss of intercostal muscle strength, and ultimately death due to pulmonary compromise.

The other four patients developed neurological deterioration, in part because of technical problems related to Harrington instrumentation. These included overdistraction, inadequate reduction, and hook impingement. Gertzbein and coworkers also reported one patient who developed a neurological deterioration secondary to a hematoma at the site of the lower hook.[56] It is clear from these reports that distraction Harrington instrumentation must be used cautiously to avoid these neurological complications. Selection of correct-size hooks

Table 7–2
**Complications in the Management of Patients with Thoracolumbar Fractures
in Different Series**

AUTHOR	NO. OF PATIENTS	PROCEDURE	NEUROLOGICAL DETERIORATION	PSEUDARTHROSIS
Aebi	30	Fixateur interne	1	—
Akbarnia	90	Steffee	—	4
Bohlman	218 (thoracic)	17 laminectomy and 8 anterior procedure	—	—
Bradford (1977)	30 (thoracic)	H-rod or anterior procedure	—	1
Bradford (1987)	59	39 H-rod	4	—
		20 anterior	1	—
Cotler	44	H-rod, 5 anterior	—	1
Denis	52	13 H-rod	—	1
		39 no surgery	6	—
Dickson	95	H-rod	—	4
Edwards	135	Rod-sleeve	2% transient paresthesia	3%
Esses	48	Fixateur interne	—	—
Flesch	40	H-rod	1	4
Jacobs	100	59 H-rod	—	—
		34 no surgery	—	—
Kaneda	27	Anterior instrumentation	—	4
Kostuik	49	Anterior instrumentation	—	2
McAfee	70	Anterior fusion	—	2
McEvoy	53	31 H-rod	—	1
		22 no surgery	3	—
Olerud	20	Transpedicular instrumentation	—	—
Osebold	63	H-rod	—	4
Roy-Camille	123	Transpedicular instrumentation	2	—
Willen	50	26 H-rod	—	1
		24 no surgery	—	—

AUTHOR	DEFORMITY	IMPLANT PROBLEMS	MISCELLANEOUS COMPLICATIONS
Aebi	2	2	
Akbarnia	7	15	3 respiratory, 7 UTI, 1 DVT, 2 PE, 1 death, and 1 hematoma
Bohlman	—	—	76 UTI, 29 pneumonia, 9 PE, 70 pressure sores, and 2 GI hemorrhage
Bradford (1977)	1	1	5 pressure sores, 2 DVT
Bradford (1987)	1	6	4 UTI, 1 decubitus
	—	1	2 UTI, 1 wound problem, 1 retrograde ejaculation
Cotler	—	7	—
Denis	1	1	—
	5	—	Skin problems with casts
Dickson	8	19	2 infections, 5 pain, and 2 deaths

Table 7–2
**Complications in the Management of Patients with Thoracolumbar Fractures
in Different Series** *Continued*

AUTHOR	DEFORMITY	IMPLANT PROBLEMS	MISCELLANEOUS COMPLICATIONS
Edwards	—	3.7% hook failure 2 broken rods	18% UTI, 4.5% decubitus, 4% DVT, 1.5% pneumonia, and 1 infection
Esses	2	6	1 infection, 1 UTI
Flesch	4	5	7 decubitus, 2 DVT, 1 pneumonia, 1 infection, 1 cardiac arrest
Jacobs	—	1	2 PE (1 death), 1 infection
	—	—	2 PE, 1 pneumonia, 1 DVT, and 2 decubitus
Kaneda	—	—	4 hematoma, 2 UTI
Kostuik	—	—	—
McAfee	3	—	1 pneumonia, 1 pneumothorax 2 neuropraxia, 1 meningitis
McEvoy	1	—	2 PE, 1 infection, 1 DVT, 6 UTI, 1 decubitus
	2	—	3 UTI, 1 decubitus, 1 pain
Olerud	2	2	—
Osebold	10	6	22 UTI, 23 decubitus, 6 DVT, 3 PE, and 1 arrythmia
Roy-Camille	—	—	7 deaths, 2 PE, 6 infections
Willen	1	5	1 decubitus, 1 DVT, 12 UTI, and 1 hemothorax
	*	—	12 UTI, 2 DVT

DVT = deep vein thrombosis, PE = pulmonary embolism, UTI = urinary tract infection
*Many developed increasing deformity

that closely match the thickness of the lamina and proper placement of the hooks are important in order to prevent hook impingement on the thecal sac and nerve roots. Distraction must be done slowly, particularly when the anterior longitudinal ligament is suspected of being torn. If a kyphotic deformity is also present, extension maneuver should be done prior to distraction, as the cord or roots may be stretched over the retropulsed bone at the apex of the deformity.[34] During extension maneuver, great caution should be taken to avoid canal penetration of the fractured lamina. An intraoperative roentgenogram should also be taken to document proper reduction of height and kyphosis. Wiring the posterior elements of the injured vertebra together prior to distraction is helpful in selected cases to prevent the complication of overdistraction.[45] One may also use a distraction rod on one side and compression rod on the other.[38, 76] Passage of the sublaminar wires should be done in a meticulous manner as discussed under scoliosis. Spinal cord contusion and development of epidural hematoma may complicate the procedure of sublaminar wiring. Compression instrumentation may cause bulging or protrusion of the injured disc in rare cases.[86, 96] Since the advent of transpedicular instrumentation, the Scoliosis Research Society Morbidity Committee reported a 3.2 per cent incidence of neural impingements by the pedicle screws.[125] The nerve root exits around the inferomedial aspect of the pedicle. Care must be taken to correctly localize the pedicle entrance both anatomically and radiologically. If a pedicle screw is too large, a "blow-out" fracture of the pedicle may result and may cause nerve root irritation. Preoperative CT evaluation is helpful in measuring the inside diameter of the pedicle.

Neurological deterioration may also result following direct decompression via laminectomy, posterolateral approach, or anterior corpectomy. Laminectomy is known to cause more instability and neurological deterioration and is considered an undesirable method of decompression in thoracolumbar fractures by most authors. Laminectomy is rarely required unless the fractured lamina is pushed into the spinal canal or the lamina is fractured with dural laceration.[20] The posterolateral approach is a safer route for neural decompression. Excision of the transverse process and the pedicle allows the surgeon to remove or impact the retropulsed fragment without retracting the spinal cord. In the lumbar region the nerve roots can be gently retracted during decompression, but postoperative nerve root dysfunction may still result owing to the retraction. The anterior approach is probably the best route of decompression, particularly in an incomplete cord injury at or above L1 level. Anterior exposure allows the surgeon to remove the pedicle and remove the retropulsed fragment more directly. Nonetheless, great caution should be exercised when using a power burr to prevent contusion or dural laceration.[13, 16] Magnification glasses, a high-intensity light, and a diamond burr are helpful during any decompression procedure.

Postoperative neurological deterioration may also be due to fixation problems.[13, 96] An anterior strut graft may dislodge into the spinal canal. Proper technique of strut grafting has been stressed.[21] The graft dislodgement is more common in three-column injuries, and posterior stabilization is important in these cases. If graft dislodgement is suspected in a patient with neurological deterioration, roentgenograms, tomograms, or CT scans should be ordered to immediately diagnose and treat the problem. Neurological deterioration may be secondary to instrument and fusion problems such as hook dislodgement, broken rods, and recurrence of deformity.[59, 96] Accurate diagnosis of neural impingement and prompt treatment are necessary to restore the patient's neurological function.

A rare but possible etiology of neurological deterioration is ischemic insult to the spinal cord. Injury to the artery of Adamkiewicz and ligation of segmental vessels during anterior approach pose a risk to spinal cord circulation. Excessive blood loss should be prevented as accompanying hypotension puts the spinal cord at more risk for circulatory compromise.

Somatosensory-evoked potential (SSEP) monitoring may be helpful in patients with intact neural function or with incomplete spinal cord injury.[107, 109] However, this is not a foolproof method because of false negatives or positives. In the future, motor-evoked potential monitoring may become useful in patients who undergo anterior decompression.

Neurological problems that are less devastating than motor or sphincter loss may be radicular pain, sensory deficit, or spinal fluid leakage. Nerve root decompression should be considered at the time of initial surgery in patients who complain of radicular pain preoperatively. For example, a patient with an L1 burst fracture may complain of radiating pain down to the groin. The L1 nerve root can be decompressed either anteriorly or posteriorly at the time of initial surgery. Most patients who develop radiculopathy postoperatively can be managed with nonsteroidal anti-inflammatory medications. Those patients with persistent radiculopathy should have a myelogram or CT scan for diagnosis of nerve root impingement. Inadequate decompression, bone graft migration, or hook misplacement may be the cause of persistent radiculopathy. Postoperative sensory deficits rarely cause significant problems and generally improve with time. Spinal fluid leakage can be potentially fatal if meningitis develops as a consequence. Patients with spinal fluid leakage should receive prophylactic antibiotics and should be put on bedrest. If a dural tear has been found during surgery, the dura should be repaired primarily, and the wound should be closed tightly without drains.[36] If leakage occurs after surgery, a subcutaneous or subarachnoid catheter will relieve spinal fluid leakage through the wound and permit wound and dural healing in many cases.[20] Patients should be taken back to surgery to repair the dura if fluid leakage does not stop within a few days.

PSEUDARTHROSIS

Pseudarthrosis continues to be a problem in spinal surgery despite advances in spinal instrumentation. At present, there is no substitute for meticulous decortication, facet excision, and massive bone grafts in achieving fusion success. The iliac crest is the best source of autogenous bone. The iliac bone is biomechanically superior to the ribs, particularly for anterior strut grafting. Allografts may be used for augmentation if the autogenous grafts are insufficient. Stable constructs with appropriate instrumentation are also important. Adequate postoperative external immobilization should not be ignored, as early instrument failures and pseudarthrosis may ensue otherwise.

Pseudarthrosis is often asymptomatic and difficult to detect with routine radiographs. Loss of correction, instrument failure, and persistent pain are warning signs of pseudarthrosis. Pseudarthrosis may be detected by plain roentgenograms, especially on oblique views. Tomograms or computed tomography may define the pseudarthrosis much better. In treating pseudarthrosis, one should first examine the cause. Occult or subclinical infection may be present. Stability may have been compromised by inadequate spinal instrumentation or the lack of postoperative external immobilization. Pseudarthrosis should be repaired if there is an associated loss of fixation, recurrence of deformity, or persistent pain. Re-exploration of pseudarthrosis is not a simple procedure. Complete exposure and thorough removal of fibrous tissues are necessary. Autogenous iliac bone grafts should be packed meticulously, and additional stabilization may be necessary as well.

Pseudarthrosis and graft problems may result following anterior grafting procedures.[6] Graft dislodgement is largely prevented by careful attention to technical details.[6, 21] Following the anterior procedure, a posterior fusion with a compression instrumentation helps to further compress the anterior graft and to increase the overall fusion rate. Graft fracture or collapse is more common with mechanically inferior grafts such as ribs. We routinely use the tricortical iliac crest for anterior strut grafting.

INSTRUMENT PROBLEMS

Hook dislodgement or rod breakage may be immediate or late postoperative complications. Hook dislodgement is the most frequently reported complication of posterior instrumentation for spinal injury (Fig. 7–5). The incidence is about 6 per cent.[34] Hook dislodgement typically involves a proximal distraction hook that displaces from the thoracic facet joint. Laminar fracture or rod-hook disengagement may also occur. Poor placement of the hook, poor hook design, excessive distraction, laminar fracture, and poor contouring are among the main causes of early hook failures.[34] In addition, the rod should span at least three vertebrae above the site of injury to decrease the tendency of the upper hook to back out during flexion.[115] Hooks for L5 and sacral fixations dislodge more frequently.[34] Pedicular screws provide more reliable fixation in this region. The bifid hook has been found to be superior to plain or ribbed hooks in resisting laminar fracture on distraction.[49] Recently, Edwards' anatomical hooks and the Jacobs' locking device have been available to solve these problems. Additional stability of the hooks can be obtained by the use of sublaminar wires on the rods.[17, 56, 105, 129] To prevent hook-rod disen-

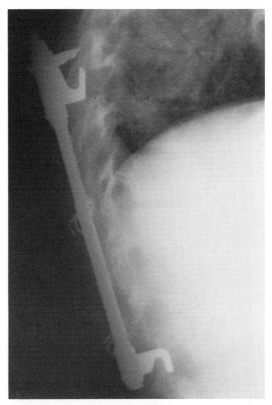

FIGURE 7–5. Upper hook dislodgement in a patient who underwent J-rod insertion.

gagement, Edwards and Levine recommend leaving 1 cm. of rod projecting beyond the hook.[34] Proper postoperative external immobilization and avoidance of the prone position are also important. Treatment of hook dislodgement is to replace the hook and to correct the underlying problem in order to maintain the initial curve correction.

Instrument failure after several months usually indicates the presence of pseudarthrosis. Broken rods, migrating rods, broken wires, and hook dislodgement are well documented in the literature. Instrument failure in the presence of pseudarthrosis usually requires surgery, especially if loss of correction is noted. Fatigue fractures of the Harrington rod occur at the rachet-rod junction, which is biomechanically the weakest part of the rod (Fig. 7–6A,B). Late instrument failure with solid arthrodesis in an asymptomatic patient needs no treatment.

Another complication that may be associated with instrumentation is pain related to the prominence of the implant. Bursitis or skin erosion may develop. This is particularly common in a thin patient. Proper rod contouring

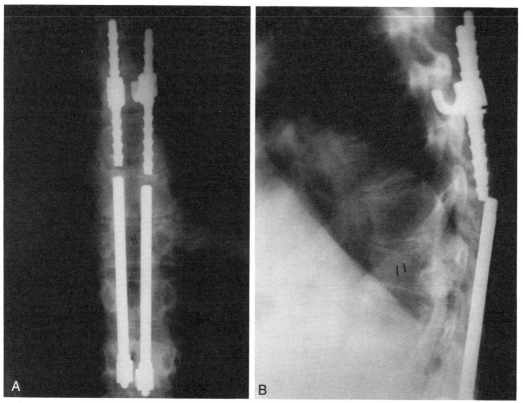

FIGURE 7–6. *(A,B)* Fatigue fracture of Harrington rods secondary to pseudarthrosis (notice that the rachet-rod junction is close to the fracture site).

is important in this regard. We routinely approximate the skin prior to closure to examine any prominence caused by the implant. Surgical removal of the offending implant may be necessary in some cases.

POST-TRAUMATIC DEFORMITIES

Post-traumatic deformities can develop following thoracolumbar spine injuries.[85] Scoliosis and kyphosis develop commonly below a spinal cord injury, particularly in younger patients.[83, 95] Mayfield and associates reported on the cases of 40 children who had sustained a spinal cord injury: 92 per cent developed scoliosis, 16 per cent developed kyphosis, and 20 per cent developed excessive lumbar lordosis.[95] The development of spinal deformity after spinal cord injury is therefore expected in patients who had injuries prior to the adolescent growth spurt. Careful observation and management by bracing or surgery are required in these patients.

Post-traumatic deformities frequently develop at the site of the injury following either conservative treatment or surgery.[89] Burst fractures with collapse of more than 50 per cent frequently result in post-traumatic deformities if treated conservatively.[100] Conservative treatment of initial traumatic kyphosis of greater than 20 degrees is also prone to failure.[99] If conservative treatment is chosen for patients with an unstable fracture, prolonged bedrest for at least eight weeks, application of a well-molded unilateral pantaloon cast, and frequent radiographic examinations are required to prevent the development of post-traumatic kyphosis. As mentioned before, implant failures and pseudarthrosis may be responsible for the development of the angular deformity. Laminectomy frequently causes kyphosis following surgery and should be avoided in patients with a thoracolumbar fracture. Recurrence of the deformity is also possible after premature removal of metal implant.[60, 69, 108, 140] We do not routinely remove the implant unless there is specific reason to do so. The status of fusion must be carefully determined prior to hardware removal. Treatment of post-traumatic kyphosis is difficult at best. Most cases require a combined anterior and posterior procedure or anterior fusion with instrumentation.[80, 93, 99, 120, 139] If the deformity is relatively flexible, posterior instrumentation and fusion may be sufficient.

Loss of lumbar lordosis can be a significant problem as in patients with a flat back syndrome who had spinal fusion down to the low lumbar region for scoliosis.[3, 3a, 60, 82] Distraction instrumentation in the low lumbar region should be avoided for this reason. Patients with loss of lumbar lordosis present with muscular pain in the upper back and lower cervical area, pain in the knees, inability to stand erect, and gait abnormalities. The most effective method of treatment for the flat back syndrome is prevention. If surgery is required in the low lumbar region, pedicular fixation devices are probably most beneficial in restoring normal lumbar lordosis. For these reasons, we prefer using a distraction instrumentation spanning three vertebrae above and two vertebrae below the site of injury at the thoracolumbar region (T11–L1), but we currently use pedicular instrumentation spanning only one above and one below the site of injury in the low lumbar region. Surgical techniques for corrective osteotomy for symptomatic loss of lumbar lordosis are exacting. Complications are frequent, including neurological injury, pseudarthrosis, and instrument failure.[82] In general, anterior release is done, followed by posterior osteotomy and compression instrumentation to achieve better correction and improve fusion rate.

CHRONIC PAIN

Patients who sustained a thoracolumbar fracture with or without neurological insult may continue to have pain from several possible sources. The first type of pain is caused by root compression from a displaced bony fragment, bone graft migration, hardware impingement, healing callus, or progressive deformity.[11, 18] Symptoms and signs of nerve root compression, a positive electromyogram, or a positive imaging study suggest the source of nerve root compression. If conservative treatment fails to relieve the pain, late decompression of the affected nerve may be necessary.

The second type of pain comes from the site of the injury. Development of pseudarthrosis, implant failure, or post-traumatic deformity is frequently responsible. Patients who had long instrumentation without fusion along the entire length of the rods may suffer from pain caused by arthritic changes in the facet joints.[73] As mentioned before, distraction instrumentation and fusion in the low lumbar region frequently cause flat back syndrome.

Another type of pain occurs in patients with complete spinal cord injuries. This type of pain is poorly localized and associated with paresthesia or spasm. Rehabilitation, use of transcutaneous electrical nerve stimulator,[118] rhizotomy, or electrical electrode implants may be helpful in selected cases.

MISCELLANEOUS COMPLICATIONS

Other complications that may develop in patients with thoracolumbar fractures include respiratory, urinary, integumentary, and metabolic problems (see Table 7–1). These problems are particularly common in patients with a spinal cord injury.

Respiratory complications may include atelectasis, pneumonia, pleural effusion, pneumothorax, chylothorax, hemothorax, acute respiratory distress syndrome, respiratory failure, pulmonary thromboembolism, and fat embolism. Many pulmonary complications may be prevented by regular chest therapy with postural drainage, percussion of chest wall, assisted coughing, use of spirometer, and intermittent positive pressure breathing apparatus. A pneumothorax may occur during either an anterior or posterior surgery. The pleura may be violated if the surgeon dissects too deeply between the transverse processes. Chylothorax may follow anterior surgery of the spine. Leakage in the lymphatic system should be recognized during surgery, and the stump should be ligated both proximally and distally. Treatment of chylothorax consists of chest tube drainage and decreasing the patient's fat intake. Pulmonary embolism is one of the most common causes of sudden death. Antithrombotic stockings of pneumatic compression devices should be used in all patients. Some authors advocate prophylactic use of heparin.[32, 46] Above all, early mobilization of the patient is the key to the prevention of pulmonary embolism or other pulmonary complications.

Urinary tract infection is the most common complication in the patient with a thoracolumbar injury. The bladder, the kidney, or the epididymis may become infected. Intermittent catheterization is preferred over indwelling catheterization to lower the incidence of urinary tract infection, particularly in the patient with a spinal cord injury.

Decubitus ulcers, the most preventable of all complications afflicting paraplegics, are avoided by turning the patient every two hours and carefully inspecting the skin over the bony prominences.[32] Rotatory beds are quite helpful in terms of skin care. Skin complications may also arise secondary to irritation from casts or braces. Aggressive treatment of pressure sores at early stages is important in preventing cellulitis, soft tissue necrosis, and deep infection.

Gastrointestinal complications are also common in patients with thoracolumbar fractures. Bleeding ulcers in the stomach may develop, particularly in patients who receive systemic corticosteroids. Postoperative ileus may occur following surgery, particularly after anterior procedures. Ileus is usually managed with nasogastric suction and delaying oral feeding until bowel sounds return. Acute cholecystitis has been seen following spinal surgery. The patient presents with an acute abdominal pain in the right upper quadrant in the early postoperative period. Prompt diagnosis with cholecystogram is necessary, and surgery may be required.

Proper fluid and electrolyte maintenance is important in patients undergoing major spinal surgery. Hypercalcemia and hyperphosphatemia are frequently seen after the patient has been in bed for a few weeks.[46] Increased bony resorption after prolonged immobilization is probably responsible for these conditions. Symptoms of hypercalcemia may include anorexia, nausea, and vomiting. Many patients with trauma may become nutritionally deficient because of increased stress and catabolism. Nutritional therapy with nasogastric feeding or parenteral hyperalimentation is important.

Wound dehiscence or infection may occur following surgery and may prolong the patient's hospitalization. Temperature, white blood cell count, and the sedimentation rate are frequently elevated in patients with wound infection. Wound infection is usually picked up by careful examination of the wound. Aspiration of the wound should be done in doubtful cases. If the appearance or aspiration of the wound suggests an infectious process, the patient should be taken to the operating room. Thorough debridement and irrigation should be performed. The fascia should be opened unless the infection is clearly localized to the superficial layer only. Instrumentation should not be removed. The wound can be closed primarily with a suction-irrigating system or left open for delayed primary closure. The patient is at a higher risk of developing an infection of the spine when infection is associated with low-velocity-missile injury to the colon.[121] All patients who undergo spine surgery after spinal fractures should receive prophylactic antibiotics.

SUMMARY

In summary, there is great controversy in the treatment of patients with thoracolumbar fracture. Nonetheless, complications associated with the treatment of fractures of the thoracolumbar spine can be minimized several ways:

1. A thorough initial clinical, neurological, and radiographic evaluation prevents delayed diagnosis, missed associated injuries, and neurological deterioration.

2. The mechanism of injury, canal compromise, and neurological status should be clearly delineated in order to render proper treatment.

3. Achieving a stable surgical construct is the main goal in unstable thoracolumbar injuries, whereas restoring the canal diameter is most important in thoracolumbar injuries that are associated with incomplete cord syndrome.

4. Attention to surgical details prevents common complications such as neural injury, pseudarthrosis, instrument problems, and deformities.

REFERENCES

1. Aebi, M., Etter, C., Kehl, T., et al.: Stabilization of the lower thoracic and lumbar spine with the internal spinal skeletal fixation system. Spine 12:544–551, 1987.
2. Akbarnia, B. A., Forgarty, J. P., and Tayob, A. A.: Contoured Harrington instrumentation in the treatment of unstable spinal fractures. Clin. Orthop. 189:186, 1984.
3. Akbarnia, B. A., Gaines, R., Keppler, L., et al.: Surgical treatment of fracture dislocations of thoracolumbar and lumbar spine using pedicular screw and plate fixation. Presented at the 23rd Annual Meeting of the Scoliosis Research Society, Baltimore, 1988.
3a. An, H. S., Simpson, M. J., Ebraheim, N. A., et al.: Burst fractures of low lumbar spine. Presented at the 56th AAOS, Las Vegas, 1989.
4. An, H. S., Perlmutter, M., Cotler, J. M., et al.: Multiple level injuries of the spine, involving the cervical spine. Accepted for presentation at the Annual American Spinal Injury Association, Orlando, Florida, May 1990.
5. Anden, U., Lake, A., and Norwall, A.: The role of the anterior longitudinal ligament in Har-

rington rod fixation of unstable thoracolumbar spinal fractures. Spine 5:23–25, 1980.

6. Bauman, T., and Garfin, S. R.: Complications associated with anterior grafting. In: Garfin, S. R. (ed.): *Complications of Spine Surgery.* Baltimore, Williams & Wilkins, 1989, pp. 248–277.

7. Bedbrook G. M.: Spinal injuries with tetraplegia and paraplegia. J. Bone Joint Surg. 61B:26, 1979.

8. Bedbrook, G. M.: Treatment of thoracolumbar dislocation and fractures with paraplegia. Clin. Orthop. 112:27, 1975.

9. Benson, D. R.: Unstable thoracolumbar fractures, with emphasis on the burst fractures. Clin. Orthop. 230:14, 1988.

10. Blauth, M., Tscherne, H., and Haas N.: Therapeutic concept and results of operative treatment in acute trauma of the thoracic and lumbar spine: The Hanover experience. J. Orthop. Trauma 1(3):240–52, 1987.

11. Bohlman, H. H.: Late progressive paralysis and pain following fractures of the thoracolumbar spine: A report of 10 patients. J. Bone Joint Surg. 58A:723, 1976.

12. Bohlman, H. H., and Eismont, F. J.: Surgical techniques of anterior decompression and fusion for spinal cord injuries. Clin. Orthop. 154:57–67, 1981.

13. Bohlman, H. H, Freehafer, A., and Dejak, J.: The results of treatment of acute injuries of the upper thoracic spine with paralysis. J. Bone Joint Surg. 67A:360, 1985.

14. Bohlman, H. H.: Treatment of fractures and dislocations of thoracic and lumbar spine. J. Bone Joint Surg. 67A:165, 1985.

15. Bradford, D. S., Akbarnia, B. A., Winter, R. B., et al.: Surgical stabilization of fracture and fracture dislocations of the thoracic spine. Spine 2:185–196, 1977.

16. Bradford, D. S., and McBride, G. G.: Surgical management of thoracolumbar spine fractures with incomplete neurologic deficits. Clin. Orthop. 218:201–216, 1987.

17. Bryant, C. E., and Sullivan, J. A.: Management of thoracic and lumbar spine fractures with Harrington distraction rods supplemented with segmental wiring. Spine 8:532, 1983.

18. Burke, D. C.: Pain in paraplegia. Paraplegia 10:297–313, 1973.

19. Burke, D. C., and Murray, D. D.: The management of thoracic and thoraco-lumbar injuries of the spine with neurological involvement. J. Bone Joint Surg. 58B:72–78, 1976.

20. Cammisa, F.P., Jr., Eismont, F.J., and Green, B.A.: Dural laceration occuring with burst fractures and associated laminar fractures. J. Bone Joint Surg. 71A:1044–52, 1989.

21. Cotler, H. B., Cotler, J. M., Stoloff, A., et al.: The use of autografts for vertebral body replacement of the thoracic and lumbar spine. Spine 10:748–756, 1985.

22. Cotler, H. B., Kulkarini, M. V., and Bondurant, F. J.: Magnetic resonance imaging of acute spinal cord trauma. Preliminary report. J. Orthop. Trauma 2:1–4, 1988.

23. Cotler, J. M., Vernace, J. V., and Michalski, J. A.: The use of Harrington rods in thoracolumbar fractures. Ortho. Clin. North Am. 17:87, 1986.

24. Court-Brown, C. W., and Gertzbein, S. D.: The management of burst fractures of the fifth lumbar vertebrae. Spine 12:308, 1987.

25. Denis, F.: The three column spine and its significance in the classification of acute thoracolumbar spine injuries. Spine 8:817, 1983.

26. Denis, F: Spinal instability as defined by the three column spine concept in acute spinal trauma. Clin. Orthop. 189:65, 1984.

27. Denis, F., Armstrong, G. W. D., Serals, K., et al.: Acute thoracolumbar burst fractures in the absence of neurological deficit: A comparison between operative and nonoperative treatment. Clin. Orthop. 189:142, 1984.

28. Denis, F., Ruiz, H., and Searls, K.: Comparison between square-ended distraction rods and standard round-ended distraction rods in the treatment of thoracolumbar spinal injuries. Clin. Orthop. 189:162, 1984.

29. Dewald, R. L.: Burst fractures of the thoracic and lumbar spine. Clin. Orthop. 189:150, 1984.

30. Dick, W., Kluger, P., Mageral, F., et al.: A new device for internal fixation of thoracolumbar and lumbar spine fractures. The "Fixateur Interne." Paraplegia 23:225, 1985.

31. Dickson, J. H., Harrington, P. R., and Erwin, W. D.: Results of reduction and stabilization of the severely fractured thoracic and lumbar spine. J. Bone Joint Surg. 60A:799–805, 1978.

32. Donovan, W. H., and Dwyer, A. P.: An update on the early management of traumatic paraplegia (nonoperative and operative management). Clin. Orthop. 189:12–21, 1984.

33. Edwards, C., and Levine, A.: Early rod-sleeve stabilization of the injured thoracic and lumbar spine. Orthop. Clin. North Am. 17:121, 1986.

34. Edwards, C. C., and Levine, A. M: Complications associated with posterior instrumentation in the treatment of thoracic and lumbar injuries. In: Garfin, S. R. (ed.): *Complications of Spine Surgery.* Baltimore, Williams & Wilkins, 1989, pp. 164–199.

35. Edwards, C. C., Rosenthal, M. S., Gellad, F., et al.: The fate of retropulsed bone following thoracolumbar burst fractures: Late stenosis or resorption. Presented at the 23rd Annual Meeting of the Scoliosis Research Society, Baltimore, 1988.

36. Eismont, F. J., Green, B. A., Berkowitz, B. M., et al.: The role of intraoperative ultrasonography in the treatment of thoracic and lumbar spine fractures. Spine 9:782–787, 1984.

37. Erickson, D. L., Leider, L. L., Jr., and Brown, W. E.: One-stage decompression-stabilization for thoracolumbar fractures. Spine 2:43–56, 1977.

38. Esposito, P. W., Alexander, A. H., and Lichtman, D. M.: Delayed overdistraction of a surgically treated unstable thoracolumbar fracture. A case report. Spine 10:393–396, 1985.

39. Esses, S. I.: The AO spinal internal fixator. Spine 14(4):373–378, 1989.

40. Farcy, J. P., Weidenbaum, M., Michelsen, C. B., et al.: A comparative biomechanical study of spinal fixation using Cotrel-Dubousset instrumentation. Spine 12:877–881, 1987.

41. Ferguson, R. L., and Allen, B. L., Jr.: A mechanistic classification of thoracolumbar spine fractures. Clin. Orthop. 189:77, 1984.

42. Fidler, M.W.: Remodeling of the spinal canal after burst fracture. A prospective study of two cases. J. Bone Joint Surg. 70B:730–732, 1988.

43. Fidler, M. W.: Posterior instrumentation of the spine. An experimental comparison of various possible techniques. Spine 11:367–371, 1986.

44. Flesch, J. R., Leider, L. L., Erickson, D. L., et al.: Harrington instrumentation and spine fusion for unstable fractures and fracture dislocation. J. Bone Joint Surg. 59A:143, 1977.

45. Floman, Y., Fast, A., Pollack, D., et al.: The simultaneous application of an interspinous compressive wire and Harrington distraction rods in the treatment of fracture-dislocation of the thoracic and lumbar spine. Clin. Orthop. 205:207–15, 1986.

46. Foo, D.: Management of acute complications of spinal cord injury. Spine State of the Art Reviews 3:211–219, 1989.

47. Frankel, H. L., Hancock, D. O., and Hyslop, G.: The value of postural reduction in the initial management of closed injuries of the spine with paraplegia and tetraplegia. Paraplegia 7:179, 1969.

48. Frederickson, B. E., Yuan, H. A., and Miller, H.: Burst fractures of the fifth lumbar vertebrae. J. Bone Joint Surg. 64:1088, 1982.

49. Freedman, L. S., Houghton, G. R., and Evans, M.: Cadaveric study comparing the stability of upper distraction hooks used in Harrington instrumentation. Spine 11:579–582, 1986.

50. Gaines, R. W., Breedlove, R. F., and Munson, G.: Stabilization of thoracic and thoracolumbar fracture-dislocations with Harrington rods and sublaminar wires. Clin. Orthop. 189:195, 1984.

51. Garfin, S. R., Mowery, C. A., Guerra, J., Jr., et al.: Confirmation of the posterolateral technique to decompress and fuse thoracolumbar spine burst fractures. Spine 10(3):218–232, 1985.

52. Garth, W. P., Jr., and Van Patten, P. K.: Fractures of the lumbar lamina with epidural hematoma simulating herniation of a disc. A case report. J. Bone Joint Surg. 71A(5):771–772, 1989.

53. Gertzbein, S. D., and Court-Brown, C. M.: Flexion-distraction injuries of the lumbar spine. Clin. Orthop. 227:52–60, 1988.

54. Gertzbein, S. D., Court-Brown, C. M., Jacobs, R. R., et al.: Decompression and circumferential stabilization of unstable spinal fractures. Spine 13(8):892–895, 1988.

55. Gertzbein, S. D., Court-Brown, C. M., Marks, P., et al.: The neurological outcome following surgery for spinal fractures. Spine 13:641, 1988.

56. Gertzbein, S. D., MacMichael, D., and Tile, M.: Harrington instrumentation as a method of fixation in fractures of the spine. J. Bone Joint Surg. 64B:526–529, 1982.

57. Gumley, G., Taylor, T. K. F., and Ryan, M. D.: Distraction fractures of the lumbar spine. J. Bone Joint Surg. 64B:520–525, 1982.

58. Gupta, K.L., Kapila, A., Nasca, R.J., et al.: Post-traumatic lumbar extra-arachnoid mass with radiculopathy responding to conservative therapy in a patient with bilateral laminar fractures. Spine 13(8):945–948, 1988.

59. Hales, D. D., Dawson, E. G., and Delamarter, R.: Late neurological complications of Harrington-rod instrumentation. J. Bone Joint Surg. 71A:1053–1057, 1989.

60. Hasday, C. A., Passoff, T. L., and Perry, J.: Gait abnormalities arising from iatrogenic loss of lumbar lordosis secondary to Harrington instrumentation in lumbar fractures. Spine 8:501, 1983.

61. Hashimoto, T., Kaneda, K., and Abumi, K.: Relationship between traumatic spinal canal stenosis and neurologic deficits in thoracolumbar burst fractures. Spine 13(11):1268–72, 1988.

62. Hazel, W.A., Jr., Jones, R.A., Morrey, B.F., et al.: Vertebral fractures without neurological deficit. A long-term follow-up. J. Bone Joint Surg. 70A(9):1319–21, 1988.

63. Herndon, W.A., and Galloway, D.: Neurologic return versus cross-sectional canal area in incomplete thoracolumbar spinal cord injuries. J. Trauma 28(5):680–683, 1988.

64. Holdsworth, F.: Fractures, dislocations and fracture-dislocations of the spine. J. Bone Joint Surg. 52A:1534, 1970.

65. Jacobs, R. R., Asher, M. A., and Snider, R. K.: Thoracolumbar spine injuries. A comparative study of recumbent and operative treatment in 100 patients. Spine 5:463, 1980.

66. Jacobs, R. R., and Casey, M. P.: Surgical management of thoracolumbar spinal injuries. Clin. Orthop. 189:22–35, 1984.

67. Jacobs, R.R., and Montesano, P. X.: Development of the locking hook spinal rod system. Orthopedics 11(10):1415–1421, 1988.

68. Jacobs, R. R., Schlaepfer, F., Mathys, R., et al.: A locking hook spinal rod system for stabilization of fracture-dislocations and correction of deformities of the dorsolumbar spine. Clin. Orthop. 189:168–177, 1984.

69. Jodoin, A., Gillet, P., Dupuis, P. R., et al.: Surgical treatment of post-traumatic kyphosis: A report of 16 cases. Can. J. Surg. 32(1):36–42, 1989.

70. Johnson, J. R., Leatherman, K. D., and Holt, R. T.: Anterior decompression of the spinal cord for neurological deficit. Spine 8:396–405, 1983.

71. Jones, R. F., Snowden, E., Coan, J., et al.: Bracing of thoracic and lumbar spine fractures. Paraplegia 25:386, 1987.

72. Kachooie, A., Bloch, R., and Banna, M.: Post-traumatic dorsal pseudomeningocele. J. Can. Assoc. Rad. 36(3):262–263, 1985.

73. Kahanovitz, N., Bullough, P., and Jacobs, R. R.: The effect of internal fixation without arthrodesis on human joint cartilage. Clin. Orthop. 189:204–208, 1984.

74. Karlstrom, G., Olerud, S., and Sjostrom, L.: Transpedicular segmental fixation: Description of a new procedure. Orthopedics 11:689–700, 1988.

75. Kaneda, K., Abumi, K., and Fujiya, M.: Burst fractures with neurologic deficits of the thoracolumbar-lumbar spine: Results of anterior decompression and stabilization with anterior instrumentation. Spine 9:788–795, 1984.

76. Keene, J.S., Wackwitz, D.L., Drummond, D.S., et al.: Compression-distraction instrumentation of unstable thoracolumbar fractures: An-

atomic results obtained with each type of injury and method of instrumentation. Spine *11*(9):895–902, 1986.

77. King, A. G.: Burst compression fractures of the thoracolumbar spine. Orthopedics *10*: 1711, 1987.

78. Kinnard, P., Ghibely, A., Gordon, D., et al.: Roy-Camille plates in unstable spinal conditions. A preliminary report. Spine *11*(2):131–135, 1986.

79. Kostuik, J. P.: Anterior fixation for fractures of the thoracic and lumbar spine techniques, new methods of internal fixation results. Spine 8:512, 1983.

80. Kostuik, J.P., and Matsusaki, H.: Anterior stabilization, instrumentation, and decompression for post-traumatic kyphosis. Spine *14*(4):379–386, 1989.

81. Krompinger, W. J., Frederickson, B. E., Mino, D. E., et al.: Conservative treatment of fractures of the thoracic and lumbar spine. Orthop. Clin. North Am. *17*:161, 1986.

82. LaGrone, M. O., Bradford, D. S., Moe, J. H., et al.: Treatment of symptomatic flatback after spinal fusion. J. Bone Joint Surg. 70A:569, 1988.

83. Lancourt, J. E., Dickson, J. H., and Carter, R. E.: Paralytic spinal deformity following traumatic spinal cord injury in children and adolescents. J. Bone Joint Surg. 63A:47–53, 1981.

84. Larson, S. J., Holst, R. A., Hemmy, D. C., et al.: Lateral extracavity approach to traumatic lesions of the thoracic and lumbar spine. J. Neurosurg. 45:628–637, 1976.

85. Leidholt, J. D., Young, T. J., Hahn, H. R., et al.: Evaluation of the later spinal deformities with fracture-dislocations of the dorsal and lumbar spine in paraplegics. Paraplegia 7:16, 1969.

86. Levine, A. M., Bosse, M., and Edwards, C. C.: Bilateral facet dislocations in the thoracolumbar spine. Spine *113*:630–640, 1988.

87. Levine, A. M., and Edwards, C. C.: Complications in the treatment of acute spinal injury. Orthop. Clin. North Am. *17*:183–203, 1986.

88. Levine, A. M., and Edwards, C. C.: Low lumbar burst fractures. Reduction and stabilization using the modular spine fixation system. Orthopedics *11*:1427, 1988.

89. Lindahl, S., Willen, J., and Irstam, L: Unstable thoracolumbar fractures. A comparative radiologic study of conservative treatment and Harrington instrumentation. Acta Radiol. Diagn. 26(1):67–77, 1985.

90. Lowe, J., Kaplan, L., Liebergall, M., et al.: Serratia osteomyelitis causing neurological deterioration after spine fracture. A report of two cases. J. Bone Joint Surg. *71*B(2):256–258, 1989.

91. Luque, E., Cassis, H., and Ramirez-Wiella, G.: Segmental spinal instrumentation in the treatment of fractures of the thoracolumbar spine. Spine 7:312, 1982.

92. Maiman, D. J., Larson, S. J., and Bonzel, E. C.: Neurologic improvement associated with late decompression of the thoracolumbar spinal cord. Neurosurgery *14*:302, 1984.

93. Malcolm, B. W., Bradford, D. S., Winter, R. B., et al.: Post-traumatic kyphosis. J. Bone Joint Surg. 63A:891–899, 1981.

94. Marshall, L. F., Knowlton, S., Garfin, S. R., et al.: Deterioration following spinal cord injury. A multicenter study. J. Neurosurg. 66:400–404, 1987.

95. Mayfield, J. K., Erkkila, J. C., and Winter, R. B.: Spine deformity subsequent to acquired childhood spinal cord injury. J. Bone Joint Surg. 63:1401–1411, 1981.

96. McAfee, P. C., and Bohlman, H. H.: Complications of Harrington instrumentation for fractures of the thoracolumbar spine. J. Bone Joint Surg. 67A:672–686, 1985.

97. McAfee, P. C., Bohlman, H. H., and Yuan, H. A.: Anterior decompression of traumatic thoracolumbar fractures with incomplete neurological deficit using retroperitoneal approach. J. Bone Joint Surg. 67A:89, 1985.

98. McAfee, P. C., Werner, F. W., and Glisson, R. R.: A biomechanical anaylsis of spinal instrumentation systems in thoracolumbar fractures. Comparison of traditional Harrington distraction instrumentation with segmental spinal instrumentation. Spine *10*(3):204–217, 1985.

99. McAfee, P. C., Yuan, H. A., and Lasda, N. A.: The unstable burst fracture. Spine 7:365, 1982.

100. McEvoy, R. D., and Bradford, D. S.: The management of burst fractures of the thoracic and lumbar spine: Experience in 53 patients. Spine *10*:631–637, 1985.

101. McGahan, J.P., Benson, D., Chehrazi, B., et al.: Intraoperative sonographic monitoring of reduction of thoracolumbar burst fractures. Am. J. Roent. *145*(6):1229–1232, 1985.

102. Meinecke, F. W.: Frequency and distribution of associated injuries in traumatic paraplegia and tetraplegia. Paraplegia 5:196, 1968.

103. Montalvo, B. M., Quencer, R. M., Green, B. A., et al.: Intraoperative sonography in spinal trauma. Radiology *153*:125–134, 1984.

104. Morgan, T.H., Wharton, G.W., and Austin, G.N.:The results of laminectomy in patients with incomplete spinal cord injuries. Paraplegia 9:14, 1971.

105. Munson, G., Satterlee, C., Hammond, S., et al.: Experimental evaluation of Harrington rod fixation supplemented with sublaminar wires in stabilizing thoracolumbar fracture-dislocations. Clin. Orthop. *189*:97–102, 1984.

106. Myer, P. R.: Complications of treatment of fractures of the dorsolumbar spine. In: Epps, C. H. (ed.): *Complications in Orthopaedic Surgery*, 2nd ed, Vol 2. Philadelphia, J. B. Lippincott Company, 1986, p. 713.

107. Myer, P. R.: *Surgery of Spine Trauma*. New York, Churchill Livingston, 1989.

108. Myllynen, P., Bostman O., and Riska, E.: Recurrence of deformity after removal of Harrington's fixation of spine fracture. Seventy-six cases followed for 2 years. Acta Orthop. Scand. 59(5):497–502, 1988.

109. Nash, C. L., Schatzinger, L. H., Brown, R. H., et al.: The unstable stable thoracic compression fracture. Spine 2:261–265, 1977.

110. Nicoll, E. A.: Fractures of the dorso-lumbar spine. J. Bone Joint Surg. *31*A:376, 1949.

111. Olerud, S., Karlstrom, G., and Sjostrom, L.: Transpedicular fixation of thoracolumbar vertebral fractures. Clin. Orthop. 227:45, 1988.

112. Oro, J., Watts, C., and Gaines, R.: Vertebral

body impactor for posterior lateral decompression of thoracic and lumbar fractures. J. Neurosurg. 70(2):285–286, 1989.

113. Osebold, W. R., Weinstein, S. L., and Sprague, B. L.: Thoracolumbar spine fractures: Results of treatment. Spine 6:13–34, 1981.

114. Osti, O. L., Fraser, R. D., and Cornish, B. L.: Fractures and fracture-dislocations of the lumbar spine. A retrospective study of 70 patients. Intern. Orthop. 11(4):323–329, 1987.

115. Purcell, G. A., Markolf, K. L., and Dawson, E. G.: Twelfth thoracic-first lumbar vertebral mechanical stability of fractures after Harrington-rod instrumentation. J. Bone Joint Surg. 63A: 71–78, 1981.

116. Quencer, R. M., Montalvo, B. M., Eismont, F. J., et al.: Intraoperative spinal sonography in thoracic and lumbar fractures: Evaluation of Harrington rod instrumentation. Am. J. Roent. 145(2):343–349, 1985.

117. Reid, D. C., Henderson, R., Saboe, L., et al.: Etiology and clinical course of missed spine fractures. J. Trauma 27:980–986, 1987.

118. Richardson, R. R., Meyer, P. R., and Cerullo, L. J.: Transcutaneous electrical neurostimulation in musculoskeletal pain of acute spinal cord injuries. Spine 5:42–45, 1980.

119. Riska, E. B., Myllynen, P., and Bostman, O.: Anterolateral decompression for neural involvement in thoracolumbar fractures. J. Bone Joint Surg. 69B:704–708, 1987.

120. Roberson, J. R., and Whitesides, T. E., Jr.: Surgical reconstruction of late post-traumatic thoracolumbar kyphosis. Spine 10:307–312, 1985.

121. Romanick, P. C., Smith, T. K., Kopaniky, D. R., et al.: Infection about the spine associated with low-velocity-missile injury to the abdomen. J. Bone Joint Surg. 67A:1195–1201, 1985.

122. Rossier, A. B., and Cochran, T. P.: The treatment of spinal fractures with Harrington compression rods and segmental sublaminar wiring: A dangerous combination. Spine 9:796, 1984.

123. Roy-Camille, R., Saillant, G., and Mazel, C.: Internal fixation of the lumbar spine with pedicle screw plating. Clin. Orthop. 203:7, 1986.

124. Roy-Camille, R., Saillant, G., and Mazel, C.: Internal fixation of the lumbar spine with pedicle screw plating. Orthop. Clin. North Am 17:147, 1986.

125. Scoliosis Research Society: Morbidity and Mortality Committee Report. Park Ridge, Illinois, Scoliosis Research Society, 1987.

126. Soreff, J., Axdorf, R., Bylund, P., et al.: Treatment of patients with unstable fractures of the thoracic and lumbar spine. Acta Orthop. Scand. 53:369–381, 1982.

127. Stauffer, E. S.: Internal fixation of fractures of the thoracolumbar spine. J. Bone Joint Surg. 66A:1136–1138, 1984.

128. Steffee, A. D., Discup, R. S., and Sitkowksi, D. J.: Segmental spine plates with pedicle screw fixation. Clin. Orthop. 203:45, 1986.

129. Sullivan, J. A.: Sublaminar wiring of Harrington distraction rods for unstable thoracolumbar spine fractures. Clin. Orthop. 189:178–185, 1984.

130. Svensson, O., Aaro, S., and Ohlen, G.: Harrington instrumentation for thoracic and lumbar vertebral fractures. Acta Orthop. Scand. 55:38, 1984.

131. Tearse, D. S., Keene, J. S., and Drummond, D. S.: Management of non-contiguous vertebral fractures. Paraplegia 25:100–105, 1987.

132. Tencer, A. F., Allen, B. L., Jr., and Ferguson, R. L.: A biomechanical study of thoracolumbar spinal fractures with bone in the canal. Part I. The effect of laminectomy. Spine 10(6):580–585, 1985.

133. Tencer, A. F., Allen, B. L., Jr., and Ferguson, R. L.: A biomechanical study of thoracolumbar spinal fractures with bone in the canal. Part II. The effect of flexion angulation, distraction, and shortening of the motion segment. Spine 10(6):586–589, 1985.

134. Trent, G., Armstrong, G. W. D., and O'Neil, J.: Thoracolumbar fractures in ankylosing spondylitis. Clin. Orthop. 227:61–66, 1988.

135. Vincent, K. A., Benson, D. R., and McGahan, J. P.: Intraoperative ultrasonography for reduction of thoracolumbar burst fractures. Spine 14(4):387–390, 1989.

136. Weinstein, J.N., Collalto, P., and Lehmann, T.R.: Long-term follow-up of nonoperatively treated thoracolumbar spine fractures. J. Orthop. Trauma 1:152, 1987.

137. White, A. A., and Panjabi, M. M.: *Clinical Biomechanics of the Spine.* Philadelphia, J. B. Lippincott Company, 1978.

138. Whitecloud, T. S., III, Butler, J. C., Cohen, J. L., et al.: Complications with the variable spinal plating system. Spine 14(4):472–476, 1989.

139. Whitesides, T. E., and Shah, S. G.: On the management of unstable fractures of the thoracolumbar spine. Spine 1:99, 1976.

140. Willen, J., Lindahl, S., and Norwall, A.: Unstable thoracolumbar fractures: Comparative clinical study of conservative treatment and Harrington instrumentation. Spine 10:111–122, 1985.

EIGHT

Infection in Spine Surgery

Richard A. Balderston, M.D.

Kalman Blumberg, M.D.

The complication of spinal infection in the treatment of patients with spinal disorders is a potentially life-threatening situation. All patients who undergo a spinal operation have a risk of postoperative infection at the operative site. This chapter will first describe the characteristics of pyogenic vertebral osteomyelitis caused by hematogenous spread and then delineate the aspects of infection in the postoperative period.

HISTORY

Spinal sepsis existed in antiquity, and its pathological sequelae have been well described in Egyptian mummies. In the fourth century BC Hippocrates described draining sinuses from both the back flank and groin as well as progressive kyphotic deformities in spinal sepsis patients. It took until the eighteenth century for Pott to fully summarize the clinical presentation and natural history of tuberculous infection of the spine. By the nineteenth century experimental osteomyelitis had been produced in animals with the intravenous injection of staphylococci. Also in the nineteenth century antiseptic measures introduced primarily by Lister improved postoperative infection rates.

The surgical treatment of spinal sepsis consisted primarily of laminectomy until the twentieth century; however, by the 1930s the se-

quelae of laminectomy, including late kyphotic deformity and inability to control the infectious process, were widely known. Hibbs and Albee recommended spinal fusion with autogenous bone graft as a treatment method for tuberculous spondylitis in 1911.[29] By the 1930s, with the introduction of antibiotic and antituberculous chemotherapeutic agents, the modern era of the treatment of spinal infection had begun.

EPIDEMIOLOGY

Over the last several decades, the epidemiology of vertebral osteomyelitis has slowly evolved. Early studies[16, 19] emphasized the high incidence of mycobacterium tuberculosis as the causative organism; however, the incidence of Pott's disease has declined in those areas of the world where living standards have improved. In underdeveloped countries tuberculosis remains a significant public health problem.

Pyogenic vertebral osteomyelitis, on the other hand, has increased in incidence. Digby[9] reported a yearly incidence of 1 case per 250,000 in England. Men are more often affected than women, by a ratio of approximately 3 to 1. Owing to multiple factors, the age of patients with spinal infection has been gradually increasing. The problem of intravenous drug abuse has increased the risk of gram-negative organisms including pseudomonas.[37, 44] Most investigators are following the HIV population closely; as yet, the clinical syndromes associated with spinal infection have not been significantly different in this unfortunate group of patients.

ETIOLOGY

Infection of the spine may occur by direct inoculation or by transport in the vascular system. The vascular anatomy of the spine may have a significant relationship to the bacterial seeding site. Batson's original studies of the venous plexus that bears his name entailed the injection of radiopaque dye into the pelvic veins of animals as well as human cadavers.[3, 4] These studies indicated that when abdominal pressure was elevated, the venous return from the pelvis travelled posteriorly into the venous plexus of the vertebral column. This valveless venous reservoir would then re-empty into the inferior vena cava and azygous systems as the pressure diminished and return flow was allowed. Batson theorized that the paravertebral venous reservoir functioned to allow continued venous return in the presence of changing abdominal and thoracic pressures. The motivating factor of his investigation was the well-known paradox of the presence of vertebral metastatic disease in patients who did not have demonstrable lung metastases. If metastatic tumor was spread only by arterial flow, the lungs should act as a filter and have significant metastatic involvement.

Wiley and Trueta injected micropaque barium solution into the cadavers of humans and rabbits to investigate the arterial system of the vertebral column.[46] In these studies they were able to postulate that the arterial supply coincided nicely with the distribution of the commonly seen infectious sites within vertebral bodies. This arterial flow, they felt, better explained the presence of micro-organisms at the level of the vertebral body end-plates. Owing to the tortuous flow of the arterioles, an area of micro-organism deposition may occur.

The vascular anatomy of the spine changes with age. In the pediatric population the blood supply to the vertebral disc has been well demonstrated. By age 20, the blood supply to the nucleus pulposus is obliterated, and blood supply to the disc is only to the annulus fibrosis. Primary disc space infection is a syndrome seen only in the pediatric age group. In adult patients, bacteria always lodge in the vertebral bodies close to the end-plates and secondarily invade the disc. Early changes of disc space narrowing have been shown to correlate with the disc's response to the products of inflammation that accumulate in the vertebral body and diffuse into the disc space.[6, 7, 22, 25]

The sites that most commonly function as a source of infection include the skin and genitourinary tract.[18] Other types of infection that can seed the spine include pharyngeal infections, pneumonia, empyema, cholangitis, abdominal abscess, and other sites of osteomyelitis. Of course, direct inoculation of the venous system by patients themselves as they practice drug abuse is also common.[37, 44]

Contiguous infections can directly invade the spine. Examples of this clinical syndrome include rare cases of empyema, retroperitoneal abscess, and pharyngeal infection. In addition, the vertebral column can be directly inoculated with bacteria from outside the body. Such circumstances include penetrating injuries by knife or bullet, discectomy and other spinal surgery, needle biopsy, chymopapain injection, percutaneous discectomy, or spinal fluid tap.

RISK FACTORS FOR INFECTION

Any patient with an existing infection is at risk for the development of a secondary spinal osteomyelitis. As has been mentioned before, patients who inject drugs intravenously are at higher risk than the general population for developing spinal sepsis. Patients who have had even minor genitourinary tract manipulation in the form of cystoscopy have a risk of developing thoracolumbar infectious involvement. Also, patients with a history of steroid use, alcoholism, malignancy, and diabetes mellitus are at increased risk compared with the general population.

Any condition that diminishes the body's response to infection creates a situation in which spinal osteomyelitis may arise. With the advent of newer chemotherapeutic agents for the treatment of HIV infection, spinal osteomyelitis may become a significant problem.

CLINICAL EVALUATION

HISTORY

The commonly reported delay in diagnosis of vertebral osteomyelitis is usually because the physician fails to consider this clinical entity.[9, 13] Confusion occurs because of a lack of differentiating symptoms and signs, often uncharacteristic x-ray findings, and the unfortunate use of prediagnostic antibiotics. There is not a characteristic specific history for vertebral osteomyelitis, but most patients present with back pain and a prior flulike syndrome. The back pain is persistent and occurs with bedrest and at night. As with patients who have degenerative disc disease, the pain is mechanical. However, analgesics rarely provide significant relief. Usually the pain is localized to the axial skeleton, but rarely, radicular symptoms will be present as well. Weight loss, anorexia, and malaise are also common presenting features.

The physician must inquire as to a history of previous infection. In addition, the common concomitant factors of recent genitourinary manipulation, diabetes mellitus, cancer, alcoholism, and steroid medication should also be sought[9] (Table 8–1).

PHYSICAL EXAMINATION

The most common physical finding is severe paravertebral muscle spasm and tenderness with diminished range of motion. However, given what would appear to be a severe roentgenographic presentation, point tenderness to either palpation or percussion may be surprisingly unstriking. Neurological deficit in the form of weakness of the lower extremities without hyper-reflexia may indicate epidural abscess in the lumbar spine.[2] Motor weakness in the lower extremities with hyper-reflexia

may indicate the presence of epidural extension in the thoracic spine. Eismont has determined a higher predisposition to neurological deficit in patients with diabetes mellitus, rheumatoid arthritis, advanced age, and a more cephalad level of infection.[10]

Patients with pain on passive motion of the hip joint may have involvement of the psoas muscle by retroperitoneal extension of the infection. Abdominal dysesthesia may be related to irritation of the thoracic spinal nerves as they leave the spinal canal at the level of the infectious process. The clinical signs of meningeal irritation, including pain with neck flexion and other maneuvers that stretch the meninges, may indicate epidural abscess.[16] The entire epidermis must be examined to determine if a subcutaneous abscess is a possible seeding source. Patients may have high fever and other signs of toxemia, including tachycardia and hypotension.

LABORATORY INVESTIGATION

In most cases the laboratory work-up of vertebral osteomyelitis is nonspecific. The leukocyte count may be elevated in cases with acute onset, but most commonly it is not elevated or only slightly elevated. The erythrocyte sedimentation rate is usually elevated with a value over 40 mm. per hour. Blood cultures may be positive, especially in patients who have an acute presentation. Urine cultures should always be taken because the genitourinary tract is a significant source of spinal infection. Depending on the patient's present immunological status, a tuberculin skin test may or may not be useful.

RADIOLOGY

The classic roentgenographic findings of pyogenic vertebral osteomyelitis depend on the stage of the disease. Early findings at two weeks usually reveal disc space narrowing owing to digestion of the nucleus pulposus by enzymes produced from the acute inflammatory response. This occurs on plain films prior to vertebral body rarefaction because of the large percentage of bone that must be removed before plain films will show a significant difference. By six weeks the vertebral bodies adjacent to the narrowed disc demonstrate decreased radiodensity. A few weeks later a reactive increase in radiodensity will occur as new woven bone is laid down on necrotic trabeculae (Fig. 8–1). Further new bone for-

Table 8–1
Vertebral Osteomyelitis: History, Physical Examination, and Laboratory Findings

HISTORY
Localized back pain
Anorexia/weight loss
GU manipulation
Skin infections
Diabetes mellitus
Malignancy
Alcohol/steroid use

PHYSICAL EXAMINATION
Paraspinal muscle spasm
Tenderness
Decreased ROM
Neurological deficit

LABORATORY
WBC: slight elevation
ESR: >40 mm./hr.

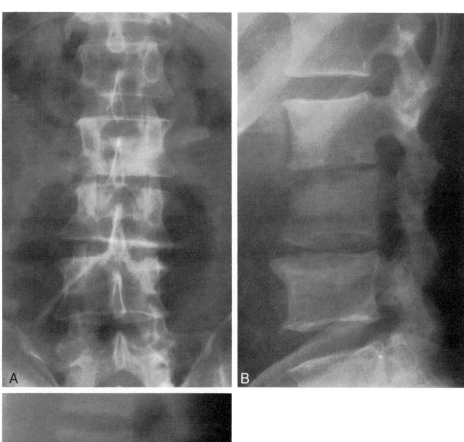

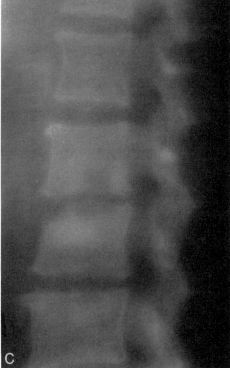

FIGURE 8–1. (*A*) LD is a 50-year-old male who recently underwent a genito-urinary procedure. This anteroposterior (*B*) and lateral plain radiograph reveals early infection with loss of disc space height, rarefaction of the adjoining vertebral bodies, and loss of end-plate definition at the L2–L3 interspace. (*C*) This lateral tomogram a few weeks later reveals increased radiodensity of the L3 vertebral body and continued loss of lordosis at this level.

mation will occur at 2 to 3 months, eventually leading to intervertebral body fusion at 6 to 24 months.

Vertebral osteomyelitis due to infection with mycobacterium tuberculosis follows a different type of course with roentgenographic findings significantly different from those of pyogenic vertebral osteomyelitis.[19] Plain films may not reveal disc space narrowing until late in the disease process. Loss of radiological density occurs as in pyogenic disease, but reactive new bone formation is often mild or absent. Fusion of the vertebral bodies is much less commonly seen in tuberculosis infections. A large soft-tissue mass may form with calcifications that can be found on x-ray and CT scan. This roentgenographic finding is relatively specific for tuberculosis. Serial roentgenographic evaluations may show the rapidity with which pyogenic vertebral osteomyelitis affects the vertebral bodies and disc space in contradistinction to tuberculosis. In general, pyogenic infections of the spine involve the lumbar area, whereas the average level for vertebral body involvement in tuberculosis is at the thoracolumbar junction.

The use of technetium-99 bone scan has improved the early diagnostic capabilities of the treating physician. The bone scan will be positive long before plain film changes occur. Other sites of infection will also be recognized with this useful technique. Modic and associates found a gallium scan to be more accurate than a technetium-99 scan with greater sensitivity and specificity.[32]

The CT scan may show bony changes earlier than plain roentgenographs.[7] In addition, the CT scan shows paravertebral soft-tissue masses and abscesses that can produce canal encroachment (Fig. 8–2).

Perhaps the most impressive means of diagnosing vertebral osteomyelitis is MRI scanning. Modic and associates described the typical changes of vertebral infection, which include decreased signal intensity of the vertebral disc space and two adjoining vertebral bodies on T1 weighted images.[32] On T2 weighted images, the adjoining vertebral bodies have an increased signal intensity, as does the disc space (Fig. 8–3). The MRI has been shown to have a sensitivity of 96 per cent, a specificity of 93 per cent, and an accuracy of 94 per cent. In addition, the magnetic resonance imaging scan provides excellent information with respect to canal involvement and soft-tissue abscess formation (see Fig. 8–2).

DIAGNOSTIC CONFIRMATION—CULTURE AND BIOPSY

In most cases of vertebral osteomyelitis, the cornerstone of management depends on an accurate bacteriological diagnosis. As has been mentioned, pre-existing sites of infection must be evaluated and cultured. This process would entail the aspiration of any skin abscesses and the procurement of a urine culture. If the patient is toxic and has high fever, blood cultures may be helpful in the identification of the organism responsible.

Closed needle biopsy is the study of choice initially to obtain bacteriological confirmation.[5, 40] With a paraspinal soft-tissue mass, a thinner needle may be used to obtain culture material. However, if the lesion is well confined to bone without significant destruction, the yield by such a procedure diminishes. Use of the CT scan or fluoroscopic guidance is mandatory for needle insertion. CT guidance of a fine needle insertion in the cervical spine has been shown to be relatively safe and effective. Stoker and Kissim found the success rate for needle biopsy of the spine to range from 60 to 96 per cent.[40] In a review of 30 biopsies of the thoracic spine, Bender demonstrated an accuracy of 90 per cent.[5] Two of 28 patients sustained a pneumothorax.

Larger diameter needle techniques, including the Craig needle, can be safely used in the lumbar spine under fluoroscopic control. Obtaining tissue from the L5-sacrum is more difficult because of the presence of the iliac crest. The experience of the pathologist and radiologist is critical for success of these closed techniques.

If closed techniques are not possible and the infectious source cannot be determined from other areas, open biopsy may be necessary. In general, anterior approaches to the spine are required for culture.[26] The posterior approach, including a laminectomy, is performed only in the case of epidural abscess or in the rare instance of primary involvement of the posterior elements only. If surgical debridement is not a high priority, costotransversectomy is the procedure of choice in lesions of the thoracic spine.

The chances of obtaining a positive culture are significantly elevated if the patient has not been treated with antibiotics prior to biopsy. The false-negative rate significantly increases with the use of prebiopsy antibiotics. In those cases in which the history, physical examina-

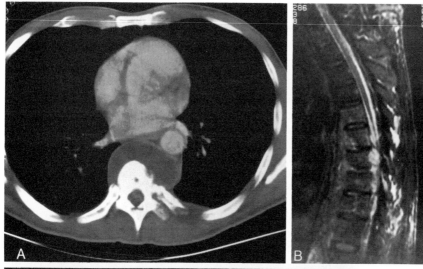

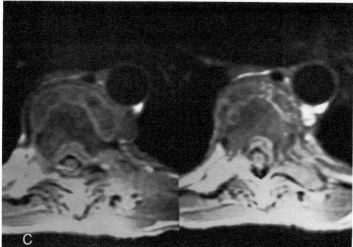

FIGURE 8–2. (*A*) This chest CT reveals early bony destruction with a large surrounding abscess cavity displacing the mediastinal contents. There is also canal encroachment with epidural abscess. (*B*) In the same patient the sagittal magnetic resonance image of T2 reveals multiple level involvement. A large anterior abscess cavity and severe spinal cord compression are demonstrated. (*C*) These transverse plane MRI scans also show a large anteriorly situated abscess cavity with a surrounding halo of edema. High-grade canal encroachment is again demonstrated.

tion, and laboratory and radiological parameters point strongly toward infection but the cultures are negative, the diagnosis must be made on histological findings. Evidence of acute or chronic inflammation should direct treatment toward the most likely organism. Although not specific, if histology demonstrates granulomatous inflammation with caseating necrosis, one should suspect tuberculosis. Brucellosis and fungal infection may also occur, although they are much rarer; skin and other immunological testing can assist in the differentiation of these organisms.

TREATMENT

The cornerstones of treatment of vertebral osteomyelitis include rest and immobilization,

intravenous antibiotics, and, rarely, surgery. Immobilization reduces pain and assists in the achievement of spontaneous fusion. Formal strict bedrest has been used, but modern treatment includes an ambulatory outpatient regimen that is allowed with the use of bracing. Diminution of pain and roentgenographic evidence of fusion mark the end of the need for brace treatment.

Intravenous antibiotics must be started immediately after biopsy with a combination of aminoglycoside and penicillinase-resistant antibiotics. This combination of antibiotics is useful for most infections. First-generation cephalosporins may not penetrate the disc space and vertebral bone sufficiently and are therefore not first-choice drugs without specific sensitivity evaluation.[12] With culture results and antibiotic sensitivities that usually appear

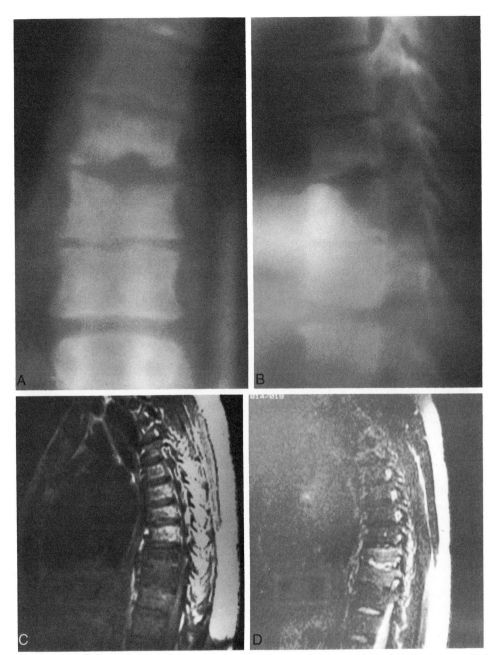

FIGURE 8–3. (*A*) Anteroposterior and lateral (*B*) tomograms of a T7 and T8 vertebral osteomyelitis. There is disc space narrowing, loss of end-plate definition, and a reactive sclerosis of the vertebral bodies. (*C*) Sagittal T1 image showing the common finding of decreased signal intensity of the vertebral disc space and two adjoining vertebral bodies. (*D*) On these T2 weighted images the involved vertebral bodies and disc space all have an increased signal intensity.

at three to five days, a more specific antibiotic may be chosen. Intravenous antibiotics are generally continued for six weeks. If a patient continues to be febrile, operative debridement may be indicated. The proper length of oral antibiotic coverage after intravenous therapy may vary from zero to six months depending on the organism and the course of the sedimentation rate. The ESR is monitored on a monthly basis once the patient leaves the hospital. With the use of a Hickman catheter many patients are able to have their intravenous antibiotic treatment as outpatients. If the patient's symptoms are not controlled or if the sedimentation rate and white cell count do not come back to normal, the antibiotic regimen must be re-evaluated.

Fortunately, with the above regimen, surgery is rarely indicated. The indications for surgical biopsy, debridement, strut grafting, or instrumentation include the following:

1. Increasing osseous involvement.
2. Increasing paraspinal abscess formation.
3. Neurological deficit.
4. Septic course with clinical toxicity, not improved by antibiotics.
5. Failure of needle biopsy to obtain necessary culture data.
6. Failure of long-term antibiotics to eradicate the infection.
7. Progressive kyphotic deformity secondary to vertebral destruction.

In patients for whom needle biopsy has not provided confirmation, the anterior approach is usually chosen for debridement. At that time autogenous graft is added to hasten the hoped-for result of spontaneous interbody fusion. Choices of donor site include fibula, iliac crest, and resected rib in cases in which the thoracic approach is used. In addition, a rib graft can be placed that is fully vascularized and simply rotated on the vascular pedicle. Most surgeons agree that the tricortical iliac crest is probably the donor site of choice, as the graft itself can provide immediate stability because of its cortical structure and early union because of its cancellous component.

If more than two vertebral bodies are involved in the process, anterior grafting is usually followed by posterior instrumentation to achieve immediate stability. Posterior instrumentation may include the Harrington or Cotrel-Dubousset devices.

In patients who have a neurological deficit secondary to canal encroachment, anterior decompressive surgery is performed. Previously, myelography was necessary to evaluate the extent of canal encroachment, but at our institution, the magnetic resonance imaging scan is the diagnostic procedure of choice to evaluate the extent of involvement of the bony canal as well as the possible involvement of the meninges themselves. In general, if more than one vertebral body has to be removed owing to spinal cord compression, posterior instrumentation is necessary for stability in addition to the anterior structural bone graft.

Patients with progressive kyphotic deformity usually require a combined approach using anterior debridement and bone grafting followed by posterior instrumentation. Given the chronic nature of the progressive deformity, anterior surgery alone is usually not adequate. This situation is usually caused by the failure of intravenous antibiotics to control the infectious process with continued bony destruction of the anterior and middle columns.

Laminectomy, especially of the cervical, thoracic, or thoracolumbar junction, for the treatment of vertebral body osteomyelitis is to be condemned. The usual result from such an ill-advised intervention is progressive kyphotic deformity with failure to eradicate the infection. Adequate debridement of the vertebral body cannot be achieved from a posterior approach.

COMPLICATIONS

Neurological deficit, abscess and fistula formation, spinal deformity, respiratory infection, GI bleeding, and death are complications associated with the infectious disease process itself. Graft complications, renal failure, allergic reactions, and wound infections may be classified as complications of treatment.

The incidence of neurological deficits ranges from 3 to 15 per cent in most unselected studies of pyogenic vertebral osteomyelitis.[8, 9, 10] Neurological deficit is usually associated with considerable bony destruction. The risk factors for progressive neurological deficit include increased age, diabetes mellitus, rheumatoid arthritis, and a more cranial level of vertebral involvement.

Abscess and fistula formation does occur with pyogenic infection but is more common with tuberculous involvement of the spine.[19] Abscess formation may be associated with severe septicemia at the time of debridement, and most authors recommend that preoperative antibiotics be given when a large abscess is drained, to avoid concomitant septicemia. Needle biopsy is indicated in patients with abscess formation to confirm the appropriate antibiotic therapy. Fistula formation may occur locally, but often the infection will appear on the skin at a site distant from the primary vertebrae involved. Psoas abscess and groin fistula, popliteal fistula, and cervical fistula are all possible sequelae.

Gastrointestinal bleeding and respiratory infection are reported complications of vertebral osteomyelitis. Griffiths and Jones reported on 3 of 28 patients with collapse of a lung base and pneumonia secondary to thoracic vertebral osteomyelitis.[15] These complications are both common causes of death in this patient population (Table 8–2).

POSTOPERATIVE SPINAL INFECTIONS

Postoperative spinal infection is a potentially catastrophic complication of spinal surgery.[28, 29, 31, 33] The potential morbidity is great. Complications may be relatively insignificant and temporary, such as superficial wound infections or stitch abscesses, with no long-term sequelae. On the other hand, vertebral osteomyelitis may result.

CLASSIFICATION

Wound infections after spinal surgery may be classified as superficial or deep. If the infection is confined to the dermis and subcutaneous tissues and does not penetrate the deep fascia, the infection is considered superficial.

Clinically superficial infections present with findings that are apparent upon inspection of the wound. The incision may become swollen, erythematous, and warm. The patient will note increased pain and tenderness. Temperature elevation may not be present, and the leukocyte count may not be elevated.

The subcutaneous tissue in obese patients may be poorly vascularized and predispose this area to infection. In addition, trauma during the surgery, which would include compression by retractors or extensive electrocoagulation, may increase the amount of necrotic tissue and predispose to an infectious process.

Infections that are present below the fascial structures are classified as deep. Acute deep infections of the spine are frequently compli-

cated by abscess formation with development of soft-tissue mass, and extension may occur to vital structures, including the pharynx and esophagus of the neck, the lungs from the thoracic spine, and the abdominal contents in the lumbar spine. In patients who have had a disc evacuation without penetration of the vertebral end-plate, the vascularity of this tissue in the adult patient is minimal and infection may occur. With increased pressure from microorganisms, infection may spread either into the vertebral bodies or peripherally about the supporting ligaments of the spine.

INCIDENCE

The overall incidence of spinal surgery complicated by postoperative infection is low. For intervertebral disc surgery without fusion, studies have reported an incidence of disc space infection ranging from 0.7 to 2.8 per cent. For patients undergoing spinal fusions that do not require instrumentation, the infection rate is somewhat higher and has ranged from 0.9 to 6 per cent. With the addition of spinal instrumentation, the incidence of infection increases. The average infection rate is 8 per cent with a range of 0.5 to 15 per cent.[29, 31, 42]

OPERATING ROOM FACTORS

For any procedure involving an approach to the spine, the rules for aseptic surgery are mandatory. Any break in strict surgical technique will increase the risk of infection in the postoperative period.

Great attention must be given to the meticulous handling of tissue. Inappropriate traction, rough handling, and inappropriate use of electrocautery will cause diminished vascularity and increased tissue necrosis, allowing for compromise of the normal infection-resistant environment. Patients who have an increased dead space, such as those with significant adipose tissue or those with a long incision, are at increased risk for infection. It would be reasonable to assume that increased operating time increases the infection rate, although two studies did not correlate prolonged operating time with an increased complication rate from infection.[31]

Foreign material will enhance the complication rate. With the increased use of metallic implants for spinal surgery, the number of postoperative infections is increasing. In addition, the use of methylmethacrylate in spinal

---

Table 8–2
Complications of Vertebral Osteomyelitis

TREATMENT ASSOCIATED
Graft/hardware
Renal failure
Allergic reactions
Wound infections

NON–TREATMENT ASSOCIATED
Neurological deficit
Abscess/fistula formation
Spinal deformity
Respiratory infection
GI bleeding
Death

procedures has been shown to significantly depress the phagocytic and migratory properties of polymorphonuclear leukocytes.

The operating room personnel themselves are a major source of postoperative wound infection.[35, 36] Proper sterile technique at the time of gowning and gloving is mandatory. Excessive operating room personnel with frequent change in personnel during the case is also a risk factor for postoperative infection.[27]

Airborne bacteria are present in all operating rooms. Bacteria are carried on particles of different sizes. Proper air exchange and filtration may assist in lowering the risk of infection.

PATIENT FACTORS

As has been mentioned in the previous sections regarding etiology and risk factors, there are a host of problems that may predispose patients to a postoperative infection. Patients who are malnourished or immunologically suppressed have an increased risk of developing infection after their surgery. Pre-existing skin or genitourinary infection at the time of the procedure may seed the operative site from these areas. Any patient who has a significant infection of another organ system should have that infection fully treated before undergoing elective spinal surgery. Patients who suffer from diabetes mellitus, malignancy, alcoholism, or steroid abuse are also at increased risk for infection in the postoperative period.

PROPHYLACTIC ANTIBIOTICS

Prophylactic antibiotics will significantly decrease the postoperative infection rate. In 1975, Horwitz and Curtin reported on 531 patients undergoing lumbar disc surgery. In their study, infection rate was diminished from 9.3 to 1 per cent with the use of prophylactic antibiotics.[20] Lonstein and associates reviewed patients undergoing spinal fusion with instrumentation. Infection rate diminished from 9.3 to 2.8 per cent in patients who were treated with perioperative prophylactic antibiotics.[29]

DIAGNOSIS

The temporal classification of wound infections in the postoperative period is acute and delayed. Acute infections occur during the patient's hospitalization and generally within one to two weeks after surgery. Acute superficial infections present with erythema, swelling, and tenderness of the surgical site. Usually there is drainage from one or more areas of the wound.

A postoperative acute deep infection is not as easily diagnosed. The wound may appear benign and may not be specifically tender to touch. However, patients will usually describe a sudden increase in pain at the operative site. In addition, they usually manifest an elevated temperature and a feeling of malaise. If neurological involvement is present, abscess formation in the epidural space may have occurred.

In either of these two circumstances, the wounds must be aspirated. Needle introduction is performed away from the surgical incision. In many instances, the superficial infection can be adequately treated with simple aspiration, culture, and antibiotic treatment.

At this time changes will not be evident on radiological examination because it will be difficult to differentiate normal postoperative changes from those associated with infection. Any patient with paralysis, dysesthesia, or root pain should be considered to have epidural abscess until proven otherwise. The rapidity of onset of symptoms can be quite striking, and treatment must be initiated as soon as possible to avoid irreversible sequelae.

POSTOPERATIVE DISCITIS

In patients undergoing intervertebral disc excision, a unique milieu is created wherein bacteria may multiply. Patients generally have a pain-free interval of a few weeks with diminished back and leg pain and an apparent successful disc excision. However, after the second week, patients present with back pain that is progressive. At this time, temperature elevation may occur, and stiffness of the paravertebral muscles will lead to a diminution in range of motion. Generally, there is a normal neurological examination. However, pain may be referred to the lower abdomen, groin, or proximal thighs. Erythrocyte sedimentation rate is always elevated. Roentgenographic findings include narrowing of the disc space followed by a loss of definition of the sclerotic line at the vertebral end-plate. The natural history of roentgenographic findings includes sclerosis with increased bone formation and occasional fusion of the adjacent vertebrae.

Unfortunately bone scanning techniques are not helpful at this time. With either a technetium or gallium scan it would be impossible to differentiate postoperative changes from those associated with infection.

The cornerstone of diagnosis remains aspiration of the disc with Gram's stain and culture. Usually, closed needle biopsy is successful with respect to establishing bacteriological diagnosis. With a positive diagnosis, intravenous antibiotics are administered. Treatment is the same as for those patients who have vertebral osteomyelitis. Our regimen includes six weeks of intravenous antibiotics with weekly monitoring of the sedimentation rate. Operative debridement is indicated if this regimen fails to control the symptoms.

ACUTE DEEP INFECTION
TREATMENT
Once the diagnosis of deep infection is suspected, needle aspiration is carried out. If the needle aspiration is positive, treatment is indicated. If needle aspiration is negative, but clinical signs progress with increased fluctuance of the wound and even mild erythema, treatment is begun.

The cornerstone of treatment is debridement in the operating room with complete exploration and irrigation. Debridement is carried down to the underlying bone graft and instrumentation. At least six liters of irrigation are used through pulsatile lavage to debride the entire wound. For deep infections we prefer to leave the wound open and close at a later date to enhance our chances of bacterial eradication.

For bone graft surgery, either autograft or allograft, we would not remove the bone graft that has initially attached to granulation tissue from the surrounding musculature. If large pieces of bone graft, usually allograft, are found to be full of pus, they are removed from the wound.

Metallic implants generally are left in place, as spinal stability during this time period is mandatory. Removal of the instrumentation device does not enhance the chances of successful treatment. If pseudarthrosis should occur after instrument removal, the chances of having persistent infection are greater.

Other authors have recommended the use of a suction irrigation system as a means of closing the wound primarily. This treatment is a reasonable one should the surgeon be trained in its usage.

DELAYED DEEP INFECTION
POSTOPERATIVE DISCITIS AND POSTOPERATIVE VERTEBRAL OSTEOMYELITIS
The treatment of delayed deep infection usually of bone and disc space is similar to the treatment for primary osteomyelitis of the spine. An accurate biopsy must be obtained, and antibiotics and immobilization are initiated.

The operative indications are the same as those for primary cases, with one exception. Should the infection continue to be significant with instrumentation in place, consideration is given to implant removal *after* the fusion has healed.

REFERENCES

1. Akbarnia, B. A.: Pyogenic infections of the spine. In: Chapman, M. W. (ed.): *Operative Orthopaedics*. Philadelphia, J. B. Lippincott, 1988, pp. 2017–2027.
2. Baker, A., Ojemann, R. G., Swartz, M. N., et al.: Spinal epidural abscess. N. Engl. J. Med. 293:463–468, 1975.
3. Batson, O. V.: The vertebral vein system: Caldwell lecture, 1956. Am. J. Roentgenol. Rad. Ther. Nucl. Med. 78:195–212, 1957.
4. Batson, O. V.: The vertebral vein system as a mechanism for the spread of metastases. Am. J. Roentgenol. Rad. Ther. 48:715–718, 1942.
5. Bender, C. E., Berquist, T. H., and Wold, L. E.: Imaging-assisted percutaneous biopsy of the thoracic spine. Mayo Clin. Proc. 61:942–950, 1986.
6. Bonfiglio, M., Lange, T. A., and Kim, Y. M.: Pyogenic vertebral osteomyelitis. Clin. Orthop. Rel. Res. 96:234–247, 1973.
7. Brant-Zawadzki, M., Burke, V. D., and Jeffrey, R. B.: CT in the evaluation of spine infection. Spine 8:358–364, 1983.
8. Collert, S.: Osteomyelitis of the spine. Acta Orthop. Scand. 48:283–290, 1977.
9. Digby, J. M., and Kersley, J. B.: Pyogenic nontuberculous spinal infection. J. Bone Joint Surg. 61B:47–55, 1979.
10. Eismont, F. J., Bohlman, H. H., Soni, P. L., et al.: Pyogenic and fungal vertebral osteomyelitis with paralysis. J. Bone Joint Surg. 65A:19–29, 1983.
11. Emery, S. E., Chan, D. P. K., and Woodward, H. R.: Treatment of hematogenous pyogenic vertebral osteomyelitis with anterior debridement and primary bone grafting. Spine 14:284–291, 1989.
12. Fitzgerald, R. H., and Thompson, R. L.: Cephalosporin antibiotics in the prevention and treatment of musculoskeletal sepsis. J. Bone Joint Surg. 65A:1201, 1983.
13. Garcia, A., and Grantham, S. A.: Hematogenous pyogenic vertebral osteomyelitis. J. Bone Joint Surg. 42A:429–436, 1960.
14. Ghormley, R. K., Bickel, W. H., and Dickson, D. D.: A study of acute infectious lesions of the intervertebral disks. South. Med. J. 33:347–353, 1940.
15. Griffiths, H. E. D., and Jones, D. M.: Pyogenic infection of the spine: A review of twenty-eight cases. J. Bone Joint Surg. 53B:383–391, 1971.
16. Guri, J. P.: Pyogenic osteomyelitis of the spine. J. Bone Joint Surg. 28:29–39, 1946.

17. Hazlett, J. W.: Pyogenic osteomyelitis of the spine. Can. J. Surg. *1*:243–246, 1958.
18. Henson, S. W., and Coventry, M. B.: Osteomyelitis of the vertebrae as the result of infection of the urinary tract. Surg. Gynecol. Obstet. *102*:207–214, 1956.
19. Hodgson, A. R., and Stock, F. E.: Anterior fusion of the spine for treatment of tuberculosis of the spine. J. Bone Joint Surg. *42A*:295–310, 1960.
20. Horwitz, N. H., and Curtin, J. A.: Prophylactic antibiotics and wound infections following laminectomy for lumbar disc herniation. J. Neurosurg. *43*:727–731, 1975.
21. Kemp, H. B. S., Jackson, J. W., Jeremiah, J. D., et al: Anterior fusion of the spine for infective lesions in adults. J. Bone Joint Surg. *55B*:715–734, 1973.
22. Kemp, H. B. S., Jackson, J. W., Jeremiah, J. D., et al.: Pyogenic infections occurring primarily in intervertebral discs. J. Bone Joint Surg. *55B*:698–714, 1973.
23. Kemp, H. B. S., Jackson, J. W., and Shaw, N. C.: Laminectomy in paraplegia due to infective spondylosis. Br. J. Surg. *61*:66–72, 1974.
24. Keon-Cohen, B. T.: Epidural abscess simulating disc herniation. J. Bone Joint Surg. *50B*:128–130, 1968.
25. King, D. M., and Mayo, K. M.: Infective lesions of the vertebral column. Clin. Orthop. Rel. Res. *96*:248–253, 1973.
26. Kirkaldy-Willis, W. H., and Thomas, T. G.: Anterior approaches in the diagnosis and treatment of infections of the vertebral bodies. J. Bone Joint Surg. *47A*:87–110, 1965.
27. Letts, R. M., and Doermer, E.: Conversation in the operating theatre as a cause of airborne bacterial contamination. J. Bone Joint Surg. *65A*:357–62, 1983.
28. Lindholm, T. S., and Pylkkanen, P.: Discitis following removal of intervertebral disc. Spine *7*:618–622, 1982.
29. Lonstein, J., Winter, R., Moe, J., et al.: Wound infection with instrumentation for scoliosis. Clin. Orthop. *96*:222–233, 1973.
30. Malinin, T. I., and Brown, M. D.: Bone allograft in spinal surgery. Clin. Orthop. *154*:68–73, 1981.
31. Moe, J. H.: Complications of scoliosis treatment. Clin. Orthop. *53*:21, 1967.
32. Modic, M. T., Feiglin, D. H., Piraino, D. W., et al.: Vertebral osteomyelitis: Assessment using MR. Radiology *157*:157–166, 1985.
33. Pilgaard, S.: Discitis (closed space infection) following removal of lumbar intervertebral disc. J. Bone Joint Surg. *51A*:713, 1969.
34. Puranen, J., Makeler, J., and Lahde, S.: Postoperative intervertebral discitis. Acta Orthop. Scand. *55*:461–465, 1984.
35. Ritter, M. A.: Surgical wound environment. Clin. Orthop. *190*:11–13, 1984.
36. Ritter, M. A., Eitzen, H. E., Hart, J. B., et al.: The surgeon's garb. Clin. Orthop. *153*:204–209, 1980.
37. Sapico, F. L., and Montgomerie, J. Z.: Vertebral osteomyelitis in intravenous drug abusers: Report of three cases and review of the literature. Rev. Infect. Dis. *2*:196, 1980.
38. Stauffer, R. N.: Pyogenic vertebral osteomyelitis. Orthop. Clin. North Am. *6*:1015–1027, 1975.
39. Stevens, D. B.: Postoperative orthopaedic infections. J. Bone Joint Surg. *46A*:96, 1964.
40. Stoker, D.J., and Kissim, C. M.: Percutaneous vertebral biopsy: A review of 135 cases. Clin. Radiol. *33*:569–577, 1985.
41. Thibodeau, A. A.: Closed space infection following removal of lumbar intervertebral disc. J. Bone Joint Surg. *50A*:400, 1968.
42. Tombard, W. W., Starkweather, P. I., and Goldman, M. H.: A study of clinical incidence of infections in the use of banked allograft bone. J. Bone Joint Surg. *63A*:244–248, 1981.
43. Wedge, J. H., Oryschak, A. F., Robertson, D. E., et al.: Atypical manifestations of spinal infections. Clin. Orthop. Rel. Res. *123*:155–163, 1977.
44. Weisseman, G. J., Wood, V. E., and Kroll, L. L.: Pseudomonas vertebral osteomyelitis in heroin addicts. J. Bone Joint Surg. *55A*:1416–1424, 1973.
45. Welch, D. M., Baker, W. J., Breightol, R. W., et al.: Indium labeled leukocytes in the evaluation of suspected inflammatory processes. J. Nucl. Med. *20*:659, 1979.
46. Wiley, A. M., and Trueta, J.: The vascular anatomy of the spine and its relationship to pyogenic vertebral osteomyelitis. J. Bone Joint Surg. *41B*:796–809, 1959.
47. Wiltberger, B. R.: Resection of vertebral bodies and bone-grafting for chronic osteomyelitis of the spine. J. Bone Joint Surg. *34A*:215–218, 1952.
48. Wood, G. W.: Spinal infections. Spine State of the Art Reviews *3*:461–493, 1989.

NINE

Complications of Surgery of the Spine in Rheumatoid Arthritis and Ankylosing Spondylitis

J. Michael Simpson, M.D.

Howard S. An, M.D.

Richard A. Balderston, M.D.

Although ankylosing spondylitis and rheumatoid arthritis are often considered together when discussing spinal deformity, they are indeed two distinct disease processes. Rheumatoid arthritis is a systemic disorder, more common in females, with a predilection to affect the smaller joints of the appendicular skeleton in a symmetrical fashion. The major clinical problems of the spine in the rheumatoid patient result from erosive changes in the cervical spine leading to pathological subluxation or dislocation.

Ankylosing spondylitis is a seronegative spondyloarthropathy affecting primarily the spine and major joints. It primarily affects males with a majority of patients being HLA-B27 antigen positive. In patients with ankylosing spondylitis, excessive stress on the upper cervical spine coupled with inflammatory changes may lead to atlantoaxial subluxation or dislocation. Severe, fixed flexion deformities of the cervical, thoracic, and lumbar spine represent the primary challenges to the spine surgeon.

RHEUMATOID ARTHRITIS

PREOPERATIVE PLANNING

Cervical spine involvement in the rheumatoid patient is reported at 25 to 95 per cent, depending on the particular study and diagnostic criteria.[4, 12, 32, 33, 37, 38] Rheumatoid syno-

vitis causes pathological changes in the ligamentous structures, articular cartilage, and bone in the form of osteoporosis, cyst formation, and erosion. The pathological processes in the cervical spine are identical to those that occur peripherally as proven by biopsy.[3, 16, 23] The specific deformity depends on the level and extent of involvement. The types of involvement in decreasing order of frequency include atlantoaxial subluxation, atlantoaxial subluxation combined with subaxial subluxation, isolated subaxial subluxation, and superior migration of the odontoid. Atlantoaxial subluxation results from erosive synovitis of the atlantoaxial, atlanto-odontoid, and atlanto-occipital joints. Subaxial destruction results from involvement of the facets, uncovertebral joints, intervertebral disc, and interspinous ligaments. Atlantoaxial impaction or pseudobasilar invagination describes the process in which the skull settles on the atlas, and atlas on the axis, resulting from erosion and bone loss in the occipitoatlantal and atlantoaxial joints, respectively.

UPPER CERVICAL PROBLEMS: ATLANTOAXIAL SUBLUXATION AND ATLANTOAXIAL IMPACTION

Atlantoaxial subluxation represents the most common and significant manifestation of rheumatoid involvement of the cervical spine. Conlon and associates[12] reported a 25 per cent incidence of radiographic atlantoaxial subluxation in a hospital population of rheumatoid patients, while Bland[4] reported 86 per cent of patients with classic rheumatoid arthritis to have radiographic evidence of cervical spine involvement. The incidence of atlantoaxial instability has been estimated at approximately 6 to 34 per cent in patients with clinical evidence of rheumatoid disease.[31, 40] The incidence has generally been shown to be higher in patients with long-standing disease, older patients, patients with severely erosive peripheral forms of the disease, and patients who have received long-term steroid treatment.[31] Smith and associates, however, did not find a significant correlation between age or duration of the disease and anterior atlantoaxial subluxation.[43] Atlantoaxial impaction, however, was found to be related to these factors. The natural history of rheumatoid patients with cervical spine involvement is one of progression.[22, 43, 48] Radiographic progression is reported at 39 to 41 per cent for anterior atlantoaxial subluxation.[43, 47] Progression of neurological symptoms, however, is less, ranging from 2 to 14 per cent.[43, 48] Significant risk factors for progression as shown by Weissman and associates are an atlantodental distance greater than 9 mm. and the presence of atlantoaxial impaction.[48]

Atlantoaxial instability in the rheumatoid patient population is generally manifested in one of two forms: anterior atlantoaxial subluxation or vertical subluxation of the odontoid (also referred to as basilar impression, atlantoaxial impaction, cranial settling, and superior migration). Posterior atlantoaxial subluxation is relatively rare and is usually associated either with fracture or erosion of the odontoid. In one series it accounted for 6.7 per cent of all atlantoaxial subluxations.[48] Lipson reports that this is not a benign condition and can cause a myelopathy by kinking the posterior cord at the cervicomedullary junction.[29]

Isolated superior migration of the odontoid is very rare. Anterior subluxation is the most common isolated deformity and may coexist with superior migration. Ranawat and associates, reporting on rheumatoid patients requiring surgical treatment, found that 70 per cent had atlantoaxial subluxation, 60 per cent had subaxial subluxation, and 16 per cent had superior migration.[38]

Lateral atlantoaxial subluxation is best appreciated on an anteroposterior radiograph when the lateral masses of C1 lie 2 mm. or more laterally on C2. Lateral subluxation is reported to account for 21 per cent of all atlantoaxial subluxations and is found more commonly in patients with cord compression.[47]

Anterior C1-C2 subluxation is assessed radiographically by measuring the atlantodental interval. This is measured from the mid-posterior margin of the anterior ring of C1 to the anterior surface of the dens. A measurement of this difference of more than 3 mm. in the adult or 4 mm. in the child on flexion/extension views is accepted as being unstable or potentially unstable (Fig. 9–1). Vertical migration of the odontoid can be radiographically assessed by several methods (Fig. 9–2). Normally, the tip of the odontoid lies 1 cm. below the anterior margin of the foramen magnum in the adult (0.5 cm. in the child). Chamberlain's line is drawn from the hard palate to the inner aspect of the posterior rim of the foramen magnum. The odontoid should not project more than 3 mm. above this line with more than 6 mm. being definitely pathological. Symptomatic basilar impression usually requires significant protrusion. McRae's line connects the front to the back of the foramen magnum. In a normal patient, the odontoid should not project beyond this line. McGregor's line connects the posterior margin of the hard palate to the posterior margin of the most caudal point of the occiput. The tip

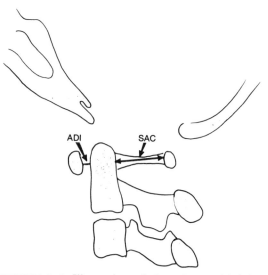

FIGURE 9–1. Illustration of the atlantoaxial joint with atlas-dens-interval (ADI) and the space available for the spinal cord (SAC). ADI > 3 mm. is abnormal in adults. (From Hensinger, R.N.: Congenital anomalies of the atlantoaxial joint. In: Sherk, H.H., et al. (eds.): *The Cervical Spine,* 2nd ed. Philadelphia, J.B. Lippincott Company, 1989, p. 237.)

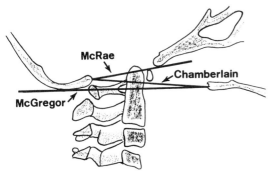

FIGURE 9–2. Illustration of lateral upper cervical spine with different lines for measuring vertical migration of the odontoid. Chamberlain's line is drawn from the posterior lip of the foramen magnum to the dorsal margin of the hard palate. McGregor's line is drawn from the upper surface of the posterior edge of the hard palate to the most caudal point of the occipital curve of the skull. McRae's line is drawn from the basion to the posterior lip of the foramen magnum. (From Hensinger, R.N., and MacEwen, G.D.: Congenital anomalies of the spine. In: Rothman, R.H., and Simeone, F.A. (eds.): *The Spine.* Philadelphia, W.B. Saunders Company, 1982, p. 190.)

of the odontoid should not project more than 4.5 mm. above this line.

Owing to the difficulty in radiographically visualizing the hard palate, Ranawat and associates devised another measurement for vertical odontoid migration (Fig. 9–3).[38] On the lateral x-ray of the cervical spine, the coronal axis of C1 is marked by connecting the centers of the anterior and posterior arches. A second vertical line is then drawn from the center of the sclerotic line of C2 (the pedicles) and extends upward along the midaxis of the odontoid until it intersects the first line. A measurement of less than 13 mm. is considered abnormal.

The method described by Fischgold and Metzger evaluates cephalad migration of the odontoid based on an anteroposterior open mouth view of the spine (Fig. 9–4).[18] Here, the digastric line (drawn from where the mastoid process joins the base of the skull) should be 1 cm. or more above the tip of the odontoid.

The clinical presentation of atlantoaxial instability in either rheumatoid arthritis or ankylosing spondylitis generally results from a combination of factors. Localized mechanical pain, secondary to the inflammatory process, and arthritic changes represent the most common presenting symptom complex. The patient will typically complain of pain and soreness of the suboccipital region with pain or discomfort radiating to the occiput. Extremes of flexion or extension of the spine tend to exacerbate the symptoms. With advanced changes in the C1–C2 articulation, neurological dysfunction may manifest itself through compression of the brain stem, spinal cord, peripheral nerve roots or vertebral artery insufficiency. Neurological symptoms are noted to a lesser degree and reported at a rate of 7 to 34 per cent.[12, 27, 45]

Patients may complain of paresthesias and

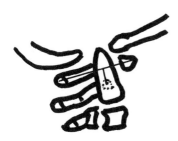

RANAWAT

FIGURE 9–3. Illustration of lateral upper cervical spine with Ranawat measurement. A horizontal line connects the centers of the anterior and posterior arches of C1. A vertical line starts at the center of the pedicles and extends superiorly along the midaxis of the odontoid. Measurement of less than 13 mm. is abnormal. (From Grantham, S.A., and Lipson, S.J.: Rheumatoid arthritis of the cervical spine. In: Sherk, H.H., et al. (eds.). *The Cervical Spine,* 2nd ed. Philadelphia, J.B. Lippincott Company, 1989, p. 567.)

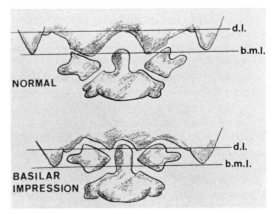

FIGURE 9–4. Illustrations of normal and basilar impression on anterior upper cervical AP tomogram with Fischgold and Metzger lines. The upper line connects the digastric grooves, and the lower line connects the lower poles of the mastoid processes. (From Hensinger, R.N., and MacEwen, G.D.: Congenital anomalies of the spine. In: Rothman, R.H., and Simeone, F.A. (eds.): *The Spine.* Philadelphia, W.B. Saunders, 1982, p. 190.)

weakness in the upper and lower extremities and occasionally may describe an electric shock sensation that traverses their entire body (Lhermitte's sign). Dizziness, suboccipital headache, dysphagia, vertigo, visual disturbances, and nystagmus are the typical symptoms that accompany vertebral artery insufficiency. Urinary retention or frequency is an important early warning sign that should not be ignored.

Some authors feel that atlantoaxial subluxation is well tolerated by many rheumatoid patients without neurological compromise. However, Mathews found that long tract signs developed in nearly one-third of patients with anterior C1-C2 subluxation and one-half of those with vertical subluxation.[33] Protective soft collars or braces may be of some limited value but generally are not well tolerated. In the patient with ankylosing spondylitis, subluxation may occur, and the joint may then become stabilized in the subluxated position without symptoms.

The indications for surgery include significant progressive neurological deterioration, intractable pain, and severe instability (greater than 9 mm.). Posterior atlantoaxial arthrodesis, using either the Gallie or Brooks technique, is indicated for patients with gross C1-C2 instability. Autogenous iliac crest graft material is preferable, but allograft material can be used in patients whose pelvic bone is too osteoporotic.

The fusion should extend to the occiput and perhaps include C3 when the patient exhibits superior migration of the odontoid. Posterior deficiency in the arch of C1 may require stabilization to the occiput to enhance the stability of the surgical construct.

Magnetic resonance imaging is helpful in patients with neurological symptoms to determine the site of cord compression. Anterior transoral decompression of the cord may be required in patients where the odontoid is causing major anterior pressure.[7, 14, 15, 36] Crockard and associates reported on this treatment modality in 14 patients with favorable results.[14] This appears to be a rational approach for patients with pure basilar invagination and narrowing of the cerebellomedullary cistern. However, this is a more hazardous approach owing to its relative unfamiliarity to the surgeon and high risk of infection. In patients where C1-C2 subluxation is coupled with anterior odontoid compression, transoral decompression followed by posterior fusion and stabilization is recommended.

SURGICAL TECHNIQUES

POSTERIOR ATLANTOAXIAL ARTHRODESIS

A halo ring is applied just prior to surgery in order to maintain traction during operation and to facilitate vest application after surgery. If traction is not required, the patient can be fitted with a posteriorly opened halo ring and the vest preoperatively. A midline incision from the occiput to the fourth cervical vertebra is made. The tips of the spinous processes are exposed and subperiosteal dissection carried out along the laminae of C2 and the posterior arch of C1. All soft tissues are then carefully removed from the bony surfaces. The arch of C1 should not be exposed more than 1.5 cm. from the midline in adults and 1 cm. in children to avoid injury to the vertebral arteries. Great care must be taken not to fracture the posterior ring of C1 while dissecting the ligamentum flavum.

Fielding and Simmons advocate the use of a modified Gallie H-graft from the iliac crest, contouring it to fit over the posterior arches of C1 and C2.[17a, 42] A doubled, U-shaped 18- or 20-gauge wire is passed under the arch of C1 from inferior to superior. A bone block is taken from the posterior iliac crest and shaped to fit between C1 and C2 as well as wires (Fig. 9–5). The loop of the wire goes over the bone block and the spinous process of C2. The ends of the wire are tightened around the graft between C1 and C2. The deep cancellous surfaces of the graft must be contoured to fit over the curved posterior surface of C1 and C2 so that the graft is in firm contact with the underlying vertebrae, immobilizing the involved segment. Additional cancellous bone chips are placed lateral to the main graft as far as possible over the laminae.

In the Brooks type of fusion, doubled, twisted 24-gauge wires are passed under the arch of C1 and then under the lamina of C2, (see Fig. 5–8). Rectangular iliac crest bone grafts (1.25 cm. by 3.5 cm.) are harvested and beveled to fit in the interval between the arch of C1 and each lamina of the axis. The wires are then tightened securing the graft in proper position.

Lipson suggests preoperative halo traction followed by posterior fusion reinforced with metal mesh, wire, and polymethylmethacrylate to enhance stability.[29] Adequate external immobilization should be carried out for approximately 12 weeks with a halo vest or cast.

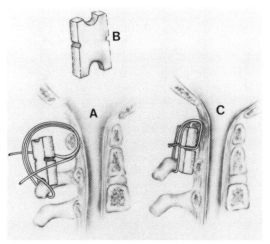

FIGURE 9–5. Gallie technique by Fielding and Simmons. *(A)* A doubled U-shaped 18- or 20-gauge wire is passed under the arch of C1 from inferior to superior. *(B)* A bone block is taken from the posterior iliac crest and shaped to fit between C1 and C2 as well as wires. *(C)* The loop of the wire goes over the bone block and the spinous process of C2. The ends of the wire are tightened around the graft between C1 and C2. (From Benson, D.R., and Anderson, D.D.: Fractures, dislocations, infections, and tumors of the atlas and axis. In: Chapman, M.W. (ed.): *Operative Orthopaedics.* Philadelphia, J.B. Lippincott Company, 1988, p. 1887.)

TRANSORAL DECOMPRESSION

In the transoral approach, the patient is supine with head placed in a hyperextended position. While routine tracheostomy is advocated by many, endotracheal anesthesia may be used as well. The soft palate is turned back on itself and held in position with a stay suture. A 5-cm. midline incision is then made in the posterior pharyngeal wall, with its center 1 cm. inferior to the palpable anterior tubercle of the atlas. The incision is carried down to bone. The posterior pharyngeal wall is then dissected subperiosteally as far lateral as the lateral masses of the atlas and axis, exposing the anterior arch of C1 and the body of C2. The anterior arch of C1 is then removed with a rongeur, exposing the odontoid process. The odontoid is then removed, preferably with a high-speed drill. Excision of a superiorly migrated and posteriorly angulated odontoid process may be difficult. Careful dissection freeing the odontoid of all soft tissue is required. If lateral C1-C2 fusion is done, articular cartilage from the C1-C2 articulation is removed and filled with wedge iliac crest graft. A single layer closure is recommended by most

to allow for drainage. Oral intake is deferred for 6 to 7 days.

POSTERIOR ATLANTO-OCCIPITAL FUSION

Significant disability may arise in the atlanto-occipital articulation of the spondylitic patient. In many patients this may represent the last available motion segment. With progressive destructive changes and undue stresses placed at a single motion segment, these patients may present with persistent pain and possible subluxation. Posterior atlanto-occipital fusion is recommended in refractory cases. Preoperative halo traction to reduce a subluxation or rotatory deformity may be warranted. As mentioned before, the fusion should extend to the occiput and perhaps include C3 when the patient exhibits superior migration of the odontoid. Posterior deficiency in the arch of C1 may require stabilization to the occiput to enhance the stability of the surgical construct.

Several techniques have been described. We prefer the method described by Wertheim and Bohlman[49] (see Fig. 5–7). A midline posterior approach is made exposing the area from the external occipital protuberance to the fourth cervical vertebra. Sharp subperiosteal dissection is completed, exposing the occiput and the cervical laminae. The external occipital protuberance is thick and represents the ideal location for passage of wires without having to go through both tables of the skull. A high-speed diamond burr is used to create a trough on both sides of the protuberance at a level 2 cm. above the foramen magnum. A towel clip is then used to create a hole in the ridge without penetrating the inner table. A 20-gauge wire is then looped through the hole and around the ridge. A second wire loop is passed around the arch of C1 and a third is passed through and around the base of the spinous process of C2. The posterior iliac crest is then exposed, and a large, thick, slightly curved graft of corticocancellous bone of appropriate width and length is obtained. The graft is then divided, and three drill holes are placed in each graft. The occiput is decorticated and the grafts anchored in place by the wires. Additional cancellous bone is then packed between the two grafts. Halo cast immobilization for 12 weeks is required.

LOWER CERVICAL SPINE PROBLEMS: SUBAXIAL SUBLUXATION

Subaxial subluxations tend to be more subtle and located at multiple levels in a given patient, producing a staircase, or stepladder, type deformity. Such subluxations can be found in 10 to 20 per cent of rheumatoid patients.[35, 40]

Five patterns of subaxial involvement have been described.[30] These include anterior subaxial subluxation, subluxation below higher fusion masses, anterior spondylodiscitis with cord compression, compression from epidural rheumatoid granulations, and apparent subaxial hyperlordosis responding to halo traction and stabilization. These may result in nerve root impingement resulting from foraminal narrowing or possibly myelopathic changes. Preoperative myelography or magnetic resonance imaging is generally required to confirm medullary or cord compression.

The indication for surgery in this particular group of patients is the development of neurological impairment and, to a lesser degree, pain. Menezes and associates suggest fusion for instabilities that are reducible.[36] Surgical treatment for subaxial subluxation usually involves wired posterior fusions, especially in the neurologically intact patient. The role of anterior fusion is unclear but may be indicated in the patient with progressive neurological loss. However, resorption and collapse of the graft have been reported in a high percentage of patients owing to the brittle nature of their bone.[38] Santavirta and associates recently suggested posterior decompression combined with posterior and posterolateral fusion for patients with progressive myelopathy.[39]

COMPLICATIONS

MORTALITY

Perioperative mortality following fusion for atlantoaxial subluxation has been reported as high as 42 per cent in early series. Recent reports have been more encouraging, possibly owing to earlier surgical intervention and improved anesthetic and perioperative management.[11, 13, 17, 24, 25, 38, 46] The perioperative mortality rate in these series averages approximately 10 per cent. In most cases these deaths were not directly attributable to the surgical procedure but reflected the systemic severity of the underlying disease process, especially with significant involvement of the patient's cardiopulmonary system.

NEUROLOGICAL DEFICIT

Neurological compromise resulting from cervical arthrosis is uncommon in the rheumatoid patient but can be devastating if it occurs. Preoperative traction to reduce the subluxation, attention to detail in surgical technique, and adequate stabilization are necessary to avoid complication. The passing of sublaminar wires is the most critical part during surgery, particularly in a patient with an incompletely reduced C1-C2 subluxation. Clark and associates reported one case of transient hemiparesis secondary to passing a sublaminar wire.[10] This resolved spontaneously except for some residual hyperreflexia. Use of intraoperative somatosensory-evoked potential monitoring is advocated.

PSEUDARTHROSIS

The difficulty in obtaining fusion of the C1-C2 articulation is illustrated by the reported different results of the various surgical procedures. In 1975, Ferlich and associates reported a 50 per cent success rate in fusing C1-C2 using a Gallie type wiring technique.[17] Bohlman achieved 10 solid fusions in 17 patients operated on for atlantoaxial subluxation.[5] Conaty and Mongan reported 67 per cent satisfactory results in 27 patients who had surgery.[11] More recently, Santavirta and associates recognized only 2 nonunions in 13 patients treated with a Gallie type of fusion.[39] Clark and associates experienced a 15 per cent rate of nonunion using a Brooks type of fusion augmented posteriorly with methylmethacrylate.[10]

Pseudarthrosis remains a problem in C1-C2 fusion in the rheumatoid patient and may be attributed to several factors. First, the posterior arch of C1 is often eroded in the rheumatoid patient. This leaves a significantly decreased surface area for bony contact with the bone graft and may lead to nonunion. Second is the difficulty in obtaining rigid fixation. Use of a halo device, especially in patients whose internal fixation is compromised by poor bone quality and erosion, is essential. The efficacy of adjunctive methylmethacrylate, with or without wire mesh, is questionable. Some feel that it may add some additional temporary support while fusion occurs. We feel that it is not necessary in all patients but should be limited to those with more severe erosive changes. Extension of the fusion mass to include the occiput is another alternative with improved fusion rates, but this procedure imparts significantly more functional impairment compared with atlantoaxial fusion.

Occipitocervical fusion has generally been more successful. Clark and associates reported union in all 16 patients treated with an occipitocervical fusion either for isolated cranial settling or for those with associated atlantoaxial or subaxial subluxation.[10] Conaty and Mongan reported only 1 nonunion in 14 patients.[11] Improved fusion rates may reflect the prolonged halo immobilization time. Other reports have not been as encouraging. Brattstrom and Granholm achieved successful fusion in 58 per cent but noted stable fibrous union in another 28 per cent.[6] Meticulous decortication, stable wire fixation, large iliac crest bone graft, and postoperative halo immobilization are all important in achieving successful fusion.

PROGRESSION OF INSTABILITY

Late subaxial subluxation below a higher cervical fusion has been reported by several authors.[9, 13] Careful preoperative radiographic evaluation is necessary to identify other areas of instability or potential instability. These areas, if identified, should be included in an extended fusion mass. Flexion/extension views of the spine and computed tomography are useful in delineating other areas of potential instability. In addition, previously asymptomatic levels may develop subluxation below already fused segments. In their series of 41 patients treated with a cervical arthrodesis, Clark and associates noted subsequent subluxation and displacement in 13 patients.[10] As a result, long-term follow-up monitoring for the development of instability is necessary.

ANKYLOSING SPONDYLITIS

PREOPERATIVE PLANNING

Ankylosing spondylitis affects primarily the spine and large joints in a predominant male population. The spine becomes inflamed, osteopenic, and eventually ossifies in a deformed position. Destructive vertebral lesions in ankylosing spondylitis encompass a spectrum of anterior lesions that have been well documented clinically and radiographically. These lesions can generally be divided into localized and extensive forms of the disease. The localized process or Romanus lesion is an anterior spondylitis that begins with a short-lived inflammatory process and results in syndesmophyte formation proceeding to ossification of the annulus fibrosus, the hallmark of ankylosing fibrosis. Andersson first documented radiological evidence of an extensive destructive discovertebral lesion in ankylosing spondylitis.[2] This type of lesion causes massive destruction of the vertebral rim and cartilaginous endplate. The underlying cause of this process is unclear. Some feel that it results strictly from an inflammatory process and hence the term spondylodiscitis. Others, however, believe in a traumatic origin. Wu and associates reported on the pathological findings in eight patients with extensive discovertebral lesions.[51] Their findings suggested that the primary pathology lies in the intervertebral disc as it is completely destroyed and replaced by fibrous scar tissue with focal areas of fibrinoid necrosis. These changes then initiate a chain of events in the disc-bone border and vertebral body, leading to progressive stiffness and ankylosis of the sacroiliac and interapophyseal joints and ossification of the annulus fibrosus and interlaminar and interspinous ligaments.

Characteristic deformities in these patients include a loss of lumbar lordosis, which may be associated with increased thoracic and cervical kyphosis. These deformities may be severe and require surgical intervention in the form of extension osteotomies. In the cervical region, atlantoaxial instability and atlanto-occipital disability are additional concerns for the spine surgeon.

In assessing any patient with ankylosing spondylitis with significant deformity, the primary site of deformity must be recognized. Careful clinical and radiographic evaluation of the cervical, thoracic, and lumbar spine and hips is essential to correctly address the patient's deformity surgically.

Ankylosing spondylitis may lead to severe flexion deformities of the spine. The ultimate goal in treatment of these patients is early recognition with adequate medical therapy in attempts to control the disease process as well as the associated deformities. However, many of these patients develop significant loss of lumbar lordosis with marked kyphosis in both the thoracic and cervical regions. Patients become grossly deformed and disabled, requiring spinal osteotomy to correct the deformity and attain a more upright stature. It is important to re-emphasize the point that the entire spine as well as the hips must be evaluated to delineate the primary site of deformity. Regardless of the area of primary deformity, accurate measurement of the deformity is necessary. Simmons believes that the most effective and reproducible measure of deformity is the chin-brow to vertical angle (Fig. 9–6). The angle is measured from the brow to the chin to the vertical with the patient standing and hips and

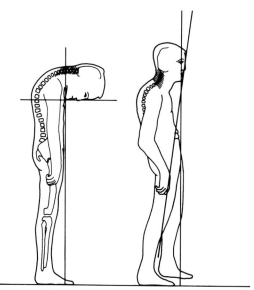

FIGURE 9–6. Illustration of chin-brow to vertical angle as a measure of the degree of flexion deformity of the spine in ankylosing spondylitis. (From Simmons, E.H.: The surgical correction of flexion deformity of the cervical spine in ankylosing spondylitis. In: Sherk, H.H., et al. (eds.): *The Cervical Spine*, 2nd ed. Philadelphia, J.B. Lippincott Company, 1989, p. 580.)

knees extended. The neck is held in the neutral or fixed position. In any patient with significant hip involvement, surgical treatment of the hips must precede correction of the kyphosis.

The indications for surgery are somewhat variable and must be individualized to meet patients' needs and expectations. The degree of deformity, patient's age, and general condition, and desire of the patient to undergo such an extensive procedure with the accompanying risk must all be considered.

OPERATIVE TECHNIQUE

CERVICAL SPINE

In a few patients with ankylosing spondylitis the primary deformity is found in the cervical spine. With severe deformity the patient may have a limited field of vision or experience difficulty in opening the mouth.

Simmons believes that a number of patients with a pre-existing, stable, painless cervical kyphosis may be converted to a painful, progressive flexion deformity following even minor trauma.[41, 42] These patients should be considered to have sustained a fracture. In Simmons' series of patients who have undergone cervical osteotomy, 36 per cent have

shown evidence of previous cervical fracture. In 31 per cent the fracture was thought to have significantly contributed to the deformity. Many of these fractures are difficult to visualize radiographically, and the patient's pain is attributed simply to the disease process. The fracture undergoes gradual erosion with collapse anteriorly, leading to a progressive flexion deformity. These fractures typically occur in the C6-T2 region with C7 and T1 being most common. Lateral tomography is advocated by most to visualize these fractures when suspected. These patients do not require an osteotomy if the diagnosis is made appropriately. Application of cranial halo and traction in line with the neck with slow restoration of the normal functional position is the treatment of choice. This should be followed with halo cast immobilization for a 4-month period. With rigid immobilization union occurs consistently over that time period. If it fails to heal, either anterior or posterior fusions may be required.

Unrecognized or untreated fractures of the cervical spine will eventually heal, and symptoms of pain will be relieved. Often the patient will be left with a fixed flexion deformity, and osteotomy will be required. Surgical correction has been associated with several reports of disastrous results and fatalities. Simmons has developed a technique, done under local anesthesia, that offers consistent, satisfactory results and relative safety.

The patient is fitted with a well-molded body jacket and halo device 1 to 2 days prior to surgery to ensure proper fit. This is a vital part of the procedure as the fused spine above and below the site of the planned osteotomy will place excessive force and possible motion at the site of the osteotomy. Secondary neurological compromise may result.

The operation is performed under local anesthesia with the patient in the sitting position in a dental type chair. This allows constant monitoring of spinal cord function and avoids major neurological complications. Nine pounds of longitudinal traction is applied through the halo along the axis of the neck. The amount of bone to be resected is determined from preoperative radiographic studies. The chin-brow to vertical angle is measured and transposed to a lateral x-ray of the cervical spine. Often a lateral tomogram is preferable. The apex of this angle is then placed at the posterior edge of the C7-T1 disc space, and the angle is centered over the posterior arch of C7. A midline incision is made over the lower cervical spine, exposing the bifid spinous process of C6, which is usually easily identified. A lateral intraoperative radiograph may be obtained if any difficulty is encountered in anatomical localization. The C7 spinous process and entire posterior arch are completely resected. The inferior portion of the C6 spinous process and the superior portion of the T1 spinous process are then removed (Fig. 9–7). The appropriate half of the arch of C6 and the superior half of the arch of T1 are then removed. Appropriate resection of the inferior portion of the spine of C6 and the upper portion of T1 with their associated laminae is then completed, based on preoperative radio-

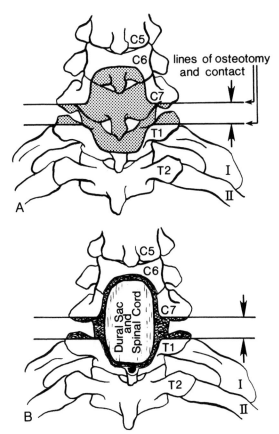

FIGURE 9–7. Illustration of laminectomy at C7-T1 junction for patients with severe flexion deformities of the cervical spine. *(A)* The entire posterior arch of C7, the inferior half of C6, and the superior half of C7 are removed. C8 nerve roots are exposed and overlying bone is removed. *(B)* After laminectomy, the spinal cord and the dural sac are visible, and the superior and inferior margins are undercut. (From Simmons, E.H.: The surgical correction of flexion deformity of the cervical spine in ankylosing spondylitis. In: Sherk, H.H., et al. (eds.): *The Cervical Spine,* 2nd ed. Philadelphia, J.B. Lippincott Company, 1989, p. 588.)

graphic planning. The inferior aspect of the C7 pedicle and the superior aspect of the T1 pedicle must be exposed and cut through in a curved fashion to protect the C8 nerve root. The nerve root should be followed laterally and all bone removed that could possibly impinge once the osteotomy is closed. This step must be performed completely and carefully.

Once the decompression is complete, the patient is sedated and the head extended through the halo device. The patient will awaken with this maneuver, and neurological function can be confirmed. The head is held in the reduced position and the halo stabilized. The bone removed during the decompression is placed posterolaterally over the apposed lateral masses and the wound is closed over suction drainage.

COMPLICATIONS

Simmons has reported on his series, which spans 20 years and includes 98 patients.[41] Neurological compromise has been noted as the most frequent complication. Thirteen patients experienced transient C8 paresthesias or signs that resolved spontaneously, while five patients had a more sustained C8 nerve root deficit. One of these underwent decompression with improvement. All patients improved with minimal residual symptoms and no gross functional loss. Additional reported neurological sequelae in this series included a Horner's syndrome, a transient lesion of the ninth and tenth cranial nerves, and one patient with mild symptoms of a central cord syndrome that developed two weeks after surgery. All of these cleared without intervention. There were no cases of permanent injury to the spinal cord.

Nonunion occurred in four patients, an incidence of 4 per cent. Three of these responded to anterior cervical fusion using Simmons' keystone strut graft. One patient required anterior and posterior grafting with posterior segmental instrumentation to obtain union.

Other reported miscellaneous complications include one fatal and one nonfatal pulmonary embolus, one intraoperative cardiac arrest, a perforated peptic ulcer, and one myocardial infarction.

LUMBAR SPINE

Patients selected for an extension osteotomy in the lumbar spine have their primary deformity in the lumbar spine with a loss of lordosis. This may be associated with an accentuated thoracic kyphosis that can be balanced through overcorrection of the lumbar deformity, returning the chin-brow to vertical angle to normal. This procedure is again associated with significant morbidity and even mortality. In the past, lumbar osteotomy has generally been associated with a mortality rate of 8 to 10 per cent and neurological compromise, including paraplegia, in the range of 30 per cent.[1, 8, 19–21, 26–28, 34, 44] An anterior osteotomy through a retroperitoneal approach is occasionally performed at the L3-L4 disc level in a patient with severe deformity in order to control the site and amount of correction more precisely. This is immediately followed by a posterior V-shaped wedge resection osteotomy. The wedge of bone to be resected is based on the preoperative lateral radiograph of the lumbar spine and the chin-brow to vertical angle. The apex of the angle is transposed to the posterior longitudinal ligament at the L3-L4 disc space, which is the center of lumbar lordosis. The ossified ligamentum flavum and the adjacent laminae are then resected upward and laterally on each side through the facet joints of L3-L4. The laminae and pedicles are undercut to prevent impingement of the dura or nerve roots. It is essential that adequate resection of bone be completed to obtain full correction of the deformity, shifting the weight-bearing axis posterior to the osteotomy site. It is also important to determine the spinal canal dimensions of the patient prior to surgery. If the canal is narrow (less than 20 mm. diameter), caution must be taken to remove adequate bone, especially superiorly. Simmons suggests leaving the central laminectomy area open to avoid compression from swelling or impingement.

The spine is then straightened and stabilized posteriorly using a compression instrumentation such as Cotrel-Dubousset system. Posterolateral fusion is performed with bone grafts. The wound is closed over suction drainage.

COMPLICATIONS

Simmons has the largest reported series of patients, having performed 100 lumbar osteotomies since 1969.[41] Eight patients developed L3 or cauda equina compression within 2 to 14 days after the surgery. All but two occurred in patients prior to the routine use of internal fixation and preoperative assessment of canal diameter. Patients with these problems were promptly re-explored, decompressed, and stabilized as already outlined. Such complications

can be minimized by thorough preoperative assessment of the spinal canal diameter by computed tomography and generous decompression, especially superiorly. It is reported that these patients generally did well following secondary decompression.

Nonunion occurred in three patients, a rate of 3 per cent. One patient without internal fixation was regrafted posteriorly and instrumented. Two other patients with internal fixation were successfully grafted anteriorly.

No patient sustained intraoperative cardiorespiratory distress. One female patient on birth control pills suffered a fatal pulmonary embolus 15 days after surgery.

One of the major complications that may occur with an osteotomy in the lumbar region is gastric dilatation and ileus. With extension of the spine through the osteotomy site, the superior mesenteric artery is stretched over the third portion of the duodenum. This may lead to gastric dilatation followed by vomiting and possible aspiration. Placement of a duodenal tube preoperatively with suction drainage is advised until the patient has re-established intestinal motility.

THORACIC SPINE

Some degree of thoracic kyphosis is commonly seen in patients with ankylosing spondylitis, but it rarely represents the only or primary site of deformity requiring correction. Most patients with a kyphotic thoracic spine will have a flattened kyphotic deformity of the lumbar spine, which can be corrected with a compensatory osteotomy in the midlumbar region, restoring balance and a normal chin-brow to vertical angle. A few patients, however, will present with thoracic kyphosis and normal or exaggerated cervical and lumbar lordosis. These patients require multiple anterior and posterior intervertebral osteotomies, instrumentation, and grafting. If the spine is incompletely ossified, some correction may be obtained with halo traction followed by multiple posterior resection osteotomies and compression instrumentation. This is followed by a second-stage anterior resection of the spondylodiscitis and strut grafting.

More commonly, the spine is rigid in the thoracic region and will first require an anterior transthoracic resection of the ossified disc spaces. These must be thoroughly curetted out and filled with autogenous iliac crest bone graft. Halo dependent traction is then applied and a second-stage posterior procedure usually performed at 10 days. Multiple wedge-shaped osteotomies are then performed posteriorly at each level, removing the ligamentum flavum and adjacent portions of laminae to allow correction upon closure of the osteotomy. Compression instrumentation and fusion are then completed.

REFERENCES

1. Adams, J.C.: Technique, dangers and safeguards in osteotomy of the spine. J. Bone Joint Surg. 34B:226, 1952.
2. Andersson, O.: Rontgenbilden vid spondylarthritis ankylopoetica. Nord. Med. 14:2000, 1937.
3. Ball, J., and Sharp, J.: Rheumatoid arthritis of the cervical spine. In: Hill, A.G.S. (ed.): Modern Trends in Rheumatology, Vol. 2. New York, Appleton-Century-Crofts, 1971, pp. 117–138.
4. Bland, J.H.: Rheumatoid arthritis of the cervical spine. J. Rheumatol. 3:319, 1974.
5. Bohlman, H.H.: Atlantoaxial dislocations in the arthritic patient: A report of 45 cases. Orthop. Trans. 2:197, 1978.
6. Brattstrom, H., and Granholm, L.: Atlanto-axial fusion in rheumatoid arthritis, Acta Orthop. Scand. 47:620, 1976.
7. Brattstrom, H., Elner, A., and Granholm, L.: Transoral surgery for myelopathy caused by rheumatoid arthritis of the cervical spine. Ann. Rheum. Dis. 32:578, 1973.
8. Briggs, H., Keats, S., and Schlesinger, P.: Wedge osteotomy of the spine with bilateral intervertebral foraminotomy. J. Bone Joint Surg. 29:1075, 1947.
9. Bryan, W.J., Inglis, A.E., Sculco, T.P., et al.: Methylmethacrylate stabilization for enhancement of posterior cervical arthrodesis in rheumatoid arthritis. J. Bone Joint Surg. 64A:1045, 1982.
10. Clark, C.R., Goetz, D.D., and Menezes, A.H.: Arthrodesis of the cervical spine in rheumatoid arthritis. J. Bone Joint Surg. 71A:381, 1989.
11. Conaty, J.P., and Mongan, E.S.: Cervical fusion in rheumatoid arthritis. J. Bone Joint Surg. 63A:1218, 1981.
12. Conlon, P.W., Isdale, I.C., and Rose, B.S.: Rheumatoid arthritis of the cervical spine: An analysis of 333 cases. Ann. Rheumat. Dis. 25:125, 1966.
13. Crellin, R.Q., MacCabe, J.J., and Hamilton, E.B.D.: Severe subluxation of the cervical spine in rheumatoid arthritis. J. Bone Joint Surg. 52B:244, 1970.
14. Crockard, H.A., Pozo, J.C., Ransford, A.O., et al.: Transoral decompression and posterior fusion for rheumatoid atlanto-axial subluxation. J. Bone Joint Surg. 68B:350, 1986.
15. Crockard, H.A., Essigman, W.K., Stevens, J.M., et al.: Surgical treatment of cervical cord compression in rheumatoid arthritis. Ann. Rheum. Dis. 44:809, 1985.
16. Eulderink, F., and Meijers, K.A.E.: Pathology of the cervical spine in rheumatoid arthritis: Controlled study of 44 spines. J. Pathol. 120:91, 1976.
17. Ferlich, D.C., Clayton, M.L., Leidholt, J.D., et al.: Surgical treatment of the symptomatic unstable cervical spine in rheumatoid arthritis. J. Bone Joint Surg. 57A:349, 1975.
17a. Fielding, J.W., Hawkins, R.J., and Ratzan, S.A.: Spine fusion for atlantoaxial instability. J. Bone Joint Surg. 58A:400, 1976.
18. Fischgold, H., and Metzger, J.: Etude radiographic de l'impression basilaire. Rev. Rheum. 19:261, 1952.
19. Goel, M.K.: Vertebral osteotomy for correction of fixed flexion deformity of the spine. J. Bone Joint Surg. 50A:287, 1968.
20. Herbert, J.J.: Vertebral osteotomy for kyphosis, especially in Marie-Strumpell arthritis. J. Bone Joint Surg. 41A:291, 1959.
21. Herbert, J.J.: Vertebral osteotomy, technique, indications and results. J. Bone Joint Surg. 31A:680, 1948.
22. Isdale, I.C., and Conlon, P.W.: Atlantoaxial subluxation: A six year follow-up report. Ann. Rheum. Dis. 30:387, 1971.
23. Kontinnen, Y., Santavirta, S., Bergroth, V., et al.: Inflammatory involvement of cervical spine ligaments in rheumatoid arthritis. Acta Orthop. Scand. 57:587, 1986.
24. Lachiewicz, P.F., Inglis, A.E., and Ranawat, C.S.: Methylmethacrylate augmentation for cervical spine arthrodesis in rheumatoid arthritis. Orthop. Trans. 11:7, 1987.
25. Larsson, S.E., Toolanen, G., and Fagerlund, M.: Medullary compression in rheumatoid atlanto-axial subluxation evaluated by computerized tomography. Acta Orthop. Scand. 57:262, 1986.
26. Law, W.A.: Lumbar spinal osteotomy. J. Bone Joint Surg. 41B:270, 1959.
27. Law, W.A.: Osteotomy of the spine. J. Bone Joint Surg. 44A:1199, 1962.
28. Law, W.A.: Osteotomy of the spine. Clin. Orthop. 66:70, 1969.
29. Lipson, S.J.: Cervical myelopathy and posterior atlanto-axial subluxation in patients with rheumatoid arthritis. J. Bone Joint Surg. 67A:593, 1985.
30. Lipson, S.J.: Rheumatoid arthritis in the cervical spine. Clin. Orthop. 239:121, 1989.
31. Martel, W.: The occipito-atlanto-axial joints in rheumatoid arthritis and ankylosing spondylitis. Am. J. Radiol. 86:223, 1961.
32. Martel, W., Duff, I.F., Preston, R.E., et al.: The cervical spine in rheumatoid arthritis: Correlation of radiographic and clinical manifestations (abstract). Arthritis Rheum. 7:326, 1964.
33. Mathews, J.A.: Atlantoaxial subluxation in rheumatoid arthritis. Ann. Rheum. Dis. 28:260, 1969.
34. McMaster, P.E.: Osteotomy of the spine for fixed flexion deformity. J. Bone Joint Surg. 44A:1207, 1962.
35. Meikle, J.A., and Wilkinson, M.: Rheumatoid involvement of the cervical spine. Ann. Rheum. Dis. 30:1541, 1971.
36. Menezes, A.H., Van Golder, J.C., Clark, C.R., et al.: Odontoid upward-migration in rheumatoid arthritis. An analysis of 45 patients with "cranial settling." J. Neurosurg. 63:500, 1985.
37. Pellici, P.O.M., Ranawat, C.S., Tsarairis, P., et

al.: Progression of rheumatoid arthritis of the cervical spine. J. Bone Joint Surg. 63A:342, 1981.

38. Ranawat, C.S., O'Leary, P., Pellici, P.M., et al.: Cervical spine fusion in rheumatoid arthritis. J. Bone Joint Surg. 61A:1003, 1979.

39. Santavirta, S., Slatis, P., Kankaanpaa, U., et al.: Treatment of the cervical spine in rheumatoid arthritis. J. Bone Joint Surg. 70A:658, 1988.

40. Sharp, J., and Purser, D.W.: Spontaneous atlanto-axial dislocation in ankylosing spondylitis and rheumatoid arthritis. Ann. Rheum. Dis. 20:47, 1961.

41. Simmons, E.H.: The surgical correction of flexion deformity of the cervical spine in ankylosing spondylitis. In: The Cervical Spine Research Society: The Cervical Spine. Philadelphia, J.B. Lippincott Company, 1989, p. 573.

42. Simmons, E.H.: Surgery of the spine in rheumatoid arthritis and ankylosing spondylitis. In: Evarts, C.M. (ed.): Surgery of the Musculoskeletal System, Vol. 2. New York, Churchill Livingstone, 1983, p. 85.

43. Smith, P.H., Benn, R.T., and Sharp, J.: Natural history of rheumatoid cervical luxations. Ann. Rheum. Dis. 31:431, 1972.

44. Smith-Peterson, M.N., Larson, C.B., and Aufranc, O.E.: Osteotomy of the spine for correction of flexion deformity in rheumatoid arthritis. J. Bone Joint Surg. 27:1, 1945.

45. Stevens, J.C., Catledge, N.E.F., Saunders, M., et al.: Atlantoaxial subluxation and cervical myelopathy in rheumatoid arthritis. Q. J. Med. 40:391, 1971.

46. Thompson, R.C., and Meyer, T.J.: Posterior surgical stabilization for atlantoaxial subluxation in rheumatoid arthritis. Spine 10:597, 1985.

47. Van Beusekim, G.T.: The neurological syndrome associated with cervical luxations in rheumatoid arthritis. Acta Orthop. Belg. 58:38, 1972.

48. Weissman, B.N.W., Aliabadi, P., Weinfeld, M.S., et al.: Prognostic features of atlantoaxial subluxation in rheumatoid arthritis patients. Radiol. 144:745, 1982.

49. Wertheim, S.B., and Bohlman, H.H.: Occipitocervical fusion. Indications, technique and long term results in thirteen patients. J. Bone Joint Surg. 69A:833, 1987.

50. Winfield, J., Cooke, D., Brook, A.S., et al: A prospective study of radiological changes in hands, feet, and cervical spine in adult rheumatoid disease. Ann. Rheum. Dis. 40:109, 1981.

51. Wu, P.C., Fang, D., Ho, E.K.W., et al.: The pathogenesis of extensive discovertebral destruction in ankylosing spondylitis. Clin. Orthop. 230:154, 1988.

Index

Note: Page numbers in *italics* refer to illustrations; numbers followed by (t) indicate tables.